The Prostate

Patrick C. Walsh, M.D., and

Janet Farrar Worthington

Illustrations by Leon Schlossberg

The Prostate

A Guide for Men and the Women Who Love Them

The Johns Hopkins University Press

Baltimore and London

To the Reader: This book is as accurate and comprehensive as we could make it. We hope it will help you understand your prostate disorder and, with your physician, develop the treatment plan that's best for you. In other words, treatment shouldn't be based solely on the contents of this book, but on your own particular needs, which you and your doctor should determine together.

© 1995 The Johns Hopkins University Press
All rights reserved. Published 1995
Printed in the United States of America on acid-free paper
04 03 02 01 00 99 98 97 96   5 4

THE JOHNS HOPKINS UNIVERSITY PRESS
2715 North Charles Street, Baltimore, Maryland 21218-4319
The Johns Hopkins Press Ltd., London

A catalog record for this book is available from the British Library.

Library of Congress Cataloging-in-Publication Data

Walsh, Patrick C., 1938–
    The prostate : a guide for men and the women who love them / Patrick C. Walsh and Janet Farrar Worthington ; illustrations by Leon Schlossberg.
        p.   cm.
    Includes index.
    ISBN 0-8018-4988-8 (hbk. : acid-free paper).—ISBN 0-8018-4989-6 (pbk. : acid-free paper)
    1. Prostate—Diseases—Popular works.   I. Worthington, Janet Farrar.   II. Title.
RC899.W35 1995   94-33397
616.6'5—dc20   CIP

To all the patients, past and present,
who inspired us to write this book,
with deep gratitude for the lessons they have
taught us—which we now share with others.

Contents

PART II. ENLARGEMENT OF THE
PROSTATE AND PROSTATITIS

Preface

My husband's father, Tom Worthington, always figured cigarettes would kill him. For years, his family had pestered him to quit smoking. Nobody expected him to die of prostate cancer, not at his age. Even when the diagnosis was made—when it was too late, when the cancer had made its fatal, metastatic leap beyond the wall of the prostate—his doctors were hopeful. "Men can live for years with prostate cancer," they assured him.

They set up a course of hormonal therapy, so successful in holding the cancer at bay in older patients. "It's a cancer driven by hormones," his family doctor said. "We'll just shut down the hormones, and the cancer will go away."

And it did. For months, serum prostate-specific antigen (PSA) tests detected no trace of the cancer in his blood. During this time, Tom, who had, as he wryly put it, "messed up his life," began fixing it again. He remarried his wife of thirty years, just months after divorcing her, saw the birth of his daughter's baby—his first grandchild—and began going to church. He believed he had been given a second chance at life; he wasn't going to blow it this time.

Then the tumor came back, with a vengeance. Within a year of his initial diagnosis, Tom was in a nursing home, castrated, hooked up to a catheter, in agonizing pain, pitifully thin, his bones so riddled with cancer that his arm snapped in two when a nurse tried to move him. Between shallow breaths, as he drifted in and out of consciousness, he told us goodbye. Then he simply stopped breathing. He was 53.

The image of Tom's suffering left an indelible imprint on his family. I'm writing about it now, in all its vivid, sad detail, because I don't want others to suffer as Tom did. My father-in-law's case, lamentably, illustrates some basic misconceptions about prostate cancer: That it is a disease only old men get. That it is uniformly slow-growing, not aggressive. That the tumor is nourished only by hormones. That hormone starvation will stop the cancer from spreading. And perhaps most important, that prostate cancer won't be missed during a routine physical exam. Tom's disease was overlooked despite two physical exams within six months, and after weeks of back pain, a common symptom.

My husband, Mark, Tom's son, is a doctor, but we were two thousand miles away. And there wasn't much he could do after the diagnosis was made. It was too late then, although we didn't know it at the time. In the end, Mark could only help by doing something Tom's own physician had failed to do—make sure Tom was in as little pain as possible, by prescribing adequate doses of painkiller to ease his horrendous suffering.

Nobody should have to die the way Tom did. It was awful. And none of us understood how rapidly his illness was progressing. None of us knew what to expect. Tom's family was desperately hungry for good information about his disease, and there just wasn't any, except for some few-and-far-between articles in the medical literature that Mark found and translated for us, and a couple of books that proved unhelpful and, worse, inaccurate.

That's how this book was born. With Patrick Walsh, M.D., Director of Urology at The Johns Hopkins Brady Urological Institute and inventor of the revolutionary "Walsh procedure" (he doesn't call it that), the now-standard operation that removes the prostate but preserves potency and continence, I wrote an article on prostate cancer for *Hopkins Medical News,* the alumni magazine for the Johns Hopkins School of Medicine, of which I was editor. Never has the magazine received more requests for reprints; clearly, we had touched a nerve. There was also an acute need, we found, for more detailed information.

A Word about the Title, and How to Use This Book

This book is written for men and women. That's because, quite frankly, Tom Worthington probably wouldn't have bought this book for himself. Many men—including my husband, father, and brother—don't like thinking about their health. Their philosophy is simple: Ignore the subject, and it will go away. So it's up to me, my mother, and the other women in the family to nag them to go to the doctor. And the men we know *really* don't want to think about anything remotely urological; they cringe at the thought of a digital rectal examination. Most men, Dr. Walsh once told me, don't even know they have a prostate—until they have a problem. The thing is, most prostate trouble can be prevented—and, if caught early enough, *all* prostate problems can be cured, even cancer. That is the message of this book, and in succeeding chapters we'll cover most aspects of the prostate in detail.

There is a lot of helpful, detailed, state-of-the-art information here—some of it so recent that your doctor may not even know about it; maybe some of this material is more than you'll even want to know, but it's there if you need it. In the prostate cancer section, for example, there are tables and charts that will help you understand what the results of certain tests mean (and which tests and treatments are useless), whether or not you have cancer that needs to be treated, the likelihood that your cancer has spread, and the best options available in planning treatment. With Tom Worthington's experience—and that of thousands of other men—in mind, we also tell you exactly what medications and symptoms to ask your doctor about, so you can help yourself or a loved one get relief from debilitating pain.

We thought about not including some of this information, and letting doctors use their own discretion about whether or not to tell you all the facts. But you have a right to know everything; after all, you're one half of the doctor-patient partnership! Also, medical care in this country is uneven. Some doctors, frankly, may not be as up-to-date as others; some, in well-meaning but misguided efforts to spare patients the burden of worry and pain, may choose not to tell the whole story. In any event, it's all here, for you to do with as you see fit.

With today's managed-care medical environment, in which some HMOs may be reluctant to provide specialist care or early screening for prostate disease, it's more crucial than ever before for patients to become their own advocates.

The reader's job is to consider this book an owner's manual of sorts, remembering, as Francis Bacon wrote four hundred years ago, that *knowledge is power.* What you learn about this troublesome gland may save someone's life, maybe even your own. And getting good information about these ailments also may preserve a man's quality of life. For prostate cancer, the days of the cure being worse than the disease are largely a thing of the past.

You can read this book two ways: from cover to cover or from summary to summary. Even though this book is as clear and easy to digest as we could make it, the prostate is not a simple thing, and its disorders are actually very complicated. Our goal here is for you to come away from this book informed, prepared and able to discuss your situation intelligently with your doctor.

However, sometimes it's a good idea to get your feet wet before you plunge in. That's why, at the end of each chapter, there's a section called "The Short Story." This section sums up the basic points you need to know about each subject covered in the book. It may help to read these sections first to get an overview and then, once you have the big picture, to go back and fill in the details by reading the rest of each chapter.

We begin with a summary of the "big three" prostate ailments, then discuss each in detail, including symptoms, diagnosis, treatment, and prognosis. We end with some information about where to get help and how to learn more.

Tom Worthington died before my husband and I had our baby. Our daughter will never know her paternal grandfather as anything more than a picture on the wall. It is my fervent hope that, with their own loved ones in mind, many more men will start getting yearly prostate examinations. And will live to enjoy their grandchildren.

Janet Farrar Worthington

Acknowledgments

This book would not have been possible without the work and experience of many people, too many to name here—we tried, but the result looked like a telephone book and had about as much personal meaning. So instead of listing all, and inevitably missing one or two, of the sources upon which we've drawn to produce this guide, we would simply like to thank those colleagues, patients, friends and family members who have helped us the very most, including:

Donald S. Coffey, Ph.D.; John D. McConnell, M.D.; Ken J. Pienta, M.D.; Alan W. Partin, M.D.; Carol Balmer, Pharm.D.; E. David Crawford, M.D.; Gary G. Schwartz, Ph.D., M.P.H.; John T. Isaacs, Ph.D.; William Isaacs, Ph.D.; Howard I. Scher, M.D.; Michael Naslund, M.D.; Jonathan I. Epstein, M.D.; Joseph E. Oesterling, M.D.; Eva Zinreich, M.D.; Mario A. Eisenberger, M.D.; Ulrike M. Hamper, M.D.; Timothy J. Wilt, M.D., M.P.H.; Louis Kavoussi, M.D.; Charles B. Wentz; Bette Rank; David Sandberg; Alex Short; R. Carmichael Tilghman, M.D.; John Anderson; and Peter Weaver.

We also acknowledge with deep gratitude the valuable contributions of these people: Peg Walsh, Mark Worthington, M.D., Barbara Downs, Ronald Farrar, Gayla Farrar, Bradley Farrar, Ann Finkbeiner, Melissa Sweeney, Howard Means, Mitchell Steiner, M.D., William Whitworth, Ruth Freishtat, Barbara Lamb, Lee Sioles, and Marilyn Shepherd.

Finally, we would like to thank Leon Schlossberg, for his superb ability to tell a story with pictures, and Jacqueline Wehmueller, our editor, for unflagging patience and support over the last two years.

Patrick C. Walsh, M.D.
Janet Farrar Worthington

Little Gland, Big Trouble

The clinical problems of the prostate defy easy answers: Why, for instance, do some men live for nearly a century without suffering from an enlarged prostate, while others, from middle age onward, need to be treated more than once? Why do some men die *with* prostate cancer and other men die *of* it—while others never get the disease? What causes the sudden swelling of the prostate, often accompanied by crippling back pain, known as prostatitis?

Prostate disorders range in degree of unpleasantness from irritating to devastating. The good news of this book is that effective treatment—and most importantly, relief of symptoms—is available for all the "big three" prostate disorders: prostate cancer; benign prostatic hyperplasia, or BPH (commonly known as enlarged prostate); and prostatitis. It's especially good to know that *prostate cancer, when caught early, is curable.* And, when detected early, prostate disorders can generally be treated without causing loss of urinary control or sexual function.

Few men who live a normal life span—about 74 years—will depart this earth unscathed by some sort of prostate ailment, ranging from painful inflammation to benign enlargement to cancer. And it's important to note that prostate disease is not an either-or situation. Having BPH, for example, does not mean that a man has "had his prostate trouble" and therefore won't also develop cancer. Nor does surgery or other treatment for BPH or prostatitis eliminate the risk of getting prostate cancer.

What this means is that after age 50, and for the rest of their lives, men need a yearly prostate check-up. This involves a digital rectal examination—when a doctor's gloved finger is inserted in the rectum to feel for a knot or lump, swelling, or anything else out of the ordinary—and something called a PSA test, a highly sensitive blood test that catches trace amounts of a protein called prostate-specific antigen. Yearly PSA tests give your doctor a continuum, a baseline reading: Any change in the PSA level means something needs to be checked out. PSA, normally secreted and disposed of by the prostate, shows up in the bloodstream in cancer and in the bothersome but generally harmless condition called BPH. (It can also be elevated briefly after an episode of prostatitis.) For thousands of men, the PSA test is boosting considerably the odds of early diagnosis for prostate cancer and BPH.

BENIGN PROSTATIC HYPERPLASIA (BPH)

For most men, during the first forty years or so of life, the prostate is on its best behavior. But after age 40, many men—an estimated 80 percent by age 80—develop benign prostatic hyperplasia (BPH), an irritating condition that causes the prostate to swell and interfere with urine flow. BPH may trigger frequent urination (several times an hour); a sense of urgency; a long wait for urine to flow; frequent awakening in the night to urinate; interruption of the urine stream (starting and stopping); and a constant feeling of fullness in the bladder. Sometimes, BPH leads to urinary tract infections; in rare cases, it can cause damage to the bladder or kidneys.

BPH develops from the inside outward, as the prostate's inner tissue starts to crowd the urethra, which runs through the encircling prostate like a straw held in someone's fist. As the inner prostate cells grow, they begin squeezing the urethra; the fist tightens. For most men with BPH, this tightening causes an irritating but still tolerable change in quality of life. However, when it progresses beyond the nuisance point—when it hinders the urinary tract, for example, or causes kidney or bladder problems—it needs to be treated.

PROSTATE CANCER

Although prostate "trouble" does seem to be a normal part of aging, *prostate cancer is not just an old man's disease.* In 1994, the American Cancer Society's

Department of Epidemiology and Statistics estimated that two hundred thousand new cases of prostate cancer would be diagnosed in the United States, and that more than thirty-eight thousand men would die of the disease. It is now the second-leading kind of cancer in men (second only to skin cancer); and, of all cancers, prostate cancer is the one whose prevalence increases most rapidly with age.

Again, there is good news: *Caught early, before it has spread, prostate cancer is curable with surgery or radiotherapy.* Better surgery has drastically reduced the operation's worst side effects, impotence and incontinence. And new research is laying careful groundwork for understanding prostate cancer and improving the hope for curative treatment even after the disease has spread.

If prostate cancer is detected early, men can be cured; they can also have a normal life. This critical message needs to be heard by doctors as well as patients. Men need to have themselves tested, and doctors need to start checking for prostate cancer earlier, and more vigilantly.

PROSTATITIS

Prostatitis refers to an inflamed, swollen, and tender prostate. This painful condition can be caused by an infection (by bacteria) or by something else— doctors don't know what causes nonbacterial prostatitis. In any case, the symptoms may include pain in the joints, muscles, lower back, and area behind the scrotum; aches, fever and chills (in acute cases); urinary trouble, including blood in the urine, pain, or burning; and painful ejaculation.

Bacterial prostatitis manifests itself in both acute (severe and requiring immediate treatment) and chronic (long-term) forms, and may be detected by bacteria in the urine; *neither form is contagious, and neither form can be transmitted to a man's sexual partner.* The treatment is to combat the bacteria and thus stop the infection. For nonbacterial prostatitis, the arsenal of treatments includes muscle relaxants. A related condition, called prostatodynia, or painful prostate, may not be an actual prostate disease but may in fact be caused by muscle spasms in the pelvis.

Next we'll take a look at how the male urinary and reproductive systems work normally, before examining what happens when the prostate—which is involved in both systems—causes trouble.

The Prostate

1

An Anatomy Primer

Your Guide to the Male Urinary and Reproductive Systems

Why start with an anatomy lesson? Say you're planning a trip: You probably consult a map, because it makes sense to know the route, the landmarks and trouble spots along the way. Because your destination doesn't exist in a vacuum, understanding and appreciating *context* is as important to your journey as the end itself.

So, if it helps, think of this chapter as your Michelin Guide to male anatomy. It's by no means exhaustive, but it does describe the context of the prostate as an important gland involved in both the urinary and reproductive systems. Knowing the prostate's role in normal anatomy may lead to a better understanding of just what happens when something goes wrong.

THE URINARY TRACT

The Kidneys

We begin with the kidneys, which lie like bean-shaped bookends, embedded in fat and fibrous connective tissue, on either side of the spine at the base of the ribs. They're located behind the pancreas and beneath the peritoneum, the large sheet of tissue lining the abdomen that encloses and protects the liver, stomach, and bowel.

The kidneys are reddish-brown, and they're not mirror images. The left kidney tends to be slightly longer, narrower, and situated a little higher than the right, which occupies somewhat cramped quarters just below the liver. The kidneys, on average, are about five inches long, three inches wide, and an inch thick. They are highly vascular: Pound for pound, the kidney handles three to five times more blood than the heart, liver and brain. An amazing 25 percent of the blood from each heartbeat flows through them, and the kidneys cleanse the blood of toxic wastes, excess water and salts. They play a pivotal role in maintaining the body's balance of fluids and electrolytes (minerals such as sodium, potassium and chloride), as well as the acid-base (pH) ratio in the body. They help metabolize vitamin D, which strengthens bones. They also manufacture renin, which helps regulate blood pressure; and erythropoietin, which regulates the body's red blood cell count.

The kidneys are the body's main filters. The system by which they cleanse the body of impurities—and, at the same time, salvage and recycle useful materials—is at once intricate and elegant. They work like a vast complex of drainage ditches, tributaries, and streams leading to a river. Each kidney contains more than a million building blocks, or tiny tubules, called nephrons. A nephron begins with a double-walled cup that contains a filtering knot (think of a tiny, wadded-up coffee filter) called a glomerulus. After this knot, the tubule's course is at first convoluted; it straightens out as it approaches the center of the kidney, then tapers and passes through a series of connecting channels to reach a large collecting duct.

This elaborate filtering network enables the kidneys to manage an incredible volume of fluid each day. The body of a man who weighs 150 pounds, for

Opposite: Here it is, the male urinary system. It starts with big filters—the kidneys, irregular, bean-shaped bookends on either side of the spine. Then come the ureters, muscular, one-way tubes that squeeze urine like liquid toothpaste from the kidneys down to the bladder, a muscle-bound holding tank. From the bladder, urine continues its downward passage via the urethra, a tube with layered, circular muscles, which tunnels through the prostate.

Generally, the prostate—a muscular, walnut-shaped gland that seems so small (about an inch and a half long) yet causes so much trouble—doesn't have much to do with urine's passage through the body. But note that it surrounds the urethra. In BPH, the growing prostate begins to choke the urethra, which can have a major impact on urine flow.

After its short, angled trip through the prostate, the urethra continues its winding course to the penis, the portal by which urine exits the body at last.

Figure 1.1. *How urine exits the body*

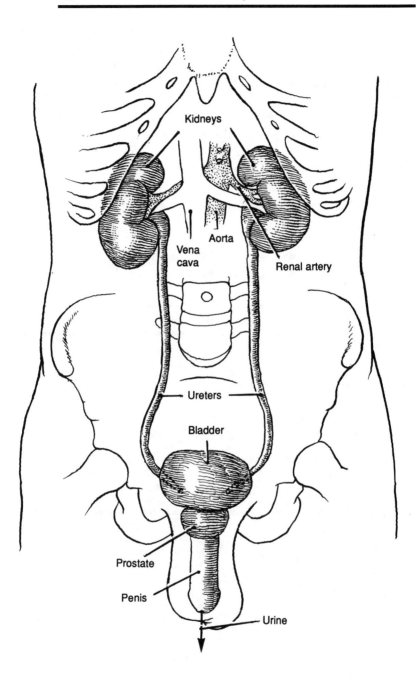

instance, contains about ten to twelve gallons of water. But his kidneys process about forty-five gallons of water a day—which means this water is constantly being refined, reabsorbed, and then processed again. If the water and minerals weren't reabsorbed, our bodies would become seriously dehydrated within a matter of hours.

So what happens to the fluid that is not reabsorbed? It continues on its way through the tubular network, to make about two quarts of urine—that's how much the average man excretes each day. By the time it reaches the collecting ducts, it's highly concentrated, and ready to be transported out of the body.

The Ureters

Urine exits each kidney through a muscular tube called the ureter. The ureters work like toothpaste tubes, squeezing, or "milking," urine from the kidneys. Each ureter is about a foot long and quite narrow—less than a half-inch wide at

---

Figure 1.2. *A closer look at the kidney*

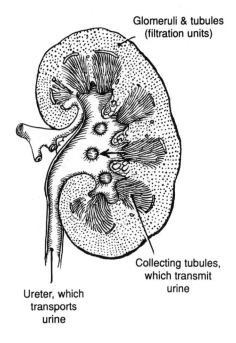

Glomeruli & tubules
(filtration units)

Collecting tubules,
which transmit
urine

Ureter, which
transports
urine

It's a system at once intricate and elegant. The kidneys cleanse the body of impurities and, at the same time, salvage and recycle useful materials. They work like a vast complex of drainage ditches, tributaries, and streams leading to a river. Each kidney contains more than a million building blocks, or tiny tubules, called nephrons. A nephron begins with a double-walled cup that contains a filtering knot (think of a tiny, wadded-up coffee filter) called a glomerulus. The tubule straightens out as it approaches the center of the kidney, then tapers and passes through a series of connecting channels to reach a large collecting duct. This elaborate filtering network enables the kidneys to manage an incredible volume of fluid each day.

What Is Urine?

Urine is what's left over after the kidneys salvage and recycle the water and useful minerals constantly passing through them. It includes tiny amounts of water, sodium, chloride, bicarbonate, potassium, and urea, the breakdown product of proteins.

Figure 1.3. *A close-up of the bladder, prostate, and urethra*

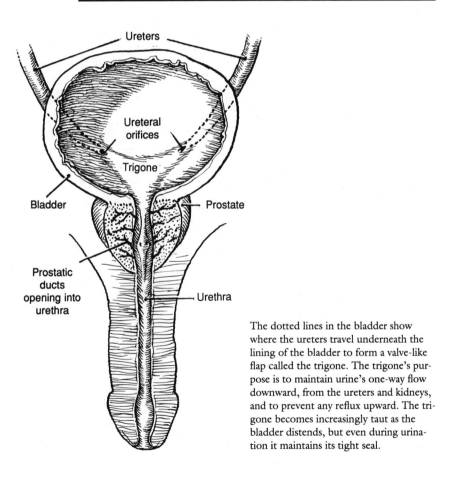

The dotted lines in the bladder show where the ureters travel underneath the lining of the bladder to form a valve-like flap called the trigone. The trigone's purpose is to maintain urine's one-way flow downward, from the ureters and kidneys, and to prevent any reflux upward. The trigone becomes increasingly taut as the bladder distends, but even during urination it maintains its tight seal.

its broadest point. Ureters are one-way conduits: Urine always flows the same way through them, whether you're standing upright or upside down. The ureters' main function is to push urine onward, and thus continue its progress through the body to the bladder.

The Bladder

The bladder is a hollow, muscle-bound reservoir that functions as a holding tank. At its fullest, it can retain about a pint of urine. In normal circumstances, the bladder marks the first point in the urinary process—after the intake of fluid, of course—at which we can exert some influence, as we choose to eliminate or hold urine. (The inability to control the elimination of urine is called incontinence.)

The bladder is designed to collapse and expand, depending on the amount of fluid it's asked to hold. A layer of connective tissue accounts for its flexibility; like a band of elastic, this mucosal lining is crinkled when the bladder is empty, but stretched and flattened when the bladder is full. Intricately woven layers and bundles of shifting muscle form a labyrinthine network that allows the bladder to contract and expel urine. A sophisticated backup system exists to protect the bladder from extreme distention and the risk of rupture: When the bladder is very full, there is a corresponding slowdown in urinary production in the kidneys.

The ureters don't cease to exist once they reach the bladder; they merely change shape. The two tubes flatten and meet to form a valve-like flap, called the trigone, at the neck of the bladder. The purpose of the trigone is to allow the free movement of urine downward from the ureters and kidneys and also to prevent any urine reflux upward—basically, to maintain the current's one-way flow. The trigone is a one-way valve that prevents urine from backing up into the kidneys as the bladder distends. Even during urination, the trigone preserves its tight seal.

With the way upward effectively blocked, urine continues its downward passage via the urethra, a tube with layered, circular muscles, which begins at the neck of the bladder and then tunnels through the prostate.

The Prostate

The prostate is a muscular, walnut-shaped gland about an inch and a half long, which sits directly under the bladder. Its main function is to manufacture part of the fluid that makes up semen, the solution that transports sperm. During orgasm (the climax of sexual intercourse), the prostate's muscles contract and force this fluid into the urethra, the main conduit for urinary and sexual fluids. (Sperm, produced by the testes, is also launched into the urethra at this time, along with fluid made by the seminal vesicles.)

Figure 1.4. *The prostate and the urethra*

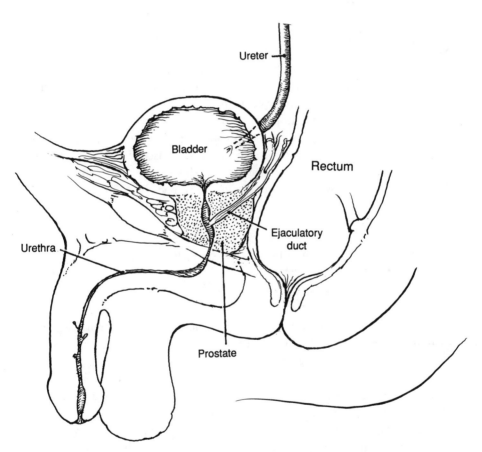

You can see why the urethra's course through the prostate, over time, can become so precarious— the prostate completely surrounds it. And when, as a man ages, the prostate grows and begins to jostle for space, the urethra becomes even more cramped—and urine has more trouble getting from the bladder through the prostate and out of the body.

The prostate changes with age: When a man reaches his mid-40s, it tends to enlarge, beginning with the innermost cells, those surrounding the urethra. In benign prostatic hyperplasia (BPH), the growing prostate begins to choke the urethra, which runs through it at a thirty-five-degree angle. This slow strangulation is why the prostate can have such an impact on urine flow. We will discuss the prostate in much greater detail in the next section, which covers the reproductive system.

The Urethra

After its short, angled trip through the prostate, the urethra continues its winding course to the penis, the portal by which urine exits the body at last. The urethra, whose total length is about eight inches, is divided into three segments—prostatic, membranous (between the prostate and penis), and penile. Like the prostate, it is involved in both the urinary and reproductive systems; it serves as a conduit not only for urine but also for secretions from the ejaculatory ducts and the prostate. The prostatic urethra, too, is equipped with a means to prevent fluid backup—a ring of smooth muscle that works with the bladder neck as a clamp during ejaculation. This clamp keeps semen from flowing the wrong way, up into the bladder, and directs its course downward, out the urethra.

THE REPRODUCTIVE SYSTEM

The Testes

The testes are a man's reproductive organs. There are two of them, each less than two inches long and about an inch wide. Each testis lies protected in the scrotum, attached like a pocket watch on a chain to a spermatic cord, which, among other things, is responsible for supplying blood to the testis.

The testes are divided into hundreds of minuscule compartments, each of which contains at least one pair of threadlike, highly convoluted tubules. If these tubules were straightened out, each would stretch to two feet in length. These tiny tubules are joined, like plumbing pipes, to straighter tubes that are the body's factories for sperm; the sperm-making process, called spermatogenesis, happens here. The testes are also the main source of the male hormone

Figure 1.5. *A closer look*

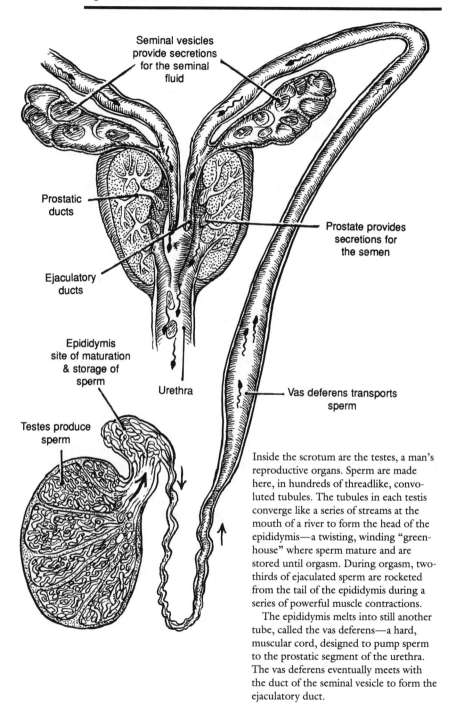

Seminal vesicles provide secretions for the seminal fluid

Prostatic ducts

Ejaculatory ducts

Epididymis site of maturation & storage of sperm

Urethra

Testes produce sperm

Prostate provides secretions for the semen

Vas deferens transports sperm

Inside the scrotum are the testes, a man's reproductive organs. Sperm are made here, in hundreds of threadlike, convoluted tubules. The tubules in each testis converge like a series of streams at the mouth of a river to form the head of the epididymis—a twisting, winding "greenhouse" where sperm mature and are stored until orgasm. During orgasm, two-thirds of ejaculated sperm are rocketed from the tail of the epididymis during a series of powerful muscle contractions.

The epididymis melts into still another tube, called the vas deferens—a hard, muscular cord, designed to pump sperm to the prostatic segment of the urethra. The vas deferens eventually meets with the duct of the seminal vesicle to form the ejaculatory duct.

testosterone, which is responsible for fertility and for secondary sexual characteristics such as post-pubertal body hair and deepening of the voice.

The Epididymis

The sperm-making tubules in each testis converge like streams at the mouth of
a river to form the head of the epididymis. In this case, the river is propor-
tionally huge and tortuous. Each twisting, winding epididymis (one on each
side), though only a millimeter wide, could be uncoiled to reach a length of
fifteen to twenty feet. The epididymis is the "greenhouse" where sperm mature and are stored until orgasm, when two-thirds of ejaculated sperm are
rocketed from the tail of the epididymis during a series of powerful muscle
contractions. The epididymis hugs the testis, clinging to one side of it before
twisting yet again and heading upward at its tail end to join still another tube
called the vas deferens.

The Vas Deferens

There is an almost immediate change in topography as the epididymis melts
into the vas deferens. This mighty tube (again, one on each side; together they
are called the vasa deferentia), is a hard, muscular cord, about eighteen inches
long and three millimeters in diameter. Its characteristic thickness—due to its
sheath of muscles, designed to pump sperm to the prostatic segment of the
urethra—means the vas deferens can easily be felt through the scrotum and
even the spermatic cord. The vas deferens winds its way to a space between the
bladder and rectum, then heads downward to the base of the prostate, where it
meets with the duct of the seminal vesicle to form the ejaculatory duct. It is
from the vas deferens that the vasectomy, a form of male contraception, gets its
name: When the vas deferens is cut, sperm cannot exit the penis through
ejaculation and instead are reabsorbed into the body.

The Seminal Vesicles

The seminal vesicles, each about two inches long, sit behind the bladder, next
to the rectum, arching over the prostate like two wings or, perhaps, like two
clusters of grapes; they appear more clumped than streamlined. Arching still
higher over them, on either side, are the vasa deferentia, which meet the

What Is Semen?

The easy answer is that semen is the ejaculate. It consists of sperm plus the secretions from the sex accessory tissues (these include the prostate and seminal vesicles), and is composed of prostaglandins, spermine, fructose, glucose, citric acid, zinc, proteins, and enzymes such as immunoglobulins, proteases, esterases, and phosphatase. Less than 1 percent of semen comes from other reproductive organs such as the testes and epididymis, which produce sperm.

Semen is not merely sperm; sperm is just a tiny fraction of the seminal fluid. So why the other secretions? In some mammals, sperm removed from the epididymis—having never made contact with secretions from the prostate and seminal vesicles—has proved capable of fertilizing an egg. Many scientists believe the varied secretions that make up semen are there as a buffer, to help sperm survive and remain active, to encourage sperm's passage in the male and female reproductive tracts, and to minimize environmental shock during intercourse. The presence of sugars such as fructose and glucose may be there to nourish the sperm, to provide energy for sperm's metabolism on its journey.

And still other secretory products—the zinc, for example, and proteases and immunoglobulins—may exist as disease fighters that cleanse the urethra, repulsing attack by harmful substances in the body that enter the urinary tract.

Semen undergoes extreme chemical transformations after ejaculation, metamorphosing from a viscous liquid to a semi-solid and back again. Usually about five minutes after ejaculation, semen coagulates into a gel-like substance; then, within about fifteen minutes it becomes a sticky liquid. In most animals, the seminal vesicles and prostate act on semen as a one-two punch: The coagulation is due to a substance made by the seminal vesicles. Then PSA, an enzyme made by the prostate, causes the coagulum to break down. The character of semen varies greatly among species. For example, in bulls and dogs (which don't have seminal vesicles), semen does ▶

> ▶ not coagulate at all. But in rats and rabbits, semen quickly coagu-
> lates to form a pellet; for these animals, PSA is crucial in helping the
> sperm reach their destination.
>
> Because semen is a body fluid, like blood, it is acted on by drugs,
> carcinogens, and pathogens (any agent that causes disease)—
> including sexually transmitted pathogens such as the HIV virus,
> which causes AIDS—to which the body is exposed. These have
> been proven to find their way into semen—and, via semen, into
> sexual partners.

seminal vesicles at V-shaped angles; these form the ejaculatory ducts, slitlike openings that feed into the prostatic urethra.

The seminal vesicles are composed of alveoli, little cul-de-sacs that bear viscous secretions—critical in ensuring the consistency of semen. (They got their name from the belief once held that the vesicles stored semen and sperm; they don't.)

Like the prostate and related tissues known as "sex accessory glands," the seminal vesicles depend on hormones for their development and growth, and for their ability to produce secretions. The seminal vesicles are highly variable among species: They're large in humans, rats, hamsters and some rabbits, but are missing altogether in dogs, cats and bears. One unusual point: The seminal vesicles, so similar to the prostate in many ways, are almost always free of abnormal growth—benign (as in BPH) as well as malignant. No one knows why.

The Prostate

The prostate is a complicated organ. In part, it is a storehouse for a series of tiny, spongy glands; the minilobes that make up these glands form fifteen to thirty secretory ducts, which empty their contents into the urethra. Buried in its fibromuscular tissue are alveoli, cul-de-sacs lined with a forest of tall, column-shaped secretory cells that drain into the urethra via a system of branching ducts and tubes.

The ingredients of the prostate's secretions, in a clear, mildly acidic fluid, are

Figure 1.6. *Regulation of the prostate: The inside story*

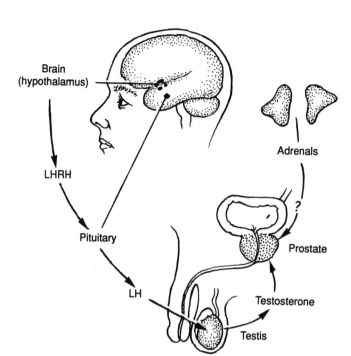

The prostate is affected from up close—by the testes—and from long-distance—by the brain. Let's begin at the top: The hypothalamus, located in the brain, makes a chemical messenger called LHRH, which is dispatched in signal pulses—like Morse code or flashes of light—to the nearby pituitary gland. These pulses tell the pituitary to transmit yet another chemical signal, called LH, which motivates the testes to make the male hormone testosterone.

Among other things, testosterone is responsible for secondary sex characteristics like post-puberty body hair and deepening of the voice, and for fertility. It is a major hormone that regulates the prostate. The adrenals also make some weak androgens; however, it's questionable whether these adrenal androgens have a significant influence on the adult prostate.

many and varied: They include citric acid, acid phosphatase, spermine, potassium, calcium and zinc. The prostate is regulated by sex hormones called androgens, which come from the testes. Foremost among these is testosterone, produced in the testes but controlled by a hormone from the pituitary gland, called luteinizing hormone. Testosterone, released from the testes, circulates in the blood. It enters cells in the prostate by diffusion, like water

Figure 1.7. *Inside a prostate cell*

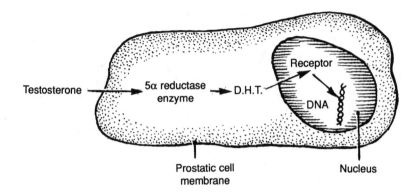

Testosterone is important to the prostate, but not in its original form; it must be transformed to an active form. It turns out that testosterone is converted by an enzyme called 5-alpha-reductase to DHT. And DHT is the major androgen, or male hormone, inside the prostate cell.

Here's how it works: Testosterone circulates in the blood. It enters cells in the prostate by diffusion, like water through a tea bag, and soon is transformed into DHT. DHT hooks up chemically with a specific protein, moves to the cellular seat of power—the nucleus—and quickly becomes a powerful force in the transmission of genetic information (DNA) from prostate cells.

through a tea bag, and soon is transformed into another chemical called dihydrotestosterone (DHT). DHT hooks up chemically with a specific protein, moves to the cellular seat of power—the nucleus—and quickly becomes a powerful force in the transmission of genetic information from prostate cells.

Some components of prostatic secretions may serve to protect the urinary tract and reproductive system from harmful substances in the body that may enter the urethra (see "What Is Semen?"). Perhaps most significant among these is prostate-specific antigen (PSA), an enzyme detectable by a blood test. In recent years, the PSA test has become a crucial addition to medicine's arsenal for detecting, and thus treating, prostate cancer and BPH (for more on this test, see Chapter 3).

For all we know about prostatic secretions, their exact role in sexual function is still an enigma. And, problems in the prostate, unlike those in most bodily systems, don't manifest themselves with symptoms easily traceable to prostate function. Urinary trouble generally is the first sign that something's not right in the prostate.

Why Have Homosexual Men Been Particularly Vulnerable to the Virus that Causes AIDS?

The prostate is naturally vulnerable to infections and inflammations (prostatitis, for example). And white blood cells, the front-line soldiers in the body's fight against infection, often travel from the prostate into the ejaculate. HIV, the virus that causes AIDS, lives in these white blood cells and is borne by them in blood and semen; men with the AIDS virus have more white blood cells in their semen than other men. But perhaps more important is that enzymes like PSA, made by the prostate, have been shown to break down the fragile tissue lining the rectum—tissue that's often traumatized already by rectal intercourse—making this area uniquely susceptible to the deadly pathogens the white blood cells bring with them.

Anatomically, the prostate is divided into five zones: *anterior,* which occupies 30 percent of the space and consists mainly of smooth muscle; *peripheral,* the largest segment, which contains three-fourths of the glands in the prostate; *central,* which holds most of the remaining glands; *preprostatic* tissue, which plays a key role during ejaculation (muscles here prevent semen from flowing back into the bladder); and *transition,* which surrounds the urethra and is the sole site of benign prostatic hyperplasia (BPH). *Most prostate cancer occurs in the peripheral zone.* Also, this is the region most likely to be tapped in a needle biopsy of the prostate.

The prostate is not the sole basis for a man's fertility or potency. Some animals that have had their prostate (or, in fact, their seminal vesicles—but not both) removed remain fertile. But growth of the prostate clearly *is* linked to sexual development: Starting at puberty, the prostate enlarges five times in size—from a weight of about 4 grams to 20 grams—by about age 20. For the next several decades, prostatitis is the most common form of prostate trouble; then, after about age 50, BPH and prostate cancer take over as the problems to worry about.

Most animals have a prostate. But only humans and dogs are prone to

Figure 1.8. *The zones of the prostate*

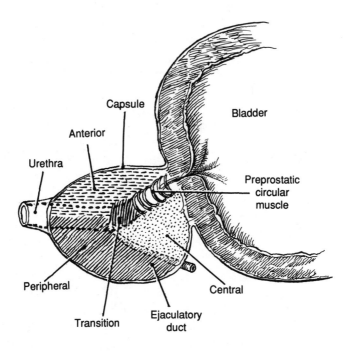

prostate trouble, and nobody knows why. What makes bulls, for instance, immune to prostate cancer? Why don't cats get BPH? Again, a mystery.

The Penis

The penis was designed for two primary functions, sexual intercourse and urination. It is a remarkable construction of nerves, smooth muscle, and blood vessels; there is no bone in the human penis (unlike the penis in some other animals, such as dogs). Instead, the penis works on hydraulic principles. Its basic structure is that of a rounded triangle; all three corners have cylindrical cavities of tissue that become engorged with blood. These are the corpora cavernosa and the corpus spongiosum. Erection involves a delicate relationship between arteries and veins: Arteries continue to pump blood into the penis, but the veins clamp down, so the blood can't recirculate, thus keeping the penis "inflated" during sexual activity. All of this is orchestrated by the rich supply of nerves that lead to and from the penis. Many of these nerves also affect the prostate, but for years, these tiny nerves were poorly understood. The sad result was that removal of the prostate almost always meant impotence. That is no longer the case.

THE SHORT STORY

To understand everything else in this book, you need a map. That's why we've started with anatomy. The prostate is a key component in two major body systems: the urinary tract and the reproductive system.

So here is a quick guide to the urinary tract:

We begin with the kidneys—the big, intricate filters that cleanse the body of toxic wastes, recycle useful materials and maintain the proper balance of water and minerals. Twenty-five percent of the blood from every single heartbeat flows through the kidneys. They're also constantly refining water—processing about forty-five gallons a day. In the average man, they produce about two quarts of urine every day.

Each kidney empties its urine into a ureter, a long, muscular pipe that squeezes, or "milks," urine from the kidneys like toothpaste through a tube. At the site where the ureter hooks up with the bladder is a simple but elegant valve that keeps urine on a one-way course—so it can't flow back into the kidneys when you urinate.

Next, we come to the bladder, a muscular reservoir that, at its fullest, can hold about a pint of urine. Urine travels from the bladder through the urethra, which runs directly through the prostate to the penis, and then to the outside world.

The prostate is strategically located at the junction between the bladder and the urethra. It is a walnut-shaped gland whose main purpose is to produce 30 percent of the fluid for semen. Secretions from the prostate also may protect men from urinary tract infections.

Now, let's take a quick look at the reproductive system:

Sperm and testosterone, the male hormone, are made in the testicles. Testosterone is the substance that makes the prostate grow at puberty; it also stimulates the prostate to manufacture its secretions. Sperm travel from the testicles to the twisting, winding epididymis, a convoluted "greenhouse" where they mature.

The epididymis connects to the vas deferens, a hard, muscular cord that winds all the way from the scrotum into the body and down to the back of the prostate. At this point, the seminal vesicles, which produce 70 percent of the fluid for semen, connect to the vas deferens to form the ejaculatory ducts, which run into the center of the prostate. When a man ejaculates, sperm rocket from the epididymis through the vas deferens and out of the ejaculatory duct, where they're mixed with the fluids from the prostate and seminal vesicles.

To make sure that the semen doesn't "back up" into the bladder, a muscular valve slams shut in the bladder neck, forcing the semen out the urethra in the penis. Soon after ejaculation, the semen coagulates. A substance called prostate-specific antigen (PSA), which is made by the prostate, then acts on the semen, causing it to become liquid again.

To understand what can go wrong with the prostate, it will probably help to study the illustrations in this chapter and the rest of the book (the illustration in the Glossary shows the male urinary and reproductive systems together). You can see from figure 1.4, for example, how the prostate encircles the urethra like a fist holding a straw—therefore, when its transition zone enlarges, in benign prostatic hyperplasia (BPH), this compresses the urethra and causes urinary problems. Also, you can see from figure 3.1 how cancer in the prostate can be detected by a digital rectal examination.

Finally, by understanding how PSA is secreted from ducts in the prostate, you'll be able to see why PSA levels increase when these ducts become obstructed, as they do in prostate cancer.

A Final Word

In medical school, before they tackle anything else, future doctors study anatomy. For months, what they're learning doesn't make much sense. But slowly the picture begins to come together. And only then, when they understand how things are supposed to work, can medical students understand what happens when something goes wrong. Think of this chapter as your crash course in anatomy. Now that you've completed it, we can begin discussing the diseases of the prostate and ways to treat them.

We turn our attention first to prostate cancer.

Part I

Cancer of the Prostate

2

Who Gets Prostate Cancer?

First, a few sobering truths: Every three minutes, a new case of prostate cancer is diagnosed in the United States. Every fifteen minutes, a man dies from it. And there's no gentle way to describe what this death is like. For too many men, death from prostate cancer is a sad end to months of excruciating pain, increasingly thin and brittle, cancer-riddled bones, awful constipation from pain-killing drugs, and miserable symptoms of urinary obstruction.

In 1994, an estimated two hundred thousand men were diagnosed with prostate cancer, and thirty-eight thousand men died because of it—about one out of every five men who developed the disease. And the numbers are getting worse. As the death rate from other illnesses is decreasing, the death rate from prostate cancer is on the rise—over the last five years, it has increased by as much as 3 percent a year. By the year 2000, the incidence of prostate cancer is expected to increase by 90 percent; prostate cancer deaths are expected to go up by 37 percent. A boy born today has a 13 percent chance of developing prostate cancer, and a 3 percent chance of dying from it. Except for skin cancer, prostate cancer is the most common cancer in men.

Hormones are one big factor in the development of the disease, although their role is not fully understood. Men who are castrated or who have pituitary failure—in which the brain no longer stimulates the testes to function—before age 40 rarely develop prostate cancer (for more on this, see Chapter 7).

Age is also a major factor. Most—more than 80 percent of the men diagnosed with prostate cancer are older, over age 65; 90 percent of the deaths are in this same group. Traditionally, less than 1 percent of prostate cancer cases have been detected in men younger than age 50, and only 16 percent have been found in men between ages 50 and 64.

The average age of diagnosis of prostate cancer is 72; the average age of death from it is 77. What does this mean? Does it mean that if you're a 52-year-old man you can breathe easy for the next twenty years? No, it doesn't. It means that, historically, prostate cancer has been diagnosed in older men. It's only recently that techniques for spotting prostate cancer early have improved significantly.

Historically, most men found out they had prostate cancer when it was advanced, and they died a few years later. (This explains why the average age of death from prostate cancer is so near the average age of diagnosis.) There is every reason to believe that, over the next few years, the average age of diagnosis is going to drop by as much as a decade—as more men are diagnosed at a point when the disease is still confined to the prostate and still curable. And there's every reason to hope that early diagnosis will reduce the number of men who die each year of the disease.

The incidence of prostate cancer increases with age more rapidly than the incidence of any other form of cancer. Epidemiologic studies show a forty-fold rise in the prevalence of prostate cancer from ages 50 to 85. With better medicine, diet and exercise, and less smoking, fewer older men are dying from other illnesses such as heart disease. So, as life expectancy increases, it's likely that prostate cancer will develop in more and more men and, *without early diagnosis and treatment,* that more and more men will die from this disease.

Another reason why more cases of prostate cancer are being diagnosed is improved diagnostic techniques. In the 1970s, more men underwent a procedure called TUR (transurethral resection of the prostate) for treatment of BPH, so more cancer was detected as a result. In a TUR procedure, excess prostate tissue is removed in fragments through the urethra; these leftover chips of tissue are routinely sent to pathologists for examination. More cases of cancer were detected as more men underwent TUR procedures. (For more on TUR and BPH, see Chapter 10.)

The 1980s saw a breakthrough in biopsy techniques—the biopsy gun, a tiny, spring-loaded needle guided by the urologist's finger during a rectal exam. This development meant that a doctor could take microscopic tissue samples throughout the prostate during a routine outpatient visit. (Before this, getting a biopsy meant a patient had to be admitted to the hospital and given an anesthetic. The biopsy gun can be used without anesthesia.) And today, the

PSA blood test and transrectal ultrasound are being used more often to diagnose cancer in the prostate (see Chapter 3).

In any event, the undeniable truth is that *prostate cancer is on the rise.* Who's at risk? That's a trickier set of statistics. Some factors, such as age, family history, and diet, clearly are very important. The roles of others, such as environment and occupation, are less certain.

DOES ENVIRONMENT MAKE A DIFFERENCE?

Here's a confounding fact: At autopsy, "incidental" prostate cancer—small clusters of cancer cells, an apparently latent form of cancer that resides in millions of men—is found in 30 percent of men of every race and culture in the world. In some men, this latent cancer never poses a danger. In others, however, it does.

There are two key statistics: 13 percent of men develop clinically significant prostate cancer at some point in their lives. And 30 percent of men have microscopic, incidental prostate cancer that's found at autopsy (which means that they lived and died and were never troubled by the cancerous cells in their prostate). The ratio of clinically significant cancer to incidental cancer is 1 to 2.5. So if you have a prostate biopsy and cancer is found, this is what you and your doctor need to find out first—which category are you in? Do you have clinically significant cancer or incidental cancer? And even if your cancer is, at the moment, in the "good" category, remember: *Incidental prostate cancer doesn't always stay that way.* Over time, in a significant number of men, this innocent-looking cancer evolves into a more malignant variety which, if not treated, will eventually prove deadly.

Studies of Japanese and American men have borne some interesting results: Incidental prostate cancer is found in as many Japanese men as American men, and both groups of men have about the same life span—74 years. *Yet hardly any Japanese men die of prostate cancer.* Why?

Prostate cancer develops in four broad stages: Initiation, promotion, progression, and metastasis, or spread of cancer. These studies of Japanese and American men suggest that whatever causes cancer *initiation* is the same in all men; the big differences seem to come in promotion, progression, and spread. These studies also suggest that at least some of the elements responsible for these last three steps—turning indolent prostate cancer into a deadly disease—are environmental.

It has been shown that, *over time, when men change their environment, they assume the cancer risk of the country where they live.* So when Japanese men, people at low risk of getting prostate cancer, move to Hawaii or California, their rate of symptomatic prostate cancer escalates—to the level of an American man's.

For years, scientists have suspected the high-fat Western diet as an obvious environmental culprit in the development of prostate cancer. But it's not that simple. For example, a high-fat diet is believed to play a big role in other diseases, like colon and breast cancer. The death and incidence rate in prostate cancer is higher among American blacks than American whites—yet the incidence of breast and colon cancer in the two groups is about the same. What accounts for this difference? And these statistics raise another question: Are black men somehow more susceptible genetically to prostate cancer than white or Asian men? We don't know. But we do know, sadly, that in this country many black men delay seeking medical care until it's too late and prostate cancer has spread.

Genetics and environment—two definite components of the prostate cancer equation. We'll examine some genetic issues first and then look at some of the environmental risks in greater detail.

DOES PROSTATE CANCER RUN IN THE FAMILY?

As with breast cancer, there seems to be a close association between a family history of prostate cancer and a man's risk of developing the disease. Big deal, you may be thinking: If prostate cancer is inevitable for so many men—if it's so common—then what difference does it make if it runs in my family? Unfortunately, *the prostate cancer that runs in families is much more likely to strike at a younger age,* when a man might not even be looking for trouble or having yearly prostate exams.

Recently, scientists at Johns Hopkins showed the undeniable link between a family history of prostate cancer and a man's probability of developing the disease (see table 2.1). This study showed that if your father or brother has prostate cancer, your risk is two times greater than the average American man's

Table 2.1 *Does Prostate Cancer Run in Your Family?*

Number of Affected Relatives	Risk
Father and/or brothers	
One	2-fold
Two	5-fold
Father/brother or Grandfather/uncle	
One	1.5-fold
Two	2.3-fold

Note: Your risk of developing prostate cancer starts at about 13 percent and goes up from there, depending on your number of affected relatives.

(which is about 13 percent). It goes up from there: Depending on the number of affected relatives you have and the age at which they develop the disease, your risk could be as high as 50 percent. Does your family history suggest hereditary prostate cancer (HPC)? You fall into this category if you have three first-degree relatives (a father or brothers) who develop prostate cancer, or two first-degree relatives, if both developed it before age 55, or if prostate cancer has occurred in three generations in your family (grandfather, father, son). *Note: HPC can be inherited from either your father or your mother.* For this reason, it's important to find out from both your father and mother about a history of prostate cancer in their brothers and father. (If neither relative is living, ask other family members, or investigate family records.) Men in families with HPC have a 50 percent chance of developing prostate cancer and are more likely to develop it at a younger age than most men. *In HPC families, men should have a digital rectal examination and PSA test every year, beginning at age 40.*

Genetic Susceptibility

Most important about these findings is that they firmly establish prostate cancer as a disease that, like breast and colon cancer, is due at least in part to genetic susceptibility.

The theory here is that cancer doesn't just happen overnight; a whole chain of genetic events must occur—picture a whole row of dominos being overturned—before a tumor can begin to grow. Some men may be born with part of the chain completed. "If you inherit some of these steps," says one molecular biologist at Johns Hopkins, "then you've shortened the time it's going to take to accumulate all of them." So inherited mutations in one or more genes probably speed up the body's journey toward cancer, and that's why these men develop their cancer at an earlier age. Environmental factors—variables such as diet—may do the rest.

This is what scientists think happens on a genetic level to make cancer possible: Mutations occur in the genes that regulate normal cell growth. When one of these genes is mutated, by whatever it is that causes cancer, the cells begin to grow at an abnormal rate. For example, some of these mutated genes, called oncogenes, when activated, become switches that work like a stuck accelerator in a car. They're mutated in such a way that they can't be turned

---

The Next Step: Targeting Genes

In a large genetic study, scientists are studying blood samples of families with hereditary prostate cancer, using highly specific DNA probes to search various chromosomes for gene mutations. They're also looking for the loss of specific chromosomal regions in prostate cancer cells, and comparing them with the normal cells of men with prostate cancer. One protein under study, called e-cadherin, is a calcium-dependent cell adhesion molecule, whose gene is located on the short arm of chromosome 16—a chromosome frequently deleted in prostate cancer. This protein appears to play an important role in cell-to-cell recognition—what tells one cell vital details about the cell next door. This gene is believed to be important in metastasis, the spread of cancer. Understanding it may one day mean being able to predict which prostate cancers will spread and become life-threatening.

"First of all," says one scientist, "we need to figure out whether losing that gene is a frequent event in metastatic prostate cancer." One eventual method of treatment, he speculates, may be simply to keep the cancer confined to the prostate—not to stop its growth, but to arrest its spread. Blocking prostate cancer's progress one day may mean, the scientist speculates: "As long as the cancer stays in the prostate, everything's all right."

off—so cells are driven to grow, and to keep right on growing. (An oncogene is a normal gene that, when expressed in an abnormal form or in excessive amounts in a cell, confers malignant potential; it is one step closer to becoming a cancer cell. Most likely, several oncogenes have to be activated, and several mutations must occur, in order for a normal cell to become cancerous.)

Other key players in the genetics of cancer are tumor-suppressor genes. These are "checkpoint" genes, calm voices of reason in a cell cycle that can easily get out of hand. Their purpose seems to be to put on the "brakes"—to control cell division. Most cancers require that one or more of these checkpoint genes be knocked out—either mutated or completely obliterated—before a cell can become malignant. Thus, the mutations that lead to the development of prostate cancer may involve a process in which the accelerator is stuck *and* the brakes have been removed, and cell growth is out of control.

Environment plus Genetics Equals . . .

The segment of cancers caused solely by environment, like that of purely inherited cancers, is believed to be small, about 5 percent. "If you knock out each end of the spectrum," says the molecular biologist, "the 90 percent of cancers in between are probably due to some sort of interaction between what you eat and smoke and get exposed to, and how your genetic predisposition handles everything."

MORE ON THE HIGH-FAT DIET

We've said that diet probably isn't enough to cause prostate cancer on its own. However, it can't be overlooked as a significant risk factor. Several studies have shown that men with high-fiber, low-fat diets are less likely to get prostate cancer. One study found prostate cancer deaths in thirty-two countries to be highly linked to fat consumption (animal fat, not vegetable fat). Another study, of 122,261 men, found a lower death rate from prostate cancer in men who ate green and yellow vegetables every day.

Vitamin A, found in yellow vegetables such as carrots, is a fat-soluble vitamin. Its influence extends far beyond its effect on our vision to encompass systems throughout the body. It is vital for the normal makeup of epithelial cells, for example (these line the prostate and are important in BPH—see Chapter 9). In laboratory experiments, scientists have linked vitamin A deficiency to the development of different kinds of tumors. In similar experiments, researchers have also been able to decrease prostate cancer with vitamin A supplements.

There have been conflicting reports about vitamin A and prostate cancer; part of the confusion may be because one kind of vitamin A—beta carotene, which comes from plants and is part of the Japanese diet—appears to *lower* risk, while another kind—that found in animals and, often, in the American diet—probably raises it.

Believe it or not, diet even has an effect on hormones such as testosterone. A diet that's low in fat and high in fiber lowers the amount of testosterone in the blood, and hormones such as testosterone play a big role in the growth of prostate cancer. One study found blood testosterone levels in young black men to be about 15 percent higher than those of young white men; a similar study found that Dutch men had higher levels of male hormones than Japanese men. Also, studies of American men have found that they have higher levels of DHT (dihydrotestosterone) metabolites than Japanese men. (DHT is the active form of male hormone in the prostate.) Some investigators interpret this to mean that more DHT may be the cause of the cancer. However, DHT is produced by the secondary organs of reproduction (such as the prostate), and Oriental men tend to have smaller hair follicles and prostates. Which is the cause and which the effect? The lower DHT may simply reflect the fact that Japanese men have inherently smaller secondary organs of reproduction, which contribute less DHT to the circulation.

Other studies found that black and white American men had higher amounts of these male hormones in their urine than black South African men, and that the level of these hormones had a lot to do with diet. When the black South African men ate a Western diet, instead of their usual vegetarian diet, their hormonal levels went up. And when black American men ate a vegetarian diet, their hormonal levels went down. Again, this seems to be more proof that a low-fat, high-fiber diet can lower any man's risk of prostate cancer.

OTHER RISK FACTORS

Locale

Does where you live affect your chances of getting prostate cancer? Actually, yes—suggest the results of a recent study of prostate cancer and geography (see figures 2.1 and 2.2).

Figure 2.1. *Geography and prostate cancer: prostate cancer deaths*

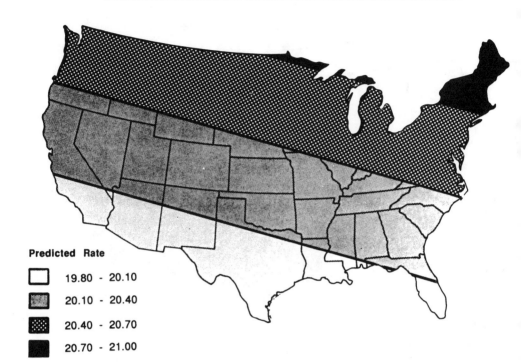

Predicted Rate

☐ 19.80 - 20.10

▨ 20.10 - 20.40

▩ 20.40 - 20.70

■ 20.70 - 21.00

In this map of the United States, the darkest regions mark the heaviest areas of death from prostate cancer (among white men, according to county records from 1970 to 1979). The lightest regions show where prostate cancer deaths are lowest. (This is a computer model showing the pattern of age-adjusted mortality rates. From Gary G. Schwartz and Carol L. Hanchette, "Geographic patterns of prostate cancer mortality," *Cancer* 70 [1992]: 2865. Reprinted with permission.)

The theory behind the study was that insufficient levels of vitamin D, a hormone known to have anticancer properties, may increase a man's risk of getting clinical prostate cancer. What's the biggest source of vitamin D? Everyday exposure to the sun's ultraviolet rays. The researchers looked at geographic distribution of the sun's ultraviolet rays and the number of prostate cancer deaths throughout the country. Their results were startling. They showed a striking north-south pattern, with the heaviest areas of prostate cancer death in the north and the lightest areas in the south. (This despite the fact that the

Figure 2.2. *Geography and prostate cancer: exposure to UV radiation*

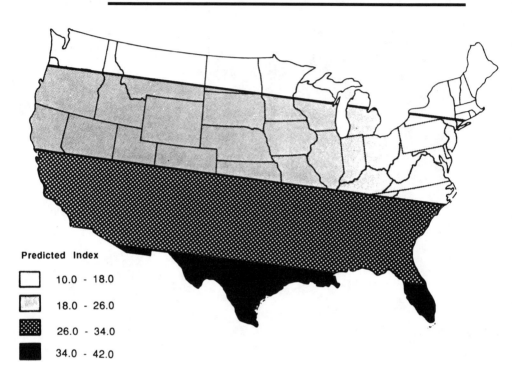

Predicted Index

☐ 10.0 - 18.0

▨ 18.0 - 26.0

▩ 26.0 - 34.0

■ 34.0 - 42.0

In this map, the lightest areas show the parts of the country getting the *least* amount of ultraviolet radiation, and the darkest areas show the parts of the country getting the most ultraviolet radiation. These areas, coincidentally, are the regions where prostate cancer deaths are lowest. These maps show that areas getting the least UV radiation had the most prostate cancer—and this suggests that UV radiation may protect men from developing clinical prostate cancer. (This is a computer model showing the pattern of UV radiation. From Gary G. Schwartz and Carol L. Hanchette, "Geographic patterns of prostate cancer mortality," *Cancer* 70 [1992]: 2865. Reprinted with permission.)

south has a higher concentration of older men than other parts of the country. Data were age-adjusted; using this method, researchers can compare different groups as if the populations had the same underlying age distribution.) But when they looked at sunlight exposure, they found just the opposite—the heaviest exposure in the south, and the least in the north. *Areas getting the least UV radiation had the most prostate cancer,* and vice versa. Their conclusion?

Ultraviolet radiation may protect men from getting clinical prostate cancer. And vitamin D, called a tumor inhibitor, somehow slows or prevents incidental prostate cancer from becoming clinical. (If you live in Alaska, or spend most of your time indoors, don't panic. More work needs to be done to confirm this theory, and as yet, having an inadequate supply of vitamin D has not been established as a definite risk factor for prostate cancer.)

These findings might help explain why prostate cancer death rates are highest in Scandinavian countries, Canada, and the United States, and lowest in Hong Kong and Japan. Also, the Japanese diet is rich in fish that contain vitamin D.

These findings also might help scientists understand why black men in this country are so susceptible to prostate cancer: People with dark skin absorb less sunlight and thus have lower levels of vitamin D. African scientists compared blood levels of vitamin D in black men in Zaire with Zairian black people living in Belgium and found significantly lower levels of vitamin D in those who had left sun-drenched Zaire.

Occupation

There's not a lot of good information on this subject, but some studies have indicated that farmers and mechanics may have a higher risk of prostate cancer. It's hard to know what to do with information from such studies, however; it's very difficult to separate what people *do* from who they *are*—their family history, their diet and habits. For example, do farmers and mechanics have more fat in their diets than others? Do they smoke more? One case-control study found that 75 percent of 40 patients with prostate cancer had a history of farming compared with 37.5 percent of control patients with BPH. (On the other hand, it could be argued that these older men were products of a generation that was much more agrarian. Who knows?)

Other studies have indicated that cadmium, a trace mineral present in cigarette smoke and alkaline batteries, may have something to do with prostate cancer. Men who are welders or who work in electroplating, over time, get exposed to high levels of cadmium; these studies suggest that cadmium exposure marginally increases a man's risk of developing prostate cancer. One explanation may be that cadmium somehow interferes with zinc, a necessary element in many of the body's activities—and men with prostate cancer have been found to have lower levels of zinc in their prostates than other men.

What does it all mean? If you're a farmer, or a mechanic, newspaper worker, plumber, welder, or worker in a rubber-producing factory (all of these have been suggested, without much proof, as occupations that raise a man's risk of getting prostate cancer), don't be alarmed. There's no evidence to indicate that you should.

Smoking

Several studies have suggested that men who smoke may be at a greater risk of developing prostate cancer. There is no *solid* evidence that proves this. For now, there seems to be only a weak association between smoking and prostate cancer. (One study, however, did suggest that men who smoke and are exposed to cadmium are at higher risk.) Having said this, it makes sense to add that smoking, which brings tobacco, nicotine (which is a powerful insecticide), and a host of toxic chemicals into every cell of the body—not just the lungs and throat—probably doesn't *decrease* a man's risk of getting prostate cancer. Conflicting reports have suggested that smoking may elevate hormone levels in men, and that this may somehow affect the prostate.

Vasectomy

A flurry of publicity recently scared millions of men and caused the government to organize major studies to investigate whether or not a link exists between vasectomy and prostate cancer. Good news: *There is no evidence that a vasectomy increases a man's risk of prostate cancer.* So why, then, does it seem that so many men who have had a vasectomy are diagnosed with prostate cancer? For one thing, a vasectomy is common, and a lot of men out there have had one. For another, as an editorial in the *Journal of the American Medical Association* pointed out, "most vasectomies are performed by urologists and most prostate cancers are diagnosed by urologists, often during procedures to evaluate genitourinary tract symptoms. Therefore, men who have undergone vasectomy may be more likely to have their prostate cancers diagnosed." In other words, because these men have a prior relationship with a urologist, they're more likely to return to a urologist for urinary symptoms and have their cancer diagnosed.

The official word on this, from the National Institutes of Health's panel on vasectomy and the risk of prostate cancer, is: If you've had a vasectomy, don't be alarmed; you're not at cancer's doorstep. "At the present time, providers shall continue to offer vasectomy . . . vasectomy reversal is not warranted to prevent prostate cancer, and screening for prostate cancer should not be any different for men who have had a vasectomy than for men who have not." The doctors on this panel felt the results of research on this subject were "inconsistent," and that the associations drawn from it were weak. They, too, cited "a strong potential for detection bias," because of "possible differences in the use of health care services by men who have had vasectomies . . . that resulted in a different rate of detection."

Anything Else?

Still other factors have been suspected, and studied, as potential risk factors for prostate cancer, including sexual behavior, viruses, socio-economic factors, other aspects of diet, and even BPH, but no strong proof has been found to link these elements to the disease.

THE SHORT STORY

How common is prostate cancer? Too common. In the United States, a man is diagnosed with prostate cancer every three minutes. Every fifteen minutes, a man dies of it. A boy born today has a 13 percent chance of developing prostate cancer, and a 3 percent chance of dying of it.

Scientists don't know precisely what causes prostate cancer, but it's clear that a number of factors are involved. First and foremost are age and hormones. Prostate cancer hardly ever develops before age 40; it becomes more common with every decade afterward. Also, it rarely develops in men who are castrated before puberty.

Genetic factors also play a role. Does prostate cancer run in your family? If your father or brother has prostate cancer, your risk of developing it is two times greater than the average American man's. Families with prostate cancer in three or more first-degree relatives (father or brother), or prostate cancer in three generations (grandfather, father, son) have a hereditary form of the disease. The significance of this is that, in these families, men have a 50 percent risk of developing the disease. Also, it's more likely to strike at a younger age—when a man might not even be looking for trouble or having yearly prostate exams.

What about environment? Clinically significant prostate cancer is rare in men who live in China or Japan. But when these men move to Hawaii or California, their rate of prostate cancer escalates—to the level of an American man's. The high-fat Western diet looms as an obvious environmental culprit, but it's not that simple. Other factors, such as vitamin A and exposure to ultraviolet light—which increases the body's levels of vitamin D—are important in determining which men develop prostate cancer.

As scientists learn more about what causes prostate cancer, perhaps someday we'll be able to turn this knowledge into positive actions—so that, maybe, one day, prostate cancer will be preventable.

3

Prostate Cancer

Screening and Diagnosis

HOW DO I KNOW IF I HAVE IT?

The more you read about prostate cancer, the more it seems that one factor is consistently underplayed—its lack of early symptoms. This is just one way in which prostate cancer differs from other diseases, many of which have early warning signs. To put it bluntly, *by the time a man has symptoms of prostate cancer, it's probably too late to cure it.* Unfortunately, when prostate cancer is in its earliest, most curable stages—before it has spread beyond the wall of the prostate—it is silent; it produces no symptoms.

That's why so much effort is being poured into screening and early diagnosis. To be sure, our understanding of prostate cancer is expanding every day, and the battle is being waged encouragingly on all fronts: *prevention, early diagnosis, effective treatment of curable disease, better management of advanced disease.* But despite many advances—at least for the immediate future—it's not likely that a breakthrough in gene therapy will enable doctors to keep prostate cancer from developing, or that scientists will make major strides in curing advanced disease. Right now, the sad truth is that there is no cure for advanced prostate cancer. Until there is, our best hope of reducing the number of deaths from prostate cancer lies in two tactics—early diagnosis and effective treatment of curable disease.

Figure 3.1. *The digital rectal exam*

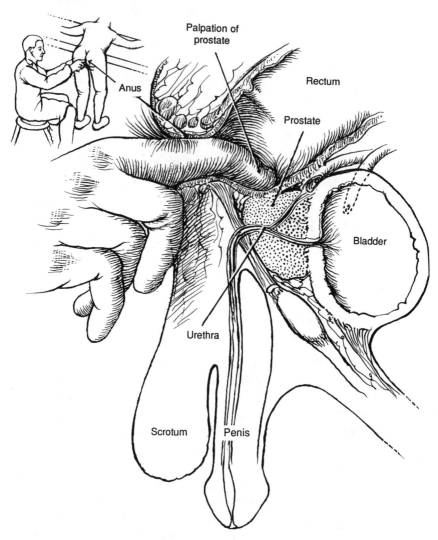

Palpation of
prostate

Rectum

Anus

Prostate

Bladder

Urethra

Scrotum Penis

(The patient is bending over the examining table.) Because of the prostate's location, it can't be seen or examined from the outside. Thus the digital rectal examination, the part of the physical men would rather do without. It's uncomfortable, but it doesn't usually hurt, is generally brief, and it can provide essential information. A doctor's gloved, lubricated finger is inserted into the rectum to feel for lumps, enlargement, or areas of hardness that could be cancer. Because BPH affects only the innermost core of the prostate, a doctor may find nothing out of the ordinary; a man may have what feels like a very small prostate, yet may be having big trouble with urinary retention. This exam also gives valuable information on the tone of the anal sphincter, which can be abnormal in men with some neurological diseases.

A Word on the Digital Rectal Exam

This is the part of the physical men would rather do without. It's uncomfortable, but it doesn't hurt, is generally brief, and it can provide essential information that simply can't be gotten any other way. You may be asked to stand next to the examining table and bend forward slightly, or your doctor may prefer that you kneel on the table or lie on your side. Note: If what you're feeling goes beyond the obvious discomfort of having someone's finger in your rectum and is clearly pain, this could be an important signal of another problem, such as prostatitis. If the exam is painful, tell your doctor.

Many men dread having this test for another reason—their doctor's bedside manner, or lack thereof. Some men even put off going to the doctor because they don't want to deal with someone who is rude, gruff, disrespectful, uncommunicative, or generally unpleasant, and this is a terrible shame. Good doctors know how to make their patients feel at ease. They talk to their patients, and treat them with respect. If your doctor's unfortunate bedside manner is keeping you away from this or any other exam, find another doctor. There are plenty of good ones out there. It's your money—and more importantly, it's your health!

Why the Digital Rectal Exam Is Not Enough

One reason so many cases of prostate cancer are not caught early is obvious: Too many men don't get regular physicals that include a *digital rectal examination* (DRE), the first step in diagnosis, when a doctor feels for a knot, lump, or anything abnormal that might be a tumor. (In men with cancer, the doctor uses the rectal exam to learn as much as possible about the cancer—does it encompass part of one lobe, one entire lobe, or both lobes of the prostate? Has the cancer spread outside the prostate, into the pelvic side wall or the seminal vesicles?)

But even for those who do get checked yearly, the digital rectal exam is not an ironclad guarantee that cancer will be found in time. As many as 40 percent of all prostate cancers begin their growth in an inopportune spot, at a point where a doctor's finger simply can't reach. Therefore, *many patients have advanced disease by the time it is diagnosed with a digital rectal exam.* Also, the digital rectal exam is only as good as the doctor performing it; it is a subjective test.

Because (unlike BPH) the disease generally begins its growth pretty far away from the urethra, most prostate cancer is fairly advanced before it leads to symptoms that men notice and worry about. But another problem is that *there really aren't any clear-cut, telltale symptoms of prostate cancer*—signs that make a doctor say, "Aha! This can only be prostate cancer!" *All of the symptoms of prostate cancer can be attributed to other causes.* Some, for example, are caused when a tumor becomes large enough to encroach on the urethra and block the urinary tract. These symptoms—frequent or urgent urination, hesitancy, interrupted or weakened flow, dribbling, trouble urinating at all, or even blood in the urine—are often mistaken for BPH. Another (although less common) symptom is the development of impotence or of less rigid erections, which can happen as cancer invades the nerves involved in erection. This, too, is accepted as something else—a sign of aging, not a cause for alarm; so is a decrease in the amount of fluid ejaculated, a problem that results when the ejaculatory ducts become blocked by the tumor. (This blockage also can cause blood in the semen.) Still other manifestations, such as severe pain in the back, pelvis, hips or thighs (which can develop as the cancer begins to attack the bone), also might be thought to spring from other causes.

Symptoms of Prostate Cancer

BPH-like symptoms (trouble urinating, frequent or urgent urination, interrupted or weakened flow, hesitancy, dribbling)
Blood in the urine or ejaculate
Severe pain in the back, pelvis, hips, or thighs
Less rigid erections or impotence
A decrease in the amount of fluid ejaculated

Why a Test like PSA Is Needed

For years, doctors have been looking for a man's version of the Pap smear—an early-warning cancer detector that spots a tumor long before it is clinically evident. In this area, no development has been more promising, or controversial, than the PSA test. Recently, you may have heard a lot, good and bad, about this test. The PSA test is not new. In years past, however, its purpose was limited; it functioned mainly as a means of monitoring already-diagnosed prostate cancer and as an indicator of tumor volume. Could its use be expanded? Could it detect cancer that had not yet been diagnosed? The answer, doctors found several years ago, was yes—*elevated levels of PSA can indeed point to the presence of cancer.* In 1992, the American Cancer Society recommended annual PSA tests for all men over age 50, and over age 40 for men at higher risk (particularly, African-American men and men with prostate cancer in the family; see Chapter 2).

However, PSA (prostate-specific antigen) is not a magic wand, pointing with resolute certainty toward prostate cancer—and that's the problem. Even doctors aren't exactly sure how best to use the test, and how to make sense of the information it provides.

Prostate-Specific, Not Cancer-Specific

PSA is an enzyme whose purpose seems to be to break down coagulated semen (this is especially useful in some animals; see "What is Semen?" in Chapter 1). PSA is made almost exclusively by the prostate; and it is prostate-specific, not cancer-specific. In other words, you can have prostate cancer and still have a low PSA level. This is why a blood test alone isn't enough, why a digital rectal exam is also a must. And, just because you have a high PSA does not necessarily mean you have prostate cancer—many men with high PSA levels don't.

However, when PSA is elevated, over a level of four nanograms per milliliter, this means you have *some sort* of prostate trouble—maybe BPH, maybe cancer, maybe an infection. Maybe the prostate has undergone some trauma, like a needle biopsy, or you've had a TUR procedure for BPH, or even a vigorous rectal exam—all of these can elevate PSA. (Conversely, taking the drug finasteride to treat BPH can artificially *lower* the PSA reading—see Chapter 10.)

Gram for gram, PSA levels in the blood are about ten times higher in cancerous tissue than benign tissue. PSA is normally secreted and disposed of

Table 3.1 *Steps for Detecting Prostate Cancer Early*

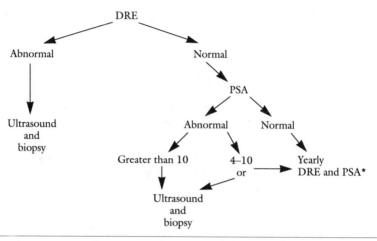

*Every six months, if your PSA is greater than 6.

through tiny ducts in the prostate. But in prostate cancer, the ductal system doesn't drain into the urethra. The PSA builds up, leaks out of the prostate and shows up in the bloodstream. That's why it has proven to be such a good marker for cancer.

But the PSA test is far from perfect. Just as high readings can signify a problem other than cancer, low readings can also be misleading. The bottom line is that *even if your PSA is low, you could still have cancer.* About a quarter of men who turn out to have prostate cancer have a low PSA level, less than 4 nanograms per milliliter. About 25 percent of men with a PSA between 4 and 10 turn out to have cancer. In men with a PSA over 10, about 65 percent are found to have cancer. (What does this mean? See table 3.1.)

The Heated Debate

If you think that all of this seems pretty uncertain, you're not alone, and this is the heart of the controversy. Recently, one group of doctors looked at PSA, transrectal ultrasound and digital rectal exam. They found these tests to be unhelpful, questioned their cost-effectiveness, and concluded that "screening for prostate cancer represents a clinical dilemma with no clear evidence to suggest decreased mortality from any diagnostic test." Critics have contended that PSA test results could prompt thousands of men to have unnecessary and expensive diagnostic procedures, which might lead to unnecessary surgery. One leading magazine told its readers that PSA "could do more harm than good by leading to premature biopsy or treatment"; that the biopsies it prompts are "an infection waiting to happen" (actually, this is not the case; see the "Biopsy" section in this chapter); and that the PSA test can be wrong "four times out of ten."

Doctors at a National Cancer Institute meeting took the PSA arguments several steps further. Many men over age 50 have cancerous cells in their prostates, they said, but just a small percentage of men die from prostate cancer. Most prostate cancer, they argued, is slow-growing and causes no problems. As one doctor told a *New York Times* reporter: "There are millions and millions of American men who have this cancer and are never ill, yet these powerful tests (PSA) are going to detect them. . . . If the PSA is elevated, the chance that it is prostate cancer is relatively small. But even if it does represent prostate cancer, there is no way to know whether testing and treatment change the outcome or improve the health of patients." Some doctors went so far as to state that men should sign informed consent agreements before getting a PSA test. "The information you get back can lead you down a cascade of interventions that can be deadly," one doctor said, citing controversial statistics from a Medicare study for incontinence, impotence, rectal injury, and death resulting from surgery to remove prostate cancer.

Whew! After such strong denunciation, why would anyone want to have a PSA test? *Because it can save lives.*

It's true, many men out there *do* have prostate cancer that doesn't do a whole lot, but just seems to percolate in the prostate without spreading. Are you one of those men? Are you willing to gamble, *with your life,* that you are? Or that you won't live long enough for your prostate cancer to spread? Ideally, doctors would be able to tell the difference between harmless and aggressive tumors, and treat only the "bad" kind of cancer. However, as a Mayo Clinic urologist recently concluded: "Since we do not have the capability to reliably distinguish aggressive tumors from those that are clinically insignificant, one must assume that any prostate cancer identified in a man *with a life expectancy of 10 years or more* is potentially life-threatening, and should therefore be treated." This doesn't mean, as some would argue, that surgery—and particularly, unnecessary surgery—is the automatic next step; it isn't, not by a long shot. (For more on treatment decisions, see Chapter 4.)

Some skeptics contend that routine PSA testing will lead to the diagnosis of those incidental cancers that are present in 30 percent of all men over age 50 (the argument being that, because these cancers are incidental, they don't require treatment or even diagnosis). As it turns out, most of the cancers diagnosed as a result of PSA testing *are* indeed significant, not incidental. A number of recent studies have confirmed this fact. In one study, of men at autopsy, no patient with an insignificant cancer had a PSA greater than 4. Other research has shown that in men with a PSA greater than 4 who undergo radical prostatectomy, their likelihood of having an insignificant tumor is 10 percent or less. And remember, some of those men with apparently harmless prostate cancer will go on to develop—and eventually die of—the real thing, clinically significant prostate cancer.

So, has PSA gotten a bad rap? It depends; much of PSA's value depends on how it's used. One big chunk of the controversy surrounding PSA revolves around the fact that many older men (over age 75) harbor prostate cancer—but most likely won't live long enough for the cancer to be a problem. Therefore, *there is no reason for men over age 75—or any man with a life expectancy less than 10 years—to have a PSA test.* Creating anxiety about what to do—what treatment decisions to make—is not helpful, humane, or necessary for these men. This makes common sense, and should eliminate many of the bitter arguments that have characterized the PSA screening debate.

Another big message from many studies is that PSA should not be used by itself, that *no treatment decision should be made on a lone PSA reading.* That PSA's partner in diagnosis must be a digital rectal exam, with ultrasound and biopsy (see below) performed in patients with abnormal findings. Also, the PSA test may spot *different* cancers than the digital rectal exam—another reason why doctors can't rely on an "either-or" approach for early detection. Together, digital rectal exam and PSA can do far more than either tactic alone. (It's like using breast exams and mammograms together to find breast cancer in women.) This was confirmed in one study of 2,634 men; investigators found that PSA and digital rectal exam were nearly equal in cancer-detecting ability, but that they didn't always find the same tumors—that if only one technique had been used, some cancers would have been missed. (They also noted that if both the digital rectal exam and PSA test were normal, transrectal ultrasound was not necessary.) In short, if digital rectal exam and PSA are used together, most clinically significant prostate cancers eventually will be found.

Bound and Free PSA

As enzymes go, PSA is kind of a tough guy. Like a feisty slugger always looking for a fight, it actively attacks proteins at every opportunity. In the bloodstream, however, PSA is usually restrained by inhibitors that prevent it from breaking down proteins; like a member of a chain gang, it is tied up, or bound.

In one promising new area of research, scientists are working to characterize the forms of PSA in the bloodstream. Is the PSA bound to the inhibitors, or is it on the loose—is it free? Currently, the tests doctors use to measure PSA detect both the bound and unbound molecules. But it might be helpful if we could tell which was which; new evidence indicates that the amount of bound PSA in the blood may be higher in men with prostate cancer than in men with BPH. If this proves to be true, one day soon it may be possible to distinguish between the PSA arising from prostate cancer and the PSA arising from BPH by measuring both its bound and free forms.

In the future, we'll see a new, more specific generation of PSA assays, tests capable of quantifying different forms of the molecule in the bloodstream. Such tests may provide useful clinical information, not only for diagnosis of prostate cancer, but also for evaluation and follow-up.

Making PSA More Meaningful

Doctors are also working to make the PSA a more meaningful and specific test. Some new approaches to PSA include:

PSA Density. This technique begins with a theory, that most men in the age group for prostate cancer also have at least some BPH, which can elevate the PSA concentration and make diagnosis more difficult. One way to distinguish between BPH and cancer, some doctors believe, is *PSA density—the blood PSA score divided by the volume of the prostate, as determined by transrectal* *ultrasound.* Basically, if you have benign disease, your PSA should not be more than 15 percent of the weight of your prostate.

In a preliminary study of sixty-one men, scientists found a difference in PSA density in prostate cancer and BPH; the average PSA density value for forty-one men with clinically localized cancer (confined to the prostate) was 0.58; for the twenty men with BPH, it was 0.04. About 83 percent of the men with prostate cancer who had a normal PSA test had an elevated PSA density score; only two men with prostate cancer had a PSA density under 0.05. The highest PSA density reading for any of the men with BPH was 0.117; most men with BPH had a PSA density level under 0.10. This study also led investigators to develop a probability curve for PSA density that helps doctors gauge a man's likelihood of having prostate cancer.

Results from this and other work suggest that PSA density may be most helpful for men with a PSA score that is higher than normal (between 4 and 10); and that if a man has a slightly elevated PSA score and a PSA density level greater than 0.15, he has a greater chance of having prostate cancer.

PSA density, concludes one study, may be "a useful tool for helping physicians decide which patients with a high normal or mildly elevated serum PSA level to subject to prostatic biopsy and which to (simply) follow."

PSA Velocity. Perhaps the most promising approach to PSA is to look at *PSA velocity—its rate of change from year to year.* The supposition is this: If cells double at a much faster rate in prostate cancer than in BPH, and if prostate cancer produces more PSA than BPH does, *it's likely that PSA's yearly rate of change will be much greater in a man with prostate cancer than in a man with BPH.* In other words: It stands to reason that if a man's PSA is going up, he has a cancer—and that cancer is probably growing.

In one study, researchers at Johns Hopkins made use of a massive data base called the Baltimore Longitudinal Study of Aging. (Since it was begun in 1958, about one thousand five hundred men have participated in this study, returning every other year for physical examinations and a battery of medical tests. Their blood samples from every checkup are stored for future studies.) The investigators looked at three groups of men who were involved in this study—those with BPH, those with prostate cancer, and a control group of men with no prostate disease. Looking at twenty years' worth of stored blood samples, investigators found that the men with prostate cancer had "significantly greater rates of change in PSA levels than those without prostate cancer *up to ten years before diagnosis.*" In other words, by tracking changes in PSA levels, they were able to detect prostate cancer years before it could be diagnosed by other means. For example, at five years before diagnosis—when PSA levels weren't appreciably different between men with BPH and men with prostate cancer—there was already a big difference in PSA velocity in men who turned out to have prostate cancer versus men who had BPH and the control group.

PSA velocity has the potential to be highly valuable in detecting prostate cancer, and in distinguishing it from BPH early—particularly now, when an increasing number of men are returning to their doctor every year for a digital rectal examination and PSA test. *PSA velocity is a fluid continuum, not a cut-and-dried, one-shot reading.* It's like having a prostate barometer—your doctor doesn't have to wait for the PSA score to reach a magic number (currently, it's 4 nanograms per milliliter). With PSA velocity, what matters is a significant change over time—an average *consistent* increase of more than 0.75 nanograms per milliliter a year, over the course of three tests separated by at least 12 to 18 months. Say over 24 months a man's PSA level went up from 1.2 to 2.3 to 3.6. Clearly, something's going on here. This obvious, steady rise could enable a doctor monitoring PSA velocity to detect clinically significant, *curable* prostate cancer in its earliest, most subtle stages, instead of waiting for the PSA level to reach the magic 4, and then doing further tests. "So the potential for PSA velocity means we can make a more accurate diagnosis of prostate cancer at *even lower levels* than the raw cutoff of 4, because it works at any level," says one of the researchers. (At present, it's unclear what rate of change is significant in men with PSA greater than 10.) Also, PSA velocity is *more specific.* If doctors use the PSA level of 4 as a cutoff point, about 40 percent of men who only have BPH undergo unnecessary biopsies. But with PSA velocity, this number is reduced; only 10 percent of men with BPH undergo an unnecessary biopsy.

Because of such studies, many doctors are excited about PSA velocity. However—although it's a big improvement over looking at a bald PSA score and trying to figure out what it means—even PSA velocity isn't a perfect system. One big point to remember: 25 percent of men with prostate cancers that are growing do *not* have a big increase in their PSA. So, just because your PSA isn't high, and just because your PSA isn't going up, that doesn't mean you don't have cancer, and it doesn't mean that your cancer isn't growing.

PSA and a Man's Age. Which brings us to PSA and age. *The theory here is this: As a man ages, his prostate gets bigger.* Therefore, why should the PSA cutoff point be the same for a 40-year-old man as for an 80-year-old man (who probably has a higher PSA level anyway, due to BPH)? In a study led by the

Mayo Clinic, doctors determined age-specific ranges for PSA: Lower than the current 4 for younger men (with a life expectancy of 25 to 30 years); and higher than 4—which probably is too severe—for older men. They recommended a cutoff of 2.5 for men aged 40–49; of 3.5 for men aged 50–59; of 4.5 for men aged 60–69; and of 6.5 for men aged 70–79.

"The age-specific reference ranges should make PSA a more selective tumor marker," the researchers said, "such that significant prostate cancers can be identified at an early, curable stage in men who are most likely to have the greatest benefit from definitive therapy . . . and unnecessary diagnostic procedures would not be performed routinely in men who are unlikely to harbor a life-threatening prostatic malignancy or benefit from therapy." (One note here is that the higher upper limit for men over age 60 may mean that some potentially curable cancers are not detected as early. The investigators plan to confront this issue in further research.)

The PLCO Study

This is another salvo in the argument about whether treatment for prostate cancer has any effect on long-term survival. Critics have stated, loudly, that "there is no evidence that definitive treatment of localized prostate cancer increases survival." However, there has been no large, well-designed study to evaluate the effectiveness of early prostate cancer treatment in prolonging lives. Moreover, there's no evidence that definitive treatment does *not* increase survival! The issue has never been properly investigated.

The PLCO study hopes to answer the question. This is a massive, multimillion-dollar study, sponsored by the National Cancer Institute, involving prostate, lung, colon and ovarian cancers. (Thus the name, PLCO.) For prostate cancer, the point is to determine whether or not screening makes a difference in life expectancy. (This also has a lot to do with the controversy surrounding the PSA test's effectiveness—see "The Heated Debate," earlier in this chapter.) Men will be screened once a year for four years, and then followed for twelve years. This is similar to the screening intervals used in a study to determine mammography's effectiveness in spotting breast cancer. However, prostate cancer is much slower-growing than breast cancer, and some doctors worry that four years isn't going to be long enough for PSA's yearly rate of change to be as meaningful as it has the potential to be.

Another worry is that the screening won't be done in the best possible way up front, and thus the follow-up, which will be expensive, will be worthless. The problem is that we don't know how best to use PSA yet. Is PSA density the way to go? PSA velocity or age-specific ranges? Scientists just don't know. So initiating a long-term study now appears, to some investigators, to be premature.

Also, in this study, treatment is up in the air—once a diagnosis is made, the treatment choice is left up to the patient and his physician. *So how can we know if PSA makes a difference in life expectancy if a man dies because he opts for no treatment or an ineffective treatment?* And finally, the age range for the study is not meaningful; it includes men up to age 74. The unfortunate fact is that many of these men probably won't be alive to see the end of the twelve-year follow-up period. It is unlikely, then, that they will live long enough to provide any new insights into the long-term effectiveness of treatment.

So it seems a shame that this massive study, which taxpayers are funding, is proceeding without a more thoughtful design.

The PIVOT Study

Another attempt to shed light on prostate cancer treatment is the national PIVOT (Prostate cancer Intervention vs. Observation Trial) study, led by a Minnesota internist and a Seattle urologist and funded by the Department of Veterans Affairs and the National Cancer Institute. Its aim is to find out which works better for clinically localized prostate cancer—radical prostatectomy with early intervention (such as radiation therapy) in case the cancer comes back, or watchful waiting, with treatment for symptoms if the cancer spreads.

"We're not looking at radiation as a primary treatment," comments the internist who's heading the study, "because studies indicate that radiation is at least not better than radical prostatectomy." Instead, the PIVOT study will "compare watchful waiting with the most frequently recommended, and probably the best, of the early intervention approaches—radical prostatectomy."

Like the PLCO study, the PIVOT study is long; it has a three-year enrollment period, and a twelve-year follow-up; 2,000 men will be able to participate. Men up to age 75 are eligible—but these older men, like the rest of the men in the study, must be healthy enough to be considered fit for surgery. Only men with prostate cancer who are considered candidates for surgery may take part in the study; they will be assigned to one of two groups—either they'll undergo a radical prostatectomy, or they will be followed closely with watchful waiting and treated as needed for specific symptoms or metastases. Many cancer centers and Veterans Administration hospitals throughout the country are participating in this study.

What's the measure of success here? It's what you might call the ultimate endpoint—death or survival. "Really, that's what the patient cares about," says the internist. "Will my disease be cured? Is my life better without the surgery? We don't know the answer to either of those questions. Those in favor of radical prostatectomy say, 'How can doctors dare not treat? They're killing people with watchful waiting!' And the watchful waiting people say that surgery doesn't prolong survival. These are two groups of intelligent, caring people, and there is information to support either of these two views."

Men in the study will be examined at least every three months the first year and every six months afterward, and periodically they will answer questionnaires about their quality of life. Their doctors will check for any evidence that prostate cancer has progressed, and they will document any changes in the patients' condition. If the patient dies, for any reason, all of this information will go to an independent review committee, which will study all the accumulated data and determine whether the man's death was definitely, probably, possibly, or definitely not due to prostate cancer.

The PIVOT study is interesting for several reasons; despite the age limit of its patients—it's hard to know how many 75-year-old men will be around for the study's conclusion—the selection criteria seem fairly strict. Men who obviously are not good candidates for surgery, the study's directors say, will not be included. Also, because of its size, the study promises highly specific results.

Transrectal Ultrasound

Like sonar on a submarine, ultrasound draws pictures using sound waves. Transrectal ultrasound can detect differences between cancerous and normal tissue in the prostate by means of a special probe, inserted in the rectum. In most cases, it allows doctors to see the entire prostate. This transrectal

---

Steps in Diagnosing Prostate Cancer

Digital rectal examination (DRE)
PSA blood test
Transrectal ultrasound
Biopsy

(through the rectum) approach is a big improvement over a lower-frequency, lower-resolution technique used several years ago, in which sound waves had to travel all the way through the abdomen to reach the prostate. Transrectal ultrasound is able to detect cancers that can't be felt in a digital rectal exam; it has been found to have a detection rate of 2.6 percent—as opposed to the 1.3 to 1.7 percent rate for digital rectal exam and the 2.2 to 2.6 percent rate for PSA. And, many men with prostate cancer detected by transrectal ultrasound (and missed by digital rectal exam) who went on to have surgery, a radical prostatectomy, to treat the cancer were found to have disease that was confined to the prostate. In other words, thanks to ultrasound, for these men the cancer was found in time to cure it.

Encouraging results. And, just as doctors had hoped PSA would become a "male Pap smear," many hoped transrectal ultrasound could be a "male mammogram," another means of screening for and detecting prostate cancer early. That hasn't happened yet. Transrectal ultrasound is neither quick nor cheap, and the results often depend on the skill of the doctor using the ultrasound equipment. So right away, these three factors rule it out as the perfect tool for routine screening—it's just not worth it to use transrectal ultrasound on everybody.

As a tool for diagnosis, ultrasound today is used as a next step—after an abnormal digital rectal exam or PSA score, or if a man has symptoms of prostate cancer or is worried because of a family history of the disease. (It rarely finds cancer in men who have had a normal PSA score and digital rectal exam, and is not necessary if both of these tests are normal.)

Perhaps its biggest drawback is that—though it's an improvement over the transabdominal approach—*transrectal ultrasound can't catch every cancer.* It misses about half the cancers greater than a centimeter in size, because to the ultrasound scanner, they sound just like regular prostate tissue. (For some reason, in some men there's no acoustic difference between normal and abnormal tissue.) And, because some normal tissue sounds just like cancer, ultrasound also mistakes many benign lesions for cancer.

What it can do: However, ultrasound *is* valuable in diagnosis. It is a great means of estimating the weight of a man's prostate—which, among other things, can help doctors get a better idea of PSA density (discussed earlier in this chapter)—and it plays a major role in directing a needle biopsy, so the right bit of tissue is tested.

Figure 3.2. *Transrectal ultrasound*

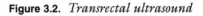

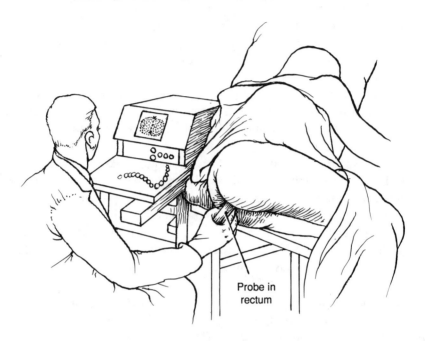

Probe in rectum

It's certainly not much fun, but transrectal ultrasound is painless, and it can be very valuable in diagnosing prostate cancer. A special probe (shown here) is inserted into the rectum, usually allowing the doctor to see the entire prostate—and often to detect cancers that can't be felt in a digital rectal exam.

As a tool for diagnosis, ultrasound today is used as a next step—after an abnormal digital rectal exam or abnormal PSA score, or if a man has symptoms of prostate cancer or is worried because of a family history of the disease. Transrectal ultrasound rarely uncovers cancer in men who have had a normal PSA score and a normal digital rectal exam, and it is not necessary for a man to have this procedure if both of these tests are normal.

Biopsy

Just a few years ago, biopsy of the prostate was done "blind"—doctors couldn't see what they were doing—and as the biopsy needle hit the prostate, the impact sometimes caused the gland to "flip" or rotate slightly, so the biopsy wasn't actually in the part of the tissue doctors thought they were reaching. Today, using transrectal ultrasound as a guide, urologists can see what they're

Figure 3.3. *Ultrasound-guided needle biopsy of the prostate*

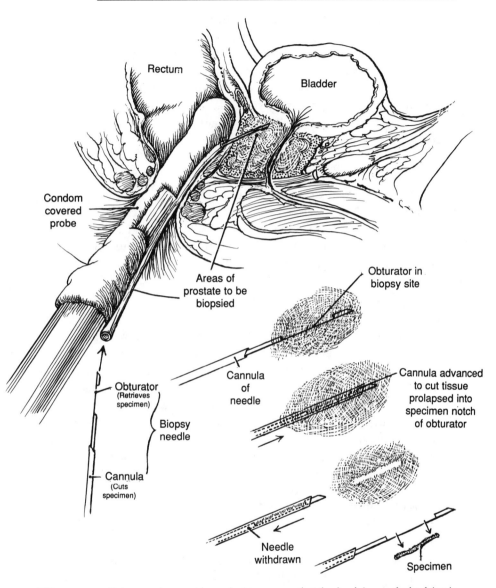

Rectum

Bladder

Condom covered probe

Areas of prostate to be biopsied

Obturator in biopsy site

Obturator (Retrieves specimen)

Cannula of needle

Cannula advanced to cut tissue prolapsed into specimen notch of obturator

Biopsy needle

Cannula (Cuts specimen)

Needle withdrawn

Specimen

Using transrectal ultrasound as a guide, urologists can see what they're doing *as they're doing it*. This is a big improvement over the biopsy techniques that were used just a few years ago. This way, a biopsy of the prostate is more accurate—and, because the needle is smaller, less painful—than ever before. The biopsy device is ingeniously designed to capture a *core* of abnormal-looking tissue (each core of tissue is about a millimeter thick), instead of just a few cells. Pathologists then study these samples under the microscope.

doing *as they're doing it*. So a biopsy of the prostate is more accurate—and, because the needle is smaller, less painful—than ever before.

Another breakthrough in biopsy technique, besides improved ultrasound technology, has been the development of the springloaded biopsy gun, a tiny device that's attached to a doctor's finger. The smaller needle means urologists can be more precise in targeting a core of abnormal tissue—even if it's surrounded by normal-looking cells. It also means that you'll feel only slight discomfort.

What about the Risk of Infection?

Despite the fact that the biopsy is taken through the rectum, infection is hardly ever a problem, if its risk is kept to a minimum—if a cleansing enema is given beforehand, and antibiotics are given both before and after the biopsy. Other temporary complications of prostate biopsy can include minor rectal bleeding and a trace of blood in the ejaculate.

Why Needle Biopsies Aren't Perfect

Despite these improvements, needle biopsy doesn't always give definitive answers. Sometimes the needle misses the cancer; sometimes what's under the microscope is almost impossible to label definitively as cancer.

Some cancers, particularly those developing in the peripheral zone of the prostate, spread laterally—like a thin sheet of plankton on the surface of the sea. So it's not uncommon that the biopsy needle goes in too deep and overshoots the target area. That's why, in an attempt to get a comprehensive picture, doctors also take several tiny samples from throughout the prostate in what's called a sextant biopsy (six biopsies, one from the top, middle and bottom of the gland on the right and left sides).

"Breast or lung cancer makes a solid nodule, just like a fist, that you usually can detect by palpation or imaging," says a Johns Hopkins pathologist who is an expert in diagnosing prostate cancer. But prostate cancer tends to infiltrate normal tissue, meandering around normal cells. Or, as another Johns Hopkins scientist explains, it spreads out like a hand, whose fingers flow into nearby tissue "like a river flooding a valley." In these cases there can be a significant amount of cancer, but not in the form of a "convenient" lump that's easy to feel or see on ultrasound.

Thus, it's not uncommon for a needle biopsy to be negative—*even though cancer is present*. This is called a false negative, and it can give both the urologist and the patient "a false optimism that the cancer isn't there," the pathologist continues. So, even if one biopsy is suspicious and a repeat biopsy is negative, "that doesn't rule out that the first biopsy *wasn't* cancer."

Imagine the difficulty of trying to capture this elusive tissue in a biopsy, using only a tiny needle. In some cases, it's like looking *with* a needle in a haystack. The thin needles used for most prostate biopsies capture tiny cores of tissue—each about a millimeter thick—which pathologists then study under the microscope.

In the easiest diagnoses, many cancer glands are found. But in tougher cases only a few are found. And this is where diagnosis gets tricky: Do these few glands mean it's only the indolent kind of cancer? Or has the biopsy captured the beginnings of more serious cancer that may require treatment? And how do you distinguish between the two?

"From the pathology standpoint, it's not quite a nightmare," says the Johns Hopkins pathologist, "but it's close. Several years ago, the only reason people were getting needles stuck in their prostate was because they had a palpable lesion. In those cases, if you found cancer—even if it were one or two glands on a needle biopsy—almost invariably, there was significant cancer in the prostate." (Clearly, diagnosis is a lot easier when cancer can be felt; by the time it reaches this point, there's usually a tumor of significant size that needs treatment.)

One man had a biopsy that was considered negative by one pathologist. His urologist sent it to this pathologist for a second opinion. "There were about four glands of cancer. We called it cancer, he had his prostate out, and there was tumor all over." But for every such patient, there's another man who turns out to have very little cancer.

Which brings us to one very tough question: Do all men who have cancer on needle biopsies need aggressive therapy? Again, the problem lies in our ability to differentiate between harmless and malevolent cancer. "If it were my family member," the pathologist confesses, "I wouldn't want to take the chance."

But eventually, the goal is *not* to treat all prostate cancers, but to predict which cancers are going to turn serious, and treat these tumors aggressively. And predict which cancers will remain indolent, and monitor them closely.

Until very recently, the technology that made early biopsy possible also made these judgment calls much tougher—pathologists had trouble correlating the amount of cancer on the needle with the amount of cancer in the entire prostate. But now, research from Johns Hopkins promises to shed fresh light—

to make needle biopsy findings much more helpful in determining a man's course of treatment.

Say a man's prostate feels normal during a digital rectal exam, but his PSA is elevated and a biopsy has found cancer cells (this is considered stage T1c disease—see table 3.2). Is this significant cancer? Should action be taken? The new research suggests that *for men with stage T1c disease,* if any cancer is found in three needle cores, or in greater than 50 percent of any one needle core, or if the Gleason score (discussed in this chapter) is 7 or higher, then it's highly likely that significant cancer is present in the prostate. On the other hand, if the cancer is Gleason 6 or less and is found in only one or two needle cores, cancer makes up less than half of these cores, *and* if the PSA density is less than 0.1 to

Table 3.2 *Two Systems for Staging Prostate Cancer*

TNM Stage	Description	Whitmore-Jewett Stage	Description
T1a	Not palpable in a DRE; found incidentally when benign tissue is removed by TUR; 5 percent or less of the removed tissue is cancerous.	A1	Same as TNM
T1b	Not palpable; found incidentally, but greater than 5 percent of the tissue removed by TUR is cancerous.	A2	Same as TNM
T1c	Not palpable; identified by needle biopsy because of elevated PSA.	—	This category is not part of the Whitmore-Jewett system.
T2a	Palpable; involves less than half of one lobe.	B1N	Palpable; involves less than half of one lobe; is surrounded by normal tissue.
T2b	Palpable; involves more than half of one lobe, but not both lobes.	B1	Palpable; involves less than one lobe.
T2c	Palpable; involves both lobes.	B2	Palpable; involves one entire lobe or more.
T3, T4	Palpable; penetrates the wall of the prostate and/or involves the seminal vesicles.	C	Same as TNM
N+	Has spread to lymph nodes.	D1	Same as TNM
M+	Has spread to bone.	D2	Same as TNM

Note: These stages can be confusing; although the newer, more explicit TNM system is becoming more popular, many doctors tend to use both systems interchangeably.

Needle Biopsies: What to Make of the Findings in Stage Tɪc Disease

Cancer is significant if . . .

It's found in three needle cores, OR
It's present in greater than half of any one needle core, OR
If the Gleason score is 7 or higher

Cancer is probably NOT significant if . . .

It's found in only one or two needle cores, AND
It makes up less than half of those needle cores, AND
The Gleason score is 6 or lower, AND
The PSA density is less than 0.1–0.15

0.15, there's a good chance that the cancer in the prostate is insignificant (that there is less than 0.2 cubic centimeters of prostate cancer, and that it is confined solely to the prostate.)

Scientists at Johns Hopkins and elsewhere are also working to develop a more scientific means of prediction than the current one, which relies heavily on the human eye. Currently, much of the interpretation of cancer simply comes down to subjective guesswork, based on how hundreds of thousands of cells look under the microscope. On the horizon may be a computerized image analysis system that measures and quantifies various cell shapes and irregularities—and, in the process, creates more lucid pictures from a murky palette.

WHERE DO I STAND?
STAGING PROSTATE CANCER

Okay, the biopsy is positive, and the diagnosis is prostate cancer. But what does this mean? The next step is to determine the stage—how far the cancer has spread—and the grade—how the cancer cells look, as an estimation of how fast they're growing.

Setting the Stage for Treatment

There are two different ways to classify prostate cancer: The Whitmore-Jewett system, and the TNM staging system. They are based on the extent to which the cancer has grown. Is it confined to the prostate? Or has it spread, and if it has, how far? Again, the staging system drives home the vital message that early diagnosis is fundamental to a cure—because prostate cancer is considered curable only in its earliest stages, when it's confined to the prostate.

The best-case scenario is when unsuspected cancer cells are not palpable (large enough for a doctor to feel during a digital rectal exam) and are found incidentally—when tissue is removed during a TUR procedure, for example (see Chapter 10), or if a doctor orders a biopsy to investigate an elevated PSA score. (In a TUR, or transurethral resection of the prostate, a procedure to treat symptoms of an enlarged prostate, overgrown prostate tissue is removed in fragments through the urethra. These bits of tissue are routinely sent to a pathologist for evaluation.) Other, less congenial cancers are found during a physical exam, when a doctor's gloved finger detects a lump or aberration—a small nodule on one or both sides of the prostate. The next category is cancer that has penetrated the wall of the prostate or invaded the nearby seminal vesicles.

Generally, the higher the letter, the worse the cancer. Cancer in the highest stages (D, N, or M) means the tumor has metastasized—a chunk of cancer has broken off and established itself in another location, generally in a nearby lymph node. The most serious stage is when cancer has infiltrated other lymph nodes and spread to distant regions, most commonly to bone. Cancer at these stages can be controlled and even kept at bay for months or even years, but not cured. And nobody, as yet, understands why this is—what critical changes take place when the cancer leaves the prostate, and why, suddenly, it defies the treatment that can be so effective in its earlier phases.

Table 3.2 presents the stages, using both systems.

The Gleason Score

Now, what does the cancer look like under the microscope? Are the cells well differentiated, or are they poorly differentiated? The architecture of normal, well-differentiated cells involves distinct, clearly defined borders. Well-differentiated cells have clear centers—think of tiny round doughnuts. When

Opposite: This illustration shows prostate cancer in all its stages, using both the TNM and the Whitmore-Jewett systems.

Figure 3.4. *What does cancer look like in the prostate?*

STAGES OF PROSTATE CANCER

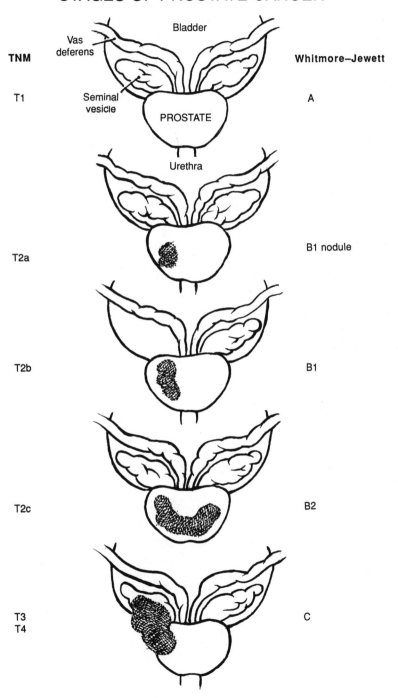

cancer cells become poorly differentiated, they seem to melt together and form solid, nasty blobs of malignancy. These cancers are the most aggressive. They run rampant, sweeping through nearby tissue and launching missiles to distant sites in the body, no longer respecting boundaries—their own, or other cells'. The results are often devastating; the fastest, most out-of-control cancer cells can kill a man within a year of their initial clinical presentation. Well-differentiated cancers tend to progress very slowly, and poorly differentiated cancers tend to spread like wildfire.

Pathologists use a system called the Gleason score to rank cell differentiation. Basically, a low Gleason score—2, 3, 4—is good. A high Gleason score—8, 9, 10—is not. What about a score right in the middle? This is another murky area, where it's hard to predict what course the cells will take.

Scientists have shown that cancers with a high Gleason score are more likely to be "margin-positive" (to have cancer that has penetrated the prostate wall to a point where it can't all be removed in surgery), more likely to have cancer in the seminal vesicles, and more likely to defy treatment than cancers with a lower score. With a higher Gleason score, there's also a higher likelihood of cancer spreading to the lymph nodes. Therefore, if a man has a high Gleason score, there is a good probability that his cancer has spread beyond the prostate wall and maybe to nearby structures.

A Word on Natural History

We've said that it's impossible to predict the course of prostate cancer. This dilemma is at the heart of the treatment debate. However, some research has shown that the *volume* of a prostate tumor has a lot to do with its behavior. Scientists who studied 100 radical prostatectomy specimens (tissue removed in surgery) found that the volume of cancer corresponded with the extent (or lack) of cell differentiation, with capsular penetration (cancer that has reached beyond the prostate wall), invasion of the seminal vesicles, and metastases to distant tissue. These researchers showed that tumors less than 1 cubic centimeter (just smaller than a half-inch) rarely metastasize, and that most tumors less than 3.5 cubic centimeters stay inside the prostate. But as a tumor gets bigger, they found, it tends to get more aggressive—and when prostate cancer is bigger than 5 cubic centimeters, its chances of being curable dwindle.

This is how prostate cancer spreads: First, of course, it grows inside the prostate. Most—about 72 percent of cancers—begin in the peripheral zone, 20 percent start in the transition zone, and 8 percent originate in the central zone. (For a look at the prostate's zones, see figure 1.8.) It reaches, and then penetrates, the prostate wall (also called the capsule). Then it continues to creep, reaching into the seminal vesicles, bladder, urethra and pelvic sidewalls. It also can expand in leaps, by metastases—invading the lymph system (channels that run throughout the body) or hitching a ride to far-off sites via the bloodstream to bone. When doctors speak of "distant metastases" of prostate cancer, they generally mean it has reached the lymph nodes, bone—the spine, ribs, or pelvic bones—or the lungs.

As prostate tumors grow, they become more heterogeneous, or poorly differentiated. Prostate cancer generally is a slow grower; in its early stages, it can take longer than four years for a tumor to double in size. Before a tumor even gets big enough for a doctor to feel—about one cubic centimeter in volume—it has to double at least thirty times. But after this, it only takes about ten more doublings for prostate cancer to become fatal—when it reaches 1 kilogram in volume.

Once again, to hammer home a point, this time of silent early growth is the ideal time to detect and strike prostate cancer.

Clinical Stage versus Pathologic Stage

This can be pretty confusing. Clinical stage is an estimate, what a doctor *believes* a man's prostate cancer to be, based on factors such as the digital rectal exam, PSA, transrectal ultrasound and needle biopsy. Pathologic stage is much more certain—and, for predicting the likelihood for cure, it's essential—because a pathologist has been able to examine actual prostate tissue and, often, tissue from the lymph nodes, not just make guesses about it based on a few cells and test results. Until recently, knowing pathologic stage was only possible when the prostate was removed. Now, however, based on table 3.3, doctors have a much better way of estimating a man's pathologic stage of cancer *before* surgery.

More on the Digital Rectal Exam and Staging

Like transrectal ultrasound, the digital rectal exam is not able to pick up microscopic cancer spread to the prostate wall and beyond. Because of this, the digital rectal exam tends to underestimate the stage of cancer. Studies have found that a significant number of cancers initially staged as T2b (B1) end up being classified as higher because of cancer that has invaded the capsule of the prostate or the seminal vesicles. For cancer with an initial clinical evaluation of T2c (B2), this degree of "understaging" ranges from 39 percent to 66 percent. One reason for this is that the digital rectal exam is subjective; it depends on the experience and perceptiveness of the doctor performing it. Another is that the digital rectal exam can only give information about the prostate gland itself—and not even all of it, at that. And it certainly can't tell anything about the nearby pelvic lymph nodes or bones. Also, if a man has had other treatment of a prostate disorder—a TUR, for instance, for BPH—this can cause the prostate to feel different on an exam, and it can throw off the digital rectal exam.

PSA and Staging

We know PSA can signal the presence of cancer. But can PSA be more specific—can it tell a doctor the *stage* of a man's tumor? Yes, it can. However, as always, PSA is tricky, and the PSA level alone doesn't tell the whole story.

As a tumor gets bigger, the PSA level generally goes up. And, as the tumor grows, it tends to be overrun by the more malignant, poorly differentiated cancer cells. These poorly differentiated cancer cells elevate PSA less per gram of tissue than well-differentiated cancer cells. Therefore, the PSA level doesn't go up in a directly corresponding way.

That's why PSA can be normal even when cancer has spread to the seminal vesicles or pelvic lymph nodes, or it can be higher than expected in men with cancer that's confined to the prostate. So, *the true meaning of PSA can't be interpreted without knowing the Gleason score.*

Scientists at Johns Hopkins have found a more accurate way to estimate the exact extent of prostate cancer, using a special table that correlates clinical stage, Gleason score, and PSA (see table 3.3).

Even though prostate cancer may appear to be confined to the prostate on examination, surgery may reveal a different story—often, the cancer turns out to be more extensive than it seemed at first. That's because insidious, microscopic bits of cancer can sneak past the prostate wall, and these can't always be found with the digital rectal exam, biopsy, transrectal ultrasound or other diagnostic methods.

Because surgery is only indicated for the cancers that truly are localized to the prostate, it would be better for everyone to know *before* the operation how extensive the cancer is.

So, how to predict which cancers may have spread beyond the prostate wall? Tables 3.3a–3.3d were developed by Johns Hopkins researchers after a study of the course of prostate cancer in 1,186 men who had radical prostatectomy.

The tables are designed to help you and your doctor predict your definitive pathological stage and best course of treatment. For example, if you have stage T2a disease, with a Gleason score of 5 and a PSA less than 4, there is an 81

Table 3.3a *Percentage of Men with Organ-Confined Disease*

Gleason Score	Clinical Stage						
	T1a	T1b	T1c	T2a	T2b	T2c	T3a
PSA ng/ml: 0.0–4.0							
2–4	100	85	92	88	76	82	—
5	100	78	81	81	67	73	—
6	100	68	69	72	54	60	42
7	—	54	55	61	41	46	—
8–10	—	—	—	48	31	—	—
PSA ng/ml: 4.1–10							
2–4	100	78	82	83	67	71	—
5	100	70	71	73	56	64	43
6	100	53	59	62	44	48	33
7	100	39	43	51	32	37	26
8–10	—	32	31	39	22	25	12
PSA ng/ml: 10.1–20							
2–4	100	—	—	61	52	—	—
5	100	49	55	58	43	37	26
6	—	36	41	44	28	37	19
7	—	24	24	36	19	24	14
8–10	—	11	—	29	14	15	9
PSA ng/ml: greater than 20							
2–4	—	—	33	20	7	—	—
5	—	—	24	32	—	3	—
6	—	—	22	14	11	4	5
7	—	—	7	18	4	5	3
8–10	—	—	3	3	1	2	2

Source: Alan W. Partin and Patrick C. Walsh, "The Use of Prostate-Specific Antigen, Clinical Stage and Gleason Score to Predict Pathologic Stage in Men with Localized Prostate Cancer," *Journal of Urology* 152 (1994):172–73. Reprinted with Permission of the American Urological Association.

percent chance that the cancer will be completely confined to your prostate. On the other hand, if your Gleason score is 8 and your PSA is 15, the likelihood drops to 29 percent. With this information and an estimation of your overall health and longevity, you and your doctor can decide whether or not it's reasonable to select curative forms of therapy, or simply to adopt a policy of watchful waiting, in which the tumor is treated only after it produces symptoms. (Note: The dashes in the tables represent lack of sufficient data to calculate probability.)

Table 3.3b *Percentage of Men with Established Capsular Penetration*

Gleason Score	Clinical Stage						
	T1a	T1b	T1c	T2a	T2b	T2c	T3a
PSA ng/ml: 0.0–4.0							
2–4	0	15	22	14	26	17	—
5	0	22	30	20	34	26	—
6	0	30	34	29	46	38	59
7	—	43	40	39	59	50	—
8–10	—	—	—	50	68	—	—
PSA ng/ml: 4.1–10							
2–4	0	22	29	19	34	27	—
5	0	29	34	28	45	34	58
6	0	45	38	38	56	49	68
7	0	58	44	49	68	59	75
8–10	—	64	48	59	77	71	87
PSA ng/ml: 10.1–20							
2–4	0	—	—	40	49	—	—
5	0	49	40	43	58	61	75
6	—	62	45	56	73	59	82
7	—	73	52	64	81	73	86
8–10	—	87	—	70	86	82	92
PSA ng/ml: greater than 20							
2–4	—	—	50	80	94	—	—
5	—	—	54	68	—	97	—
6	—	—	53	86	90	96	95
7	—	—	67	80	96	95	98
8–10	—	—	74	97	99	97	98

Source: Partin and Walsh (1994).

Acid Phosphatase

Acid phosphatase is an enzyme that, just like PSA, is secreted by the prostate gland. When a prostate becomes cancerous, the ductal system stops working properly. So, like PSA, acid phosphatase builds up in the prostate, leaks out and is reabsorbed by the bloodstream. That's why elevated acid phosphatase levels can signal that something's wrong with the prostate. There are two ways of looking at acid phosphatase: Radio-immunoassay, and enzymatic assay. The radio-immunoassay test is *not* helpful. It is often elevated in men with BPH, and therefore it gives little useful information. The enzymatic test, however, can be helpful, because, if it is elevated, it usually signifies advanced disease. But, like PSA, acid phosphatase can be tricky. There are many men with advanced disease in whom acid phosphatase is not elevated.

Table 3.3c *Percentage of Men with Seminal Vesicle Involvement*

Gleason Score	Clinical Stage						
	T1a	T1b	T1c	T2a	T2b	T2c	T3a
PSA ng/ml: 0.0–4.0							
2–4	0	1	Less than 1	1	2	2	—
5	0	3	Less than 1	2	4	4	—
6	0	6	1	5	9	9	8
7	—	12	4	9	17	17	—
8–10	—	—	—	17	29	—	—
PSA ng/ml: 4.1–10							
2–4	0	2	Less than 1	1	3	3	—
5	0	4	Less than 1	3	6	6	5
6	0	9	1	6	11	12	11
7	0	18	5	12	22	23	18
8–10	—	29	23	22	38	40	40
PSA ng/ml: 10.1–20							
2–4	0	—	—	3	4	—	—
5	0	7	Less than 1	5	8	12	11
6	—	15	1	11	19	17	18
7	—	28	6	19	33	33	31
8–10	—	55	—	29	50	53	49
PSA ng/ml: greater than 20							
2–4	—	—	Less than 1	12	30	—	—
5	—	—	Less than 1	11	—	29	—
6	—	—	2	35	40	53	31
7	—	—	9	31	73	62	55
8–10	—	—	31	81	93	73	65

Source: Partin and Walsh (1994).

When a man has an elevated acid phosphatase level but no sign of metastases—when no cancer has shown up on a bone scan, for instance, or in the lymph nodes—some doctors label this cancer D0, on the suspicion that cancer *has* spread, only on a scale that's still too small for doctors to detect on a clinical level.

The PSA test is much more sensitive, and its increasingly widespread use has led some doctors to question the value of acid phosphatase. For instance: In one study of 460 men with prostate cancer, 21 men had elevated acid phosphatase scores. But for 17 out of these 21 men, advanced cancer had been detected either by an abnormal digital rectal exam or PSA score, so the acid phosphatase test provided helpful information for only four men out of the whole group! (This is what scientists call a "low yield" of unique information.) Therefore, acid phosphatase is no longer considered a must-have test before a doctor can

Table 3.3d *Percentage of Men with Lymph Node Involvement*

Gleason Score	Clinical Stage						
	T1a	T1b	T1c	T2a	T2b	T2c	T3a
			PSA ng/ml: 0.0–4.0				
2–4	0	2	Less than 1	1	2	4	—
5	0	4	1	2	4	9	—
6	0	8	2	3	9	17	15
7	—	15	2	7	18	31	—
8–10	—	—	—	13	32	—	—
			PSA ng/ml: 4.1–10				
2–4	0	2	1	1	2	5	—
5	0	4	1	2	5	10	8
6	0	9	2	4	11	19	16
7	0	18	3	8	20	34	28
8–10	—	30	5	15	35	53	50
			PSA ng/ml: 10.1–20				
2–4	0	—	—	1	3	—	—
5	0	5	3	2	6	13	11
6	—	11	4	5	13	22	20
7	—	21	7	9	24	39	35
8–10	—	41	—	17	40	59	54
			PSA ng/ml: greater than 20				
2–4	—	—	6	2	7	—	—
5	—	—	9	3	—	29	—
6	—	—	8	9	18	53	31
7	—	—	24	11	44	62	55
8–10	—	—	41	35	76	73	65

Source: Partin and Walsh (1994).

determine the best therapy. It is most helpful in determining the extent of an advanced tumor.

More on Transrectal Ultrasound and Staging

Most studies have found transrectal ultrasound to be a rather mediocre predictor of the presence of cancer that has penetrated the prostate wall, and to be downright poor in finding cancer that has reached the seminal vesicles. In two studies, only 30 percent of tumors that had spread to the seminal vesicles could be found by ultrasound. One investigation, of thirty men undergoing radical prostatectomy, found ultrasound's sensitivity in spotting cancer that had worked its way beyond the prostate wall was a measly 5 percent. Another study, comparing ultrasound and pathological staging in 121 men, found ultrasound's overall accuracy in staging was only 66 percent—better, but still not reliable enough. And a multicenter study of 230 men found that ultrasound correctly staged 66 percent of locally advanced cancer and only 46 percent of the cancers confined to the prostate.

Ultrasound's main difficulty is its inability to "see" microscopic cancer spread. So, to sum up: *No definitive decision about a man's course of treatment should be made on the basis of ultrasound alone, and ultrasound readings shouldn't be the cause of a man's exclusion from surgery that could potentially cure his disease.*

Bone Scan (Radionuclide Scintigraphy)

In a bone scan, doctors inject into the bloodstream a radioactive tracer, a chemical that's attracted, like a magnet, specifically to bone. (This substance is harmless and soon passes out of the body.) Then, using a device called a gamma camera, doctors take pictures of the bones. Normal bone absorbs the radioactive tracer at a lower level. But in areas of new growth—of bone regeneration, as in a healing fracture, or cancer—the tracer accumulates; more is absorbed, and this surplus shows up as a "hot spot" on the image. Studies have shown that the bone scan is better at spotting metastases to bone than a physical examination and other tests—that, basically, bone scans are highly sensitive. Often it can seem that they're *too* sensitive—because they also detect new or old fractures, infection, arthritis, anything that's got to do with the bone in question. These scans can tell a bone's life story, and sometimes, in all this information, the true picture of cancer can be clouded. Sometimes, suspicious areas that show up on a bone scan may also need to be checked out with a routine X-ray, an MRI, or even a bone biopsy.

Some doctors have suggested that if your PSA is less than 10, it's unnecessary to get a bone scan. *We don't agree and, in fact, believe the bone scan to be valuable for several reasons:*

For one, even some patients with low PSA levels (men with poorly differentiated tumors, for example) nonetheless have prostate cancer that has spread to bone. A bone scan could confirm this, or rule it out. Also, the radioactive tracer used for the bone scan is excreted through the kidneys, and this is a good opportunity to check the kidneys, and make sure the cancer isn't causing any urinary obstruction.

Perhaps the strongest argument for a bone scan is that it provides an essential baseline. Say a man starts having severe back pain five years after being treated for prostate cancer, and a new bone scan shows a lesion. It is extremely useful to have an earlier bone scan for comparison, to see if the lesion has been there all along, or if its development is a new event and is something to be worried about. This may be the bone scan's most valuable benefit. For these and other reasons, we believe all men should have a baseline bone scan *when prostate cancer is diagnosed.*

Optional Imaging Tests

MRI (Magnetic Resonance Imaging). MRI is painless and noninvasive; it gives a three-dimensional scan of the body, producing images that are like slices of anatomy. It creates better pictures than CT scans (see below), but it's expensive and time-consuming (an average scan lasts about 45 minutes). Also, being inside an MRI machine, according to one patient, is "like being a sardine in a can." Some patients (5 percent or fewer) actually become claustrophobic while they lie in the machine's tube-like embrace. To help prevent this, some hospitals play soothing music while patients are being imaged. (One bit of advice for men about to undergo an MRI scan: It really helps to relax, close your eyes and, if you can, try to go to sleep.)

Currently, MRI is not a first-line tool for staging prostate cancer. In one multi-center study, transabdominal MRI (an image taken through the abdomen) correctly staged only 57 percent of men with localized prostate cancer and spotted only 60 percent of all malignant tumors. MRI tends to miss some prostate tumors and underestimate the size of others.

"In our experience," concluded two University of California researchers, "MRI does not have high enough sensitivity or specificity for extracapsular extension, seminal vesicle invasion, or lymph node metastasis to be of use in staging clinically localized prostate cancer."

However, in the future, a transrectal approach may—as in ultrasound—improve the picture. Recently, a special coil, attached to a balloon and inserted in the rectum, has been developed that gives a more detailed picture of the prostate and its surroundings. Will this help doctors distinguish organ-confined from advanced disease (or, for that matter, from BPH)? This is uncertain; preliminary data suggest that this approach is only slightly better.

So, to sum up: At present, MRI doesn't seem to be necessary in men who appear to have localized prostate cancer, based on the digital rectal exam, clinical stage and PSA.

CT (Computed Tomography). Getting a CT scan basically means having a circular series of X-ray pictures taken by a machine that goes around the body.

Then a computer puts the pictures together, generating images that, as in MRI, are like slices of anatomy. The CT tube, where a patient lies, is bigger than the tube in an MRI machine, so claustrophobia is not a problem, and this technology is faster than MRI. However, the pictures aren't as good. (One way doctors can enhance CT images is to give patients an intravenous dye; however, this can cause an allergic reaction in some people.)

When it comes to imaging the prostate, CT has turned out to be something of a dud. It can't visualize cancer in the prostate, and it's not very good at showing cancer that has spread beyond the prostate. This is mainly because CT looks for sizeable masses. It can't spot tiny invasions; and this is how most prostate cancers spread to new territories. (For example, the overwhelming majority of metastases to the lymph nodes start out on a microscopic level.)

In detecting localized spread of prostate cancer (beyond the prostate wall, or into the seminal vesicles), CT has been found to have a sensitivity of 50 percent at best. It also has an unfortunate false-positive rate in diagnosing prostate cancer in the seminal vesicles.

Chest X-ray. In 6 percent of men with prostate cancer, bits of the tumor break off and establish themselves in the lungs. In late-stage disease, this figure rises to 25 percent. So the presence or absence of cancer in a man's lungs can help doctors stage the disease.

Molecular Staging of Prostate Cancer

Medical science has devised a promising new means of hunting for prostate cancer cells in the blood. It's called molecular staging because the techniques it uses come from the high-tech field of molecular biology.

There are several ideas at work here. One is that PSA is only made by prostate cells. (This is not entirely true; PSA is also manufactured in tiny amounts at other body sites such as the urethral glands and submandibular gland.) Another is that PSA-secreting cells can be identified in the blood using a state-of-the-art technique called Polymerase Chain Reaction, or PCR. (PCR is an extremely powerful means of amplifying DNA—it works like a tiny, molecular Xerox machine, churning out countless copies of bits of genetic material.)

Before we discuss this new test, we must say that this technique should *not* be confused with simpler PSA measurements. It's a different kettle of fish altogether! Other PSA tests, which we've discussed extensively in this chapter, determine how much PSA is circulating in the plasma, the liquid part of blood. In the molecular staging technique, scientists extract cells from the blood to determine whether *those cells* can make PSA.

Some scientists have been impressed by initial reports of this test's success: In one recent study, researchers obtained blood from radical prostatectomy patients before they underwent surgery. They compared the frequency of a positive PCR test for PSA (which means cells in the blood were able to secrete PSA) to a man's pathologic stage of cancer. In this study, 87 percent of the men with positive surgical margins, and 83 percent of men with positive seminal vesicles, had a positive PCR test.

Pretty strong results! However, we must not over-interpret them. Here's why: For years, it has been known that cancer cells can be present in the blood of patients with many different types of cancer *that can still be cured.* (The cancer is curable because these cells have not yet developed the ability to survive at distant sites.) In fact, in the study mentioned above, 25 percent of patients *with curable cancer* had a positive PCR test; their test results were "false positives." And this tells us something we already knew, that just because a man has cancer cells circulating in his blood, this doesn't mean his cancer can't still be cured.

For this reason, we believe that a man's treatment decisions should not be based on this test until more is known about it. Finally, another matter for scientists to explore is the possibility that this PCR test may not even be a true measure of PSA. It may actually be measuring a molecule that bears a striking resemblance to PSA but isn't PSA.

Laparoscopic Pelvic Lymphadenectomy

Picture someone ice-fishing—cutting a tiny, inconspicuous hole, dropping a line and bringing out a big fish. That's the idea behind laparoscopic surgery. It's much less invasive than traditional surgery that involves an incision, and the benefits to patients include shorter hospitalization, quicker recovery time, less postoperative pain, and a better cosmetic result—a few tiny holes, for example, instead of a scar several inches long.

There is a growing movement in surgery to be minimally invasive—to make smaller holes, not big incisions, and, whenever possible, to use the body's natural passageways, such as the urethra, to reach internal organs (as in the TUR procedure, described in Chapter 10). One doctor describes it as "surgery through telescopes." (The concept itself is not new; use of the endoscope as a means of exploring the body dates back to the turn of this century.) This is the thinking behind the laparoscopic techniques to reach the pelvic lymph nodes in men with prostate cancer.

A man is diagnosed as having early-stage disease. Because there's no evidence that the cancer has spread, he's a candidate for curative therapy—surgery or radiation. But as we know, unfortunately, sometimes cancer has indeed spread, in tiny amounts, to the lymph nodes.

So: Is the cancer really localized? For many men who undergo radical prostatectomy (the retropubic procedure), this question is answered before surgery (see table 3.3a–3.3d); for others, it's answered on the operating table. Before even touching the prostate during a radical prostatectomy, the surgeon removes the patient's pelvic lymph nodes and sends them to pathology, where sections of the nodes are frozen and examined for cancer. If widespread cancer is found, the surgeon doesn't remove the prostate because it wouldn't do any good. But the man still must spend several days in the hospital to recover from the incision.

For this and other reasons, an increasing number of men are undergoing laparoscopic pelvic lymphadenectomy (dissection of the lymph nodes) as a means of staging prostate cancer. It has minimal side effects, a brief hospital stay (one or two days), and men can go back to work in one to two weeks. Some men are even having this done as outpatients.

Who Should Get It?   Some doctors recommend laparoscopic pelvic lymphadenectomy in men who are at higher risk of having cancer that has spread beyond the prostate. This group includes men with stage B2 or B3 disease, high Gleason scores (8, 9, 10); elevated acid phosphatase levels; or a PSA score higher than 20. It also is recommended for some men who opt for radiation therapy—particularly, those for whom open surgery would be too risky.

Who Shouldn't Get It?   Even minimally invasive surgery can be complicated and potentially dangerous in men with other health problems. These include: Men with a history of Crohn's disease, peritonitis, intestinal obstruction, heart or lung disease, impaired blood flow, or a hernia in the diaphragm. It's possible, too, that just having had previous surgery may cause complications in a laparoscopic procedure. (Indeed, if you have had any other health problems, make sure your doctor knows about it before you undergo *any* procedure!) Also, any man with apparent localized disease and a low probability of lymph node involvement (see table 3.3d) who is planning to undergo a radical retropubic prostatectomy does not need this procedure.

What Happens.   In a laparoscopic pelvic lymph node dissection, doctors make a tiny incision, about half an inch long, just beneath the navel. By means of a small needle, the abdomen is gently filled with air, to give doctors more room to work. Then, using a tiny camera and watching the procedure as it happens on a TV screen, the surgeon removes the pelvic lymph nodes. The gas is pumped out and the incision is closed.

Anesthesia.   You'll most likely be given general anesthesia, which means you'll be unconscious throughout the surgery. You'll have a nasogastric (NG) tube inserted through your nose and into your digestive tract; this helps reduce the possibility of air compression and the risk of vomiting.

Afterward.   A Foley catheter usually is kept in place only until the anesthesia is worn off and you're able to urinate on your own. The NG tube probably will be removed in the recovery room shortly after surgery. You'll be given a diet of clear liquids for a day or two.

Pros and Cons.   Despite its "kinder, gentler" technique, some doctors question the value of laparoscopic pelvic lymphadenectomy. For one thing, minimally invasive or not, it's still invasive, and it's not without side effects. These don't occur often, but they can be significant and may include injury to the bladder or bowel, internal bleeding, damage to blood vessels, gas embolism (when air, pumped into the abdomen, escapes into the bloodstream), or even, rarely, heart failure and death.

Is the procedure ultimately necessary? It has no therapeutic benefit—a doctor can't cure a man's prostate cancer by removing cancerous lymph nodes; once the cancer spreads to the lymph nodes, it always spreads to other sites, like bone, as well. Perhaps the most useful benefit of this procedure is that it can rule out surgery for a man who doesn't need it—but so can careful staging.

Also, finding that the lymph nodes are cancer-free still does not mean a man's cancer is curable. Say, for example, a man has a large, palpable cancer that invades the muscles in the pelvic side wall (stage T3 or C), a Gleason score of 8, and a PSA level of 30. Sadly, there is no reason for this man to go ahead with a lymph node dissection; his disease is already extensive, and treatment for him should be aimed at relieving symptoms and pain. To put this man through the rigors of a procedure that ultimately won't help him is neither helpful nor kind.

And finally, when surgical candidates are carefully evaluated, only about 5 percent wind up having positive lymph nodes—so a separate procedure just to determine the state of the lymph nodes is probably unnecessary in most men. Even this number may decrease as doctors begin computing the results of the digital rectal exam, PSA and the Gleason score. Methods for determining the scope of prostate cancer are constantly being refined.

However, the laparoscopic pelvic lymph node dissection *can* be useful in some instances—in a man who's scheduled to undergo a radical perineal prostatectomy, for example, instead of a retropubic operation. (With the perineal approach, the lymph nodes aren't dissected.) Also, sometimes this procedure provides more information than the frozen sections obtained during prostatectomy, and this may be helpful in determining the state of cancer in a man with a high Gleason score (8, 9 or 10).

"Minilap" (Minilaparotomy Staging Pelvic Lymphadenectomy)

A standard staging pelvic lymphadenectomy (dissection of the pelvic lymph nodes) generally is performed just before a radical prostatectomy. (This varies among doctors and hospitals; some doctors base this decision on the Gleason score.) If the lymph nodes are entirely free of cancer or—in some cases, *almost* entirely free—the surgeon proceeds with the operation to remove the prostate.

We need to clarify here: When prostate cancer has spread to the lymph nodes, it cannot be cured. However, if the cancer fits certain conditions—if cancer in the lymph nodes is microscopic and the Gleason score is lower than 8—there is still a chance that surgery will help control the disease locally. This is important for younger men who can expect to live a long time. In this case, for men younger than 70, many surgeons will still perform a radical prostatectomy, because there is a good chance that these men may live for many years before the cancer reappears elsewhere. Also, surgery in these men reduces the risk of other cancer-related problems, such as urinary obstruction or bleeding, developing later.

If disease that was thought to be localized turns out to be widespread, however, the operation generally does not continue; it wouldn't do any good. (Imagine what a blow this is to the patient; worse, even though he didn't have the full operation, he still had an incision and his lymph nodes removed; he'll have to be in the hospital for nearly a week, just to recover from this. This is why staging candidates carefully before surgery is so important—because it could help a man avoid such an ordeal.)

The laparoscopic pelvic lymphadenectomy has a reduced hospital stay (see above). But if the lymph nodes are negative, giving the green light to a radical retropubic or perineal prostatectomy, many men then go ahead and have that surgery.

The goal behind the "Minilap" is to provide the best of both worlds. It begins with an incision slightly larger than in the laparoscopic procedure. If there's cancer in the lymph nodes, the incision is closed. But if the lymph nodes are cancer-free, this incision is lengthened and the radical retropubic prostatectomy is performed under the same anesthetic. (For more on prostatectomy, see Chapter 5.)

THE SHORT STORY

How do you know if you have prostate cancer? Don't wait for symptoms to show up, because for *early* prostate cancer, there aren't any. By the time a man has noticeable symptoms of prostate cancer, it's probably too late to cure it. To make matters worse, *all* of prostate cancer's symptoms can be attributed to other causes. That's why the American Cancer Society recommends that, after age 50, men undergo a yearly digital rectal exam and take a yearly PSA test, a blood test that measures levels of PSA (prostate-specific antigen), a key enzyme made by the prostate. Men at higher risk—men who have a strong family history of prostate cancer or who are of African-American heritage—should begin this testing at age 40.

PSA is prostate-specific, not cancer-specific. You can have prostate cancer and still have a low PSA level; about 25 percent of men with prostate cancer do. And, just because you have a high PSA does not necessarily mean you have prostate cancer; many men with high PSA levels don't. It just means that you have *some sort of prostate trouble*—maybe BPH, maybe prostate cancer, maybe an infection—and that you should see a urologist to find out what kind of problem you have.

No treatment decision should be made on a lone PSA reading. PSA's partner in diagnosis must be a digital rectal exam, and then, if either is abnormal, ultrasound and biopsy should be performed. Together, the rectal exam and PSA can do far more than each tactic alone.

Should every man have a PSA test? *No.* The goal of PSA testing is to identify curable cancers in men who are probably going to live long enough to *need* to be cured. Therefore, there is no reason for most men over age 75, or any man with a life expectancy of less than ten years, to have a PSA test. Creating anxiety about what to do—what treatment decisions to make—is not helpful, humane or necessary for these men.

If something abnormal is found in the digital rectal exam, regardless of your PSA level, you should have a prostate biopsy. (This is done with the help of transrectal ultrasound; biopsies are discussed in this chapter.) If the rectal exam is normal and your PSA is greater than 4, you should also have a biopsy.

The number 4 comes up often in discussions of PSA and prostate cancer. That's because it has become something of a "magic number." Many doctors believe that a PSA level greater than 4 is abnormal, and a PSA less than 4 means everything's fine. But more and more doctors are realizing that having a strict cutoff number probably isn't the best way to use PSA, and they're beginning to use other definitions for early diagnosis of prostate cancer.

One of these is called *PSA density,* in which the PSA number is divided by the prostate size, which is estimated by transrectal ultrasound. The reason size is important is that having BPH (benign enlargement of the prostate) can make PSA higher anyway—so it's tougher for doctors to distinguish between BPH and cancer. Basically, if you have benign enlargement, your PSA should not be more than 15 percent of the weight of your prostate. If it's greater than that, advocates of PSA density believe, you should have a biopsy.

Another technique is called *PSA velocity*—its rate of change from year to year. PSA velocity is a fluid continuum, not a cut-and-dried, one-shot reading. It's like having a prostate barometer—your doctor doesn't have to wait for PSA to reach the magic number of 4. What matters instead is an average, consistent increase of greater than 0.75 nanograms per milliliter per year, over the course of three readings spaced no closer than 12 to 18 months apart. (Say a man's PSA level went up from 1.2 to 2.3 to 3.6 over 24 months—clearly, something's happening here, and it needs to be investigated.)

Finally, some investigators use *age-specific ranges for PSA*. The theory here is that, as a man ages, his prostate gets bigger. Therefore, why should the PSA cutoff point be the same for a 40-year-old man as for an 80-year-old man—who probably has a higher PSA anyway, due to BPH? Advocates of this approach recommend a cutoff of 2.5 for men in their forties, of 3.5 for men in their fifties, of 4.5 for men in their sixties, and of 6.5 for men in their seventies. Using this system, doctors hope to detect more cancers in younger men, and to prevent unnecessary biopsies in older men.

Further study should determine which of these techniques is most useful. Once a diagnosis of prostate cancer has been made, the next step is to determine the cancer's stage—in other words, how far has it spread?

What tests do you need? For most men, the only imaging study that's really necessary is a bone scan. Under some circumstances, further tests—an MRI or CT scan, or lymph node evaluation—may be advised. However, for most patients with a negative bone scan (which indicates that the cancer has not spread to the bone), information from the physical examination, the grade of the tumor (using a system called the Gleason score, which is discussed in this chapter), and the PSA findings can enable physicians to estimate the extent of cancer—and therefore, a man's likelihood of cure. And then this crucial determination helps a man select which form of treatment is best for him. (See table 3.3.) Treatment options are discussed in detail in Chapter 4.

4

I Have Prostate Cancer

What Do I Do Now?

TO TREAT OR NOT TO TREAT

Is the cancer extensive enough to require treatment? Or is it too extensive to be cured? For many doctors and patients, this is the toughest dilemma of all. Urologist Willet F. Whitmore summed it up best when he said, "Is cure necessary in those in whom it may be possible? And is cure possible in those in whom it may be necessary?"

Think about it. Two men have cancer that is localized, confined to the prostate. One man is 52, the other is 82. Should treatment be the same for both men? Of course not. The stage of a cancer, a man's age and overall health have a huge impact on treatment decisions.

Similarly, efforts to detect prostate cancer as early as possible should be targeted to men with not only the *greatest risk* of getting the disease but also the *greatest potential benefit* from treating it. Men who have other serious medical conditions, or whose life expectancy is less than ten years, will not benefit greatly from early detection and treatment of prostate cancer. Indeed, aggressive treatment in these men may not only be unhelpful, it may also produce complications that can make a man's "golden years" needlessly unpleasant.

Prostate cancer grows relatively slowly. When it is localized, it takes two or three years to double in size. And the confounding fact is that cancer can stay in the prostate indefinitely. It takes a long time and many steps involving subtle genetic changes before a normal cell, which is designed to live and die, becomes a cancer cell—before some switch is activated that makes the cell think it's immortal—and before such cells start dividing endlessly. (In high-risk men, some of these steps may be shortened. See "Who Gets Prostate Cancer?")

If localized prostate cancer is found in a 65-year-old man, for example, it could stay localized for years and he may die *with* prostate cancer, not *of* it. This is what happens to hundreds of thousands of men, and it's one of the factors that can make treatment decisions so cloudy.

But—and this is the crux of the issue—*once it escapes the prostate, cancer's growth is relentless.* It can no longer be cured. Once the cancer has spread to bone, the average life expectancy for a man is about three years.

So: If a man has localized disease, the big, blunt question is, How long is he probably going to live? Nobody wants to think about this question, but there it is. Let's go back to our 65-year-old man. He's in otherwise good health, and he can reasonably expect to live at least ten more years. His cancer is curable now. If he does nothing about it, if he opts for watchful waiting, he may miss his golden opportunity for cure. Remember, right now we have no way of estimating the biological potential of prostate cancer. We can't determine if it's harmless or deadly; we don't know *if* or *when* it will make that fatal leap beyond the prostate. Even in its earliest stages, prostate cancer doesn't always spread considerably, in logical, creeping, easy-to-predict steps. And unfortunately, men with the earliest stages of prostate cancer can have metastases before they ever even develop palpable cancer that can be felt by a doctor's gloved finger during a rectal examination.

At the other end of the spectrum is the man in his eighties. Even if his cancer is organ-confined and curable, it's not likely that he will live long enough for major treatment to be worthwhile. Older men are less resilient; aggressive treatment is much harder on them. What's the point of risking incontinence (a result of surgery) or rectal bleeding (a result of radiation) in an 85-year-old man? If his disease progresses to the point where he has difficulty with urination, there are many ways to treat such symptoms (ranging from a TUR to hormonal treatment). For most older men, the number of *years of life*—the long-term survival—is not nearly as important as the *life in those years*—the quality of life.

Conflicting Reports about What to Do

Watchful waiting is certainly not a new approach. It's been a mainstay of prostate cancer treatment for years; and today, one third of men with prostate cancer are treated with watchful waiting.

Some doctors who argue for watchful waiting refer to studies that suggest the mortality rate for men who don't get treatment is low—about the same as for men who don't have prostate cancer.

But results can be seriously misleading. One prominent Swedish study, for example, citing a "high ten-year survival rate in patients with early, untreated prostatic cancer" has been widely criticized because it's based on a group of older men, average age 72, with small, slow-growing tumors. (Only 4 percent of these men had aggressive, poorly differentiated tumors—unlike the 10 percent to 20 percent of men with localized cancer in this country who undergo therapy. So basically, this was not a typical group—many of these patients would have been followed with watchful waiting in the United States, as well.)

After ten years, 13 percent of these men had died from the cancer. *And the disease had progressed in another 50 percent of the men.* Most of these men eventually did need treatment (castration or hormonal therapy) to treat urinary obstruction, bleeding or pain.

So even in the men who haven't died *of* prostate cancer (yet) this statistic almost becomes a technicality. Certainly their lives aren't the same as those of men without prostate cancer. It's hard to enjoy old age when prostate cancer's symptoms begin to affect your quality of life. Incredibly, one of these men who "demonstrated no evidence of disease progression before death" turned out, an autopsy revealed, to have *died of prostate cancer.* How could this be? Men with end-stage prostate cancer don't usually drop dead without warning. They suffer, as do their loved ones who watch this happen. They become increasingly frail as the cancer eats away their bones. Life ebbs away over a period of time that seems at once fleeting and yet agonizingly slow. How, then, could someone die *of* this cancer and be classified as being without symptoms? This astounding statistic suggests that men in the Swedish health care system were not carefully watched and that the progression rates are probably higher than the 50 percent these investigators quoted. (It also sheds unsavory light on another statistic: Some of the most strenuous objections to aggressive treatment for prostate cancer have come from doctors in Sweden, where definitive treatment for this disease is not widespread. And—this comes as news to many—Sweden has the highest death rate from prostate cancer in the world!

In Sweden, half of the men who are diagnosed as having localized prostate cancer die from it, and 69 percent of men who live longer than 10 years also die of the disease.)

These statistics are particularly distressing to think about when you consider this: Today, when localized prostate cancer is diagnosed in men who have a lifespan longer than ten years, *the decision not to offer these men potentially curable therapy may be a death sentence.* Because in most patients, the disease is going to progress.

Recently, research published in the *New England Journal of Medicine* summarized a number of studies involving watchful waiting. In these studies, the article's authors reported, the men treated with watchful waiting were carefully selected from a large group of patients because they were felt to have slow-growing cancers that were unlikely to spread. These patients were not representative of the usual patient who walks into a doctor's office—in other words, they were almost all "best-case scenarios." Even so, ten years later, 40 percent of the men in these elite groups who had Gleason scores from 5 to 7 had developed metastases to bone, and by fifteen years, 70 percent had developed these metastases. (The survival time for patients with metastases to bone is about two to three years.) These observations drive home two points: One is that prostate cancer marches on; it continues to progress in most patients— even in those with the mildest-looking disease. And the other is that if a man with localized prostate cancer does not get effective treatment, and if he lives long enough, he will very likely die of prostate cancer.

Results of still another study show something different: In men with clinically localized prostate cancer, radical prostatectomy reduced the development of metastases and death from prostate cancer by 50 percent when compared with men who were followed with watchful waiting.

WATCHFUL WAITING

Who Should Opt for Watchful Waiting?

Now is the time for some plain speaking, so here goes: At the top of this list should be men who are too old or too ill either to undergo the rigors of treatment or to live another ten years—long enough for such treatment to be worthwhile. Also in this group should be men who don't want to experience the side effects associated with "definitive," or curative treatment; men who are diagnosed with stage T3, T4 or N+ (C or D) disease who don't yet have symptoms; men whose prostate cancer is truly incidental and not yet something to worry about (some men with stage T1a or A1 cancer, see below); and men with stage T1c disease who have low Gleason scores and low PSA densities (see below).

The advantages of watchful waiting include its initial freedom from side effects and, at first, the financial break—it's the cheapest option because there's no expensive treatment to pay for.

Watchful waiting doesn't mean "do nothing," and it doesn't mean your doctor has written you off—it means you get treatment for specific symptoms when you need it. This can mean hormone treatment or spot radiation to ease bone pain; it can mean a TUR or other procedures to bring relief when the prostate cancer becomes large enough to obstruct the urinary tract; it can mean a host of options aimed at tackling specific problems, prolonging life and easing pain.

Watchful Waiting and Curable Prostate Cancer

The benefits of watchful waiting aren't that clear for younger men with localized disease—men who probably could be cured if they act in time. The biggest disadvantage here is that what one doctor calls the "window of curability" may silently close forever while the patient is being watched.

If you have curable disease and opt for watchful waiting, you will have to live with uncertainty about the future. At present, there is no reliable way to tell when the disease is just beginning to progress, even if it hasn't yet escaped the prostate. In about 25 percent of men with growing prostate cancer, there is never a significant, telltale rise in PSA.

So if you're a man under age 70 with localized, curable prostate cancer who decides to watch and wait, think hard about this risk. You should return to your doctor at regular intervals—every six or twelve months at least—for repeat digital rectal examinations, PSA tests and, probably, yearly prostate biopsies to help doctors find out if the cancer that's in your prostate is staying put or if it's on the move. You also need to understand the risks you could be facing down the road if cancer spreads—the long-term symptoms, and the side effects and costs of treatment for advanced disease.

When Watchful Waiting May Be a Safe Gamble

You're young and healthy enough to have surgery, and your disease is certainly considered curable—in fact, it's microscopic, probably incidental prostate cancer. Why seek treatment now?

There used to be two polarized schools of thought about this: One was that all of these men needed treatment as soon as possible. "We can definitely cure it now. Time's wasting—let's get going!" some doctors said. They urged patients to have their cancer "nipped in the bud," treated when the chances of curing it were at their peak. The other group was not nearly so optimistic; these doctors believed that treatment didn't really prolong life by that many years anyway, so what was the point? (Amazingly, a number of doctors still feel this way—see "Conflicting Reports about What to Do," in this chapter.)

Beware of Extremes. One of the first lessons a doctor learns in medical school is that, "There are always two things you never say—always and never." The truth is probably somewhere in the middle.

For many years at Johns Hopkins, the approach was that if a man had cancer found at a TUR but not a tumor large enough to be felt in a digital rectal exam (men with stage T1 or A cancer), then his cancer was the incidental kind, with "low malignant potential" and not much clinical significance—the kind of cancer men die "with," not "of." And so they weren't treated.

In 1976, Johns Hopkins investigators embarked on a pioneering study using tumor volume to predict cancer patients' prognosis. They analyzed the medical histories of more than 100 of these men who were not treated, and they followed their progress for an average of seven years. Their findings: One group of these men did reasonably well; their cancer rarely progressed. But another group did not fare so well; their cancer continued to grow.

What was the difference between these two groups? The clue, investigators found, was in the percentage of cancer found in tissue removed during the TUR. (This work provided the now-standard classifications for stage T1 disease.)

When 5 *percent or less* of the tissue was cancerous, only 17 percent of the men went on to develop more advanced cancer; this is now the classification for stage T1a, or A1, disease. But when *more than 5 percent* of the resected tissue was cancerous, 68 percent of these men went on to develop cancer progression; this now is the classification of stage T1b, or A2, disease. "It is felt that the amount of cancer in almost all of these patients is significant enough to warrant therapy," says one of the investigators.

Further analysis has shown that when men with stage T1a disease undergo radical prostatectomy, about 25 percent of them turn out to have a significant amount of cancer in the prostate—the kind of cancer that's found in men with palpable tumors.

So: Some men with stage T1a cancer require treatment. Some don't. How to tell the difference? Our old friend PSA comes back to help us again. As it turns out, the level of PSA three months after TUR can be helpful in identifying the men at highest risk of cancer progression. If the PSA is less than 1.0, virtually all of the men with stage T1a (A1) disease have an insignificant amount of cancer. "And we feel that these men can probably be followed with careful digital rectal examinations and PSA tests every six months or a year," says one of the study's chief investigators.

If the PSA is greater than 10, all of these men are likely to have significant cancer remaining, and all should have definitive therapy before it's too late.

What about the patients in the middle, with PSA levels between 1.0 and 10—the range for about half the men with T1 disease? Currently, there's just no way to predict exactly how much cancer remains in the prostate—and, therefore, who will need treatment and who won't. Some doctors have advised these men to undergo a repeat TUR, but there's no real evidence to suggest that this will provide any helpful information—it's hard on the patient, to boot. Also, a repeat TUR may make it more difficult for a surgeon to perform a subsequent radical prostatectomy.

Other investigators are enthusiastic about the use of ultrasound and random needle biopsies as follow-up measures for these men, but the long-term success rate for these procedures has yet to be determined; cancer could still slip outside the prostate and not be caught in time. The safest guideline here may be the patient's age: If he's younger than 60, aggressive, curative therapy should be strongly considered.

Another group who could have insignificant cancer are men with stage T1c disease (found by needle biopsy, after an elevated PSA score). Ten percent of these men with a PSA greater than 4 have insignificant cancer. PSA density (see Chapter 3), plus the findings of the needle biopsy (see Chapter 3) can be helpful in predicting which of these men can afford to wait.

What Happens to Cancer Cells over Time

Some men who opt for watchful waiting take solace in the fact that their cancer cells are well-differentiated. *But unfortunately, just because you have well-differentiated cancer cells today does not mean they'll stay that way forever.* There are two concepts here; one is *genetic drift.* As a cancer progresses—as its cells double again and again—the DNA becomes less stable. The cancer develops new mutations; it becomes more aggressive. As the tumor progresses, well-differentiated cells deteriorate into poorly differentiated cells. The other concept is *heterogeneity,* or clonal selection. By the time a prostate cancer is large enough to be diagnosed clinically, its cell population is mixed—a diverse group of cells, all jockeying for position in one location. In this varied group are both well- and poorly differentiated cells, cells driven by hormones and cells untouched by hormones. And although an initial biopsy may find well-differentiated cancer cells, almost certainly some poorly differentiated ones have mingled in there as well. With time and further growth, these poorly differentiated cells grow at a faster rate than do their more sedate, better-differentiated counterparts. Eventually, they will outpace the stately progression of the well-differentiated cells and dominate the tumor. So a well-differentiated cancer, one that's localized to the prostate, may be only a temporary condition. And unfortunately, we can't tell which well-differentiated cancers are going to stay that way.

Cost Is a Factor, Too

In the long term, it's unclear whether watchful waiting will actually result in a decrease in health care dollars, as some studies have claimed. A 65-year-old man has a 50-percent likelihood of living fifteen years. The Swedish study mentioned above suggests that even under the best circumstances, about half of men with untreated localized disease will live to see their cancer spread beyond the prostate, requiring further treatment for advanced disease. If these men decide to have hormonal treatment, the cost of this over two years, at hundreds of dollars a month, may be more than the expense of a radical prostatectomy (which is about $12 thousand). Also, the symptoms from advanced cancer and the side effects of hormonal treatment and chemotherapy can be much worse than the side effects that can accompany treatment for early disease.

IF I DECIDE TO GET TREATMENT, WHAT ARE MY CHOICES?

For tumors that are confined to the prostate—stages T1 and T2 (A1, A2, B1 and B2)—there are two main choices: Surgery, the radical prostatectomy; and radiation therapy. Radiation also is used when the cancer has spread just outside the gland, to kill cancer cells and to shrink the prostate. High-energy X-ray beams are aimed at the prostate and sometimes at nearby lymph nodes.

Table 4.1 *Treatment Pros and Cons*

	Radical Prostatectomy	Radiation Therapy
Ideal candidate		
Age	Younger than 70	Any age
Stage	T1b, T1c, T2 (and some men with T1a disease)	T1, T2, T3, T4
Chief advantages	If cancer is confined to the prostate, this is the best way to cure	Less invasive
Chief disadvantages	Side effects: impotence 25–75% incontinence 2–5% death 0.2%	May not cure localized cancer; Side effects: rectal injury 1–2% impotence 40% death 0.2%

Which Treatment Is Better for Localized Disease?

A better question might be, "Which treatment is right for me?" There are several important considerations here: Your age and overall health, the stage of cancer, the side effects associated with different treatments, and finally—most importantly—your own wishes.

When prostate cancer is localized *in men with a life expectancy of 10 years or more,* the goal for treatment is cure. This sounds obvious, until we remember that when prostate cancer is advanced, cure is no longer an option. In other words, if we don't remove the disease or treat it effectively when it's localized —if the cancer gets outside the prostate—we can't stop it.

The big advantage of radical prostatectomy is that *there is no better way to completely eliminate cancer that is curable* (see above). The disadvantages are the side effects—namely, the risks of impotence and incontinence (see Chapter 5). And radical prostatectomy is not "a walk in the park." *It is major surgery, and the body must be in strong enough shape to handle it.*

Radiation therapy's great advantage is that it isn't surgery. But its major disadvantage, especially for the younger patient, is that *its ability to control the cancer may not last forever.* Many studies have suggested that with standard radiation treatment—external-beam therapy—there is a strong likelihood that a prostate biopsy a few years later will be positive. These studies have also suggested that the likelihood that PSA will be in the undetectable range ten years after radiation is only 10 percent. In contrast, a large study at Johns Hopkins showed that the likelihood of PSA remaining in the undetectable range ten years after surgery was 70 percent.

In choosing the treatment that's best for you, it's important to try for a balance between effectiveness and side effects. More information on each of these choices follows in this chapter, and the next chapters cover these treatments in significantly greater detail.

Radical Prostatectomy Is a Better Option For . . .

The ideal candidates for radical prostatectomy are the men most likely to benefit from it. Therefore, radical prostatectomy should only be considered in men who have cancer that appears to be confined to the prostate and therefore is potentially curable. Also, it should only be considered in men who are *young enough and healthy enough to live long enough to benefit from being cured.*

Good candidates for surgery, then, are men in their fifties or sixties, in otherwise good health, with localized prostate cancer. This includes men with stage T1b (A2), T2a (B1N), T2b (B1), and T2c (B2) cancer. It also includes some men with stage T1a (A1) cancer, and most patients with stage T1c disease.

Also, radical prostatectomy can cure cancer that has penetrated through the prostate wall *IF* the cancer is well- to moderately well-differentiated (a Gleason score of 7 or less) and if it's possible for doctors to get what's called a "clear surgical margin" so they can cut out all the tumor.

Men with stage T3 (C) disease generally are not considered candidates for radical prostatectomy. However, sometimes the interpretation of the digital rectal examination can be wrong. Sometimes, doctors overestimate the tumor's actual extent—when indeed it may not have spread beyond the prostate. Twenty-five percent of these men who undergo surgery turn out to have organ-confined cancer. (Again, tallying the results of the PSA test, Gleason score and clinical stage may help doctors avoid such overestimation. See table 3.3.)

Radical Prostatectomy Is Not a Good Option For . . .

Radical prostatectomy is not helpful for men with disease that has spread widely beyond the prostate. Nor is it ideal for older patients (men who are not likely to live longer than 10 years).

Once prostate cancer escapes the wall of the prostate to the point where it widely invades the seminal vesicles, pelvic lymph nodes or bone, it can no longer be cured. *Surgery in these men, with its side effects, including the risk of incontinence and impotence, not only fails to cure, it is an unnecessary ordeal.* The principal goal here is to control the tumor locally; this can be done with radiation, hormone therapy, or a combination of both. Ultimately, these men need palliative care—treatment that will lengthen their lives and ease their pain. With late-stage cancer, the goal is simply to do everything possible *to fight the cancer and buy more time.* The focus changes to ensuring good quality of life, rather than a cancer-free life. The main line of treatment for late-stage prostate cancer is hormone therapy and, later, chemotherapy and spot radiation to treat painful metastases.

Why is age a factor? Several reasons. One is that men in their seventies often have more advanced cancer than the clinical findings might lead a doctor to suspect. As men age, the prostate enlarges from BPH—so by the time a doctor can feel a cancerous lump in these men with their larger prostates, it's probably bigger than the cancer that can be felt in a younger man with a smaller prostate. Studies have shown that for men with T2b (B1) disease, the likelihood that the cancer is confined to the prostate is less for men in their seventies than for men in their fifties.

Also, older men are more likely to suffer side effects from surgery; they don't do as well as younger men in recovering continence and sexual function. And finally, because men over age 70 aren't likely to live as long as men twenty years younger, it's difficult to show that radical prostatectomy actually does more than radiation therapy to lengthen life in these men.

Radiation Is a Better Option For . . .

The ideal candidates for radiation treatment are patients who are older, or who are less likely to be cured by surgery.

Men who undergo radiation treatment are said to be "negatively selected" —that is, they get radiation therapy because radical prostatectomy has been ruled out as the best option for them. They are generally older men; men in poor health who aren't considered strong enough for surgery; or men who have disease that has extended beyond the prostate to the point where it can't be removed surgically (stage T3 or T4, or C).

However, others who opt for radiation treatment are men with organ-confined disease who just don't want to have surgery.

Why Not Have Both Treatments?
A Word On Combined Approaches

Although some men appear to have clinically localized cancer, there's a good chance that their cancer has spread beyond the prostate (see table 3.3).

For these men, the combination of radiation and surgery might sound like a promising option. However, it is not yet certain whether radiation after prostatectomy is ultimately helpful. Note: Radical prostatectomy is definitely not very successful in men who have undergone radiation treatment (see Chapter 6), and in the minds of many urologists, surgery after the fact is not an option. However, men who have undergone radical prostatectomy *can* go ahead and have radiation therapy later.

Some surgeons recommend hormonal treatment to shrink the prostate (and, they hope, the tumor) before radical prostatectomy, believing that this will make the cancer more curable. But, as one Johns Hopkins scientist explains, "hormone therapy is not a vacuum cleaner—it can't suck the cancer cells back into the prostate once they've escaped." There is no reason to believe that hormone treatment before radical prostatectomy will make it possible for surgeons to retrieve and eliminate cancer cells that have strayed from the prostate. Also, this approach may mislead a surgeon into thinking the cancer picture is rosier than it actually is, and thereby encourage a less-aggressive cancer operation.

The findings in surgery determine the course of the operation—more or less tissue is removed, depending on what the surgeon sees when the body is opened up. If, for example, there is any hint that the cancer has escaped the prostate along the nerve bundles that lie on either side of it, these nerves should be "widely excised"—cut out, along with as much nearby tissue as possible. But if a man has received hormonal treatment, the surgeon may be reassured—falsely—about the extent of disease. A surgeon may think, "There's no way the cancer could ever reach out this far, not after that hormone treatment I started. I'll leave these nerve bundles in and give this guy a break—now he can keep his sexual potency." As a result of such well-meaning thinking, the surgeon may leave malignant cells behind instead of doing what any good surgeon normally does in a cancer operation—cutting out as much tissue as possible in an aggressive, no-holds-barred attempt to cure the disease.

There's another extremely important fact you should know about hormone therapy: It's effective *only while a patient is on it.* The day you stop taking it is the day it stops working. Inevitably and almost immediately, the cancer cells begin growing again. If a surgeon has been timid or overconfident during surgery and not removed all the tissue that needed to be removed, the cancer is going to come back—hormones didn't kill it.

SO WHAT DO I DO?

First, educate yourself. Learn everything important there is to know about your own cancer—your clinical stage, PSA level and Gleason score. Consult table 3.3a–3.3d. Explore all your options—we've done our best to cover them all in this chapter, and specific forms of treatment are covered in greater detail in the next chapters. Get a second opinion, and a third if you need it, and talk to patients. If you can't get some names from your doctor, call a prostate cancer support group (see "Where to Get Help," at the back of this book) or another organization that specializes in prostate cancer. Be your own advocate, and take heart—there is much you can do to make sure you get the best treatment possible.

Table 3.3 can be extremely helpful to you and your doctor in making the decision about treatment. In the best cases, it can identify men who are likely to be cured. But what if the probabilities in the table suggest that cure is unlikely? Say a man has a palpable tumor involving one entire lobe of the prostate (stage T2b, or B1 disease), a Gleason score of 7, and a PSA between 10 and 20. The likelihood that his tumor is confined to the prostate is 19 percent; the probability that his cancer has penetrated beyond the prostate wall is 81 percent. He has a 33 percent chance of having cancer in the seminal vesicles, and a 24 percent chance of lymph node involvement. What should this man do? Here, age plays a major role. Say this man is in his early fifties. Even though cure is not certain, it's clear that *if he does nothing* he will probably die of his disease. Because the side effects of surgery are much milder in men this age, surgery is certainly a reasonable option, and it does offer the possibility of cure.

On the other hand, say he's in his seventies. The question here is whether a

Table 4.2 *Treatment of Prostate Cancer*

Clinical extent of disease	Stage	Options
Localized	T1, T2, A, B	Radical prostatectomy Radiation therapy Watchful waiting
Locally extended beyond the prostate	T3, T4, C	Radiation therapy Hormone therapy
Metastasized to lymph nodes and bone	N+, M+	Hormone therapy Chemotherapy Spot radiation for pain

man *who may not live long enough to die of prostate cancer* should be put through an operation with an uncertain likelihood of cure. Surgery has more side effects on people in their seventies. So, for this man, radiation therapy is a better, more reasonable option.

THE SHORT STORY

The diagnosis is official. You have prostate cancer. What do you do now? The stage of your cancer and your age and overall health all have a huge bearing on this important decision.

Prostate cancer grows relatively slowly. It can stay localized, or confined to the prostate, indefinitely—so a man can die *with* prostate cancer, and not *of* it. But once it escapes the prostate, cancer's growth is relentless. It can no longer be cured. And once it has spread to bone, a man's average life expectancy is about three years.

In studies of watchful waiting in men with small, moderately well-differentiated cancers (Gleason scores from 5 to 7) that appear to be localized to the prostate, this is what happens over time: In ten years, 40 percent of these men will have cancer that has spread to the bone; by fifteen years, 70 percent of these men will have cancer spread to bone.

What does this mean to you? Once again, we go back to your age, general health, and stage of cancer.

Say a man is in otherwise good health, and he can reasonably expect to live at least ten more years. His cancer is localized to the prostate, and therefore it's curable now. If he does nothing about it, he may miss his golden opportunity for cure. There's no way of predicting if or when cancer will make that fatal leap beyond the prostate. Even in its earliest stages, prostate cancer doesn't always spread considerately, in logical, creeping, easy-to-predict steps. And unfortunately, men with the earliest stages of prostate cancer can have metastases before they ever even develop a palpable tumor that can be felt by a doctor's gloved finger during a rectal exam.

But say a man is in his eighties. Even if his cancer is organ-confined and curable, it's not likely that he will live long enough for major treatment to be worthwhile. Older men are less resilient; aggressive treatment is much harder on them.

Watchful waiting doesn't mean your doctor has written you off—it just means you get treatment for specific symptoms if and when you need it.

So who should opt for watchful waiting? At the top of this list should be men who are too old or too ill either to undergo the rigors of treatment or to live another ten years (long enough for such treatment to be worthwhile). Also in this group should be men with cancers that are considered too advanced to cure—men with stages T3, T4, N+, C and D. (Note: This doesn't mean there is no treatment for these men. There is. Advanced cancer can still be fought; it just can't be cured.) And finally, for men with cancers that are truly incidental (some men with stage T1a and T1c disease), watchful waiting is probably a reasonable gamble.

On the other hand, the benefits of watchful waiting aren't that clear for younger men with localized disease—men who probably could be cured if they act in time. The biggest disadvantage here is that the "window of curability" may silently close forever, even as the patient is being watched. If you are in otherwise good health, have localized prostate cancer, and a life expectancy longer than ten years, you should strongly consider aggressive treatment.

Which form of treatment is best for you? There are two good choices—radical prostatectomy and radiation therapy.

Radiation therapy's great advantage is that it is not surgery. Therefore, it's an ideal form of treatment for men who are older, or who have cancer that is too advanced to cure by surgery. The big advantage of radical prostatectomy is that there is no better way to completely eliminate cancer that is curable. The best candidates for radical prostatectomy are men who are young enough and healthy enough to live long enough to benefit from being cured. Younger men also experience fewer complications from the surgery.

This book discusses all the major treatments for prostate cancer, beginning with the "gold standard"—radical prostatectomy—in Chapter 5.

5

Treating Prostate Cancer

Radical Prostatectomy

A LITTLE HISTORY

The operation to remove the prostate as a treatment for cancer was first performed in 1904, at the Johns Hopkins Hospital by a urologist named Hugh Hampton Young. Young's procedure, called a radical perineal prostatectomy, was a success: Six and a half years later, when the patient died of other causes, an autopsy showed that his prostate cancer had been cured.

In the late 1940s, another approach, called the radical retropubic prostatectomy, was developed, and like Young's operation (which still is used today, although not as often as the retropubic approach), it proved extremely effective in stopping prostate cancer in its tracks—if, that is, the cancer was confined to the prostate.

Both the radical perineal and retropubic operations had a definite down side—in the form of two devastating side effects, incontinence and impotence. Worse, radical retropubic prostatectomy also became known among urologists for the extreme bleeding that went along with it. Every surgeon who performed it would probably admit that this operation used to be performed in a sea of blood.

So, understandably, when radiation treatment for prostate cancer was introduced and popularized (see Chapter 6), doctors as well as patients welcomed this alternative therapy. (In men who receive radiation treatment, an average of 60 percent remain potent, and incontinence is not a problem.)

An Anatomical Approach to Surgery

The late 1970s saw important modifications in the retropubic approach. For the first time, the anatomy of the venous drainage surrounding the prostate was understood, and with this knowledge evolved new surgical methods to lessen the awful blood loss. The new techniques did two things: With less bleeding, the operation became safer; and with what surgeons call "a bloodless field," it became possible for surgeons actually to see what they were doing—a major improvement! In the process, critical structures could be looked for and saved that previously had been unrecognized and damaged as surgeons blindly felt their way. More precise dissection and reconstruction reduced the likelihood of troublesome urinary incontinence from as high as 15 percent to 2 percent, and even those 2 percent are not incontinent all the time.

But what about impotence? It had been widely assumed that penile nerves inevitably were damaged by the radical prostatectomy. Previously, many people thought the nerves to the erectile tissue in the penis ran through the prostate and would be damaged as a necessity when the prostate was removed. It didn't make sense, that the nerves from one organ would run through another organ, but this had always been the assumption—even in medical textbooks. One highly respected anatomy textbook, for example, reported helpfully that the nerves that enable erection were "extremely small, difficult to follow in the adult cadaver," and that their location was known "merely through experimental studies."

Meanwhile, something unusual was taking place: Gradually, as one urologist began using the new techniques, his patients began reporting that their potency had returned. What was happening? Insight came with the discovery that the nerves that run to the corpora cavernosa, the spongy, erectile bodies in the penis, sat *outside* the capsule of the prostate. Which meant that it should be possible to preserve sexual function in men undergoing this operation. Until that time, these tiny nerves had almost always been inadvertently destroyed during surgery because doctors didn't even know of, and therefore couldn't appreciate, their existence. The nerves were never removed, but were damaged and left in place.

In the early 1980s at Johns Hopkins, this new knowledge—*that these microscopic bundles of nerves on either side of the prostate could be preserved*—was first put into action. The patient, a 52-year-old psychology professor, regained his sexual function within a year after the modified, "nerve-sparing" surgery. (Actually, this term only tells part of the story, but this description has stuck, and many people use it. The operation's proper name is the anatomical radical retropubic prostatectomy.) Twelve years later, this patient is alive and cancer-free; his quality of life remains excellent.

Better understanding of the anatomical terrain also led to another important bonus: Surgeons now knew *exactly where the scalpel could and could not go*. So, depending on the extent of a man's cancer, it became possible for them either to save these nerves deliberately, or to remove more tissue by cutting these bundles away—in surgical terms, to create "wider margins of excision"— than they previously had believed possible. (Before this discovery, surgeons routinely gave this area a wider berth because they were afraid of injuring the patient's rectum.) Which means that with these anatomical techniques, surgeons now have a better chance of removing all the cancer.

Today at Johns Hopkins (the hospital is noted here because results vary worldwide, depending on a range of factors including the surgeon's skill and the selection criteria for patients), in men aged 50 to 59 who undergo anatomical radical retropubic prostatectomy, *75 percent regain potency*. (Overall, at ten years or more after surgery, only 4 percent have local recurrence of cancer, and only 7 percent develop distant metastases; and 70 percent have an undetectable level of PSA.) Important determinants in the return of sexual function include age, the stage of cancer, and the extent of nerve loss—whether one or both nerve bundles remain, or whether they had to be removed during surgery.

We used to say, "If we make a diagnosis and you're going to need surgery, it may make you incontinent and impotent." And patients said, "Hold the phone! I'd rather have the disease." Now, when we talk to patients, we tell them we have three goals: Removing all of the tumor, preserving urinary control, and preserving sexual function. Sexual function is number three because, if it is lost, there are many ways to restore it.

Men who are impotent following radical prostatectomy have normal sensation, normal sex drive, and can achieve a normal orgasm. The one element they may be lacking is the ability to have an erection sufficient for intercourse, and that can be restored by means including a vacuum erection device, injections, even a penile prosthesis. (For more on impotence, see Chapter 8.)

Are you in good hands? What to look for in a surgeon

Doctor A is a nice, personable young doctor, whose empathy for your condition appealed to you immediately.

That's great. Now what else do you know about him? Is he a board-certified urologist? What training has he had? Does he know—and use—the nerve-sparing techniques, the anatomical approach to radical prostatectomy? How many of these operations does he do a year? What success has he had in preserving potency and continence? (If he can't or won't give you his rate of success as compared to reports from other surgeons, or to results published in medical journals, this may be a red flag, and perhaps you should look elsewhere.) You should be able to get a good idea of his success rate, in numbers or percentages. And if he hasn't done very many of these operations—at least 150—you might want to find a more experienced surgeon. Look at it this way: *Do you want to be one of the patients he's learning on?*

When you're looking for a surgeon, you don't necessarily want some name-brand academician or a specialist in other areas of urologic surgery. You want to find a doctor who performs this particular operation. *Often.* Preferably, a doctor who does this operation every day, or several days a week.

Doctor B is another nice doctor, a respected, fatherly man who's been operating in this town as long as anybody can remember. Just looking at him inspires confidence.

Swell. But does he also keep up with the latest research? Does he continue his education regularly, brushing up on old surgical skills as well as mastering new techniques?

Does he operate on nearly every man he treats who has prostate cancer? (This is not a desirable quality in a surgeon.) Or does he screen his patients carefully, making every attempt to spare any man with cancer that *can't be cured by surgery* the unnecessary ordeal and expense of an operation? ▶

▶ Remember: Radical prostatectomy is a tricky operation, and *you don't want a surgeon who's "pretty good"* at it. Also, you can't assume that every urologist does this well. There are no second chances here; this is a one-shot operation. You are looking for the one surgeon who will perform the one radical prostatectomy you will ever receive in your life, the one operation that will cure your cancer. You want a surgeon who isn't going to leave some cancer behind, who knows how to control excessive bleeding so you don't wind up incontinent, impotent or both. (Note: Unexpected trouble can crop up in any operation; nobody can help that. But the unexpected is less likely to happen with an experienced surgeon.)

So ask questions. Find out how often your doctor's patients require radiation therapy after surgery, or treatment with hormones. If the number is greater than 15 percent, this suggests that the doctor either doesn't do a very good job selecting surgical candidates, or is not completely removing all the cancer during surgery. It also suggests that you need to get a second opinion. But you should get a second opinion anyway. Always get a second opinion.

THE ANATOMICAL RETROPUBIC APPROACH

Before the Operation

Are you in shape for surgery? Your doctor will want to check you out thoroughly beforehand. Surgery may be delayed if you've recently had other prostate surgery for BPH (see below), and it's generally scheduled for six to eight weeks after a needle biopsy of the prostate. These delays give the body a chance to recover from the earlier procedures. Also, imagine a surgeon's difficulty in trying to operate on inflamed, irritated tissue, where a needle has penetrated the rectal wall six times, and it hasn't yet healed properly! A few weeks' wait, though it may seem agonizing to a man who's anxious to have the cancer removed as soon as possible, can be critical in helping the surgeon preserve the delicate neurovascular bundles and avoid injury to the patient's rectum during the procedure.

Before surgery, when you give the doctor your medical history, be sure to say so if you've had any unusual problems with bleeding in the past (from dental work, for example). Also, aspirin can cause excessive bleeding; *if you are taking aspirin regularly, make sure you stop at least ten days before the operation.* Another point to discuss with your doctor: Many men who undergo radical prostatectomy need a blood transfusion during the procedure. The best blood for you to get, obviously, is your own; if your hospital allows this, it's a good idea to donate several units of your blood ahead of time. This is another good reason for the six-to-eight-week delay; it gives you plenty of time to make up your own blood bank. The night before surgery, you'll be given an enema and perhaps some laxatives, as well. Or, if you're scheduled to be admitted the day of your surgery, you may be asked to give yourself an enema or take laxatives the night before. You'll probably be told not to eat anything the night before surgery, as well.

Does It Matter If I've Already Had Prostate Surgery for BPH?

This is how some men find out they have prostate cancer—when the prostate tissue removed in a TUR procedure or open prostatectomy is evaluated by a pathologist. It's more difficult for surgeons to perform a radical prostatectomy after an open prostatectomy, but that doesn't mean it can't be done. It often is, and with greater success. You may be told to wait, however, about twelve weeks after a TUR procedure, until the inflammation from this operation has gone down.

Anesthesia

You will be anesthetized; this can happen several ways. Most likely, you'll have either spinal or epidural anesthesia; with both forms, you remain conscious and aware of the procedure, even though you can't feel it. In *spinal anesthesia,* you'll have a shot of local anesthetic injected into the small of your back through the dura, the membrane lining the spinal cord, and into the spinal fluid. Within minutes, you'll feel numb, relaxed and heavy from your waist to your toes. After surgery, you'll be asked to lie flat in bed until the numbness goes away and you can move your legs again. *This is important; sitting up too soon can cause a severe headache.*

Epidural anesthesia is like having an IV tube hooked up to your back, instead of to a vein in your arm. A local anesthetic enters the body through a tiny plastic tube, inserted between the vertebrae of your spine near the small of your back. The epidural anesthetic (often used to provide pain relief in pregnant women during labor) bathes the area outside the membrane lining the spinal cord, temporarily numbing the nerves in your lower body. Unlike spinal anesthesia, which comes in one dose, epidural anesthesia can be given continuously. The area of numbness can be adjusted; so can the degree of pain relief. After surgery, this tube can also be used to administer pain relief for the first few days. One point about epidural anesthesia: It reduces the likelihood of blood clots in the legs, perhaps by boosting blood circulation in the legs during surgery.

During Surgery: What Happens

First, let's review the territory. (It might help if, as you read this, you refer to figures 5.1–5.8.) For a surgeon, this is precarious terrain indeed: The prostate (Fig. 5.1) is located deep in the pelvis, surrounded by structures that are fragile and vulnerable to injury—the rectum, the bladder, the sphincter responsible for urinary control, some large blood vessels, and the bundles of nerves that are responsible for erection.

The operation begins with an incision through skin and muscle in the abdomen that extends from the pubic area to the navel (Fig. 5.2). Almost immediately, before the prostate is ever reached, the surgeon removes a triangle of tissue on each side of the bladder; these triangles contain important lymph nodes. This is called a *staging pelvic lymphadenectomy*—dissection of the pelvic lymph nodes, to make sure they're free of cancer. These lymph nodes are removed, then rushed to a pathologist for what's called frozen-section analysis to check for cancer; the tissue is frozen, then sliced into very thin sections to be examined under the microscope.

(Note: Some doctors only have frozen-section analysis done if a man's Gleason score is 8 or higher. One reason for this is that with lower-grade, well- to moderately well-differentiated tumors—Gleason 7 or less—the long-term prognosis of patients is different than for men with high-grade, poorly differentiated tumors. Most men with Gleason scores of 8 or higher will have metasta-

Figure 5.1. *The radical retropubic prostatectomy, step by step*

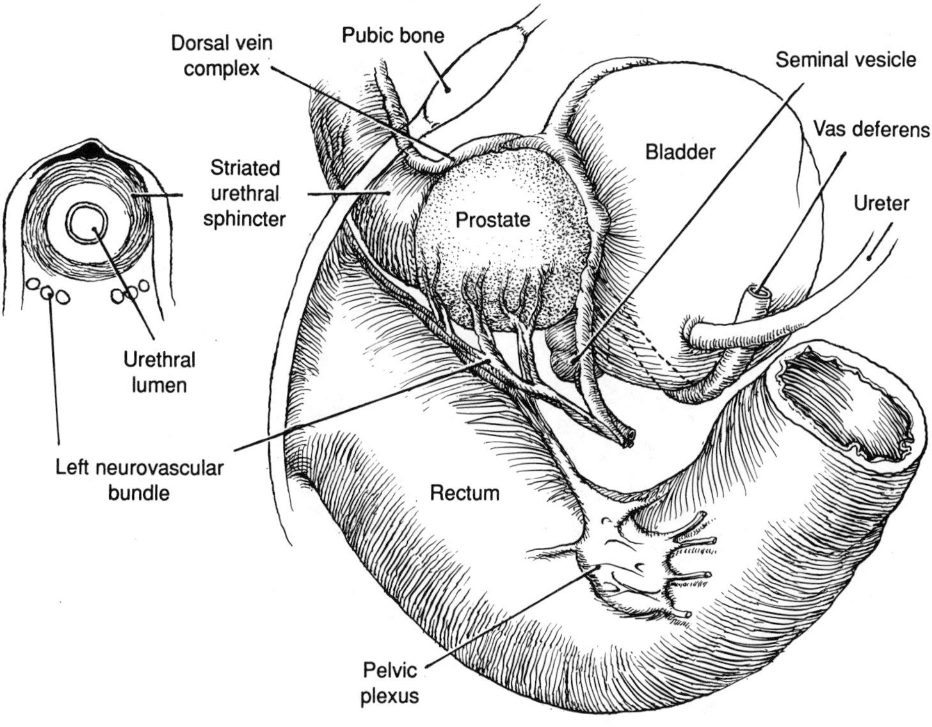

You're looking at the prostate and surrounding terrain—the rectum and bladder, key nerves, veins and the urethral sphincter, a tube-shaped structure that helps control urine. You can also see one of the two neurovascular bundles, the package of nerves critical for erection, which sit on either side of the prostate. Figures 5.1–5.8 reprinted from Patrick C. Walsh, "Radical Prostatectomy: A Procedure in Evolution," *Seminars in Oncology* 21 (1994):662–71. Used by permission, W. B. Saunders Company.

ses to bone within the first four years after surgery; therefore, removing the prostate ultimately does not benefit these men. But with Gleason scores of 7 or lower—*even when there is a tiny bit of cancer in a lymph node*—60 percent of men have no sign of metastases on bone scans ten years later. This doesn't mean the cancer won't eventually come back in these men, but that it can take years longer to return when the tumor is of a lower, better-differentiated grade. So, because these men can live for many years, they often benefit from having

Figure 5.2. *The radical retropubic prostatectomy* (continued)

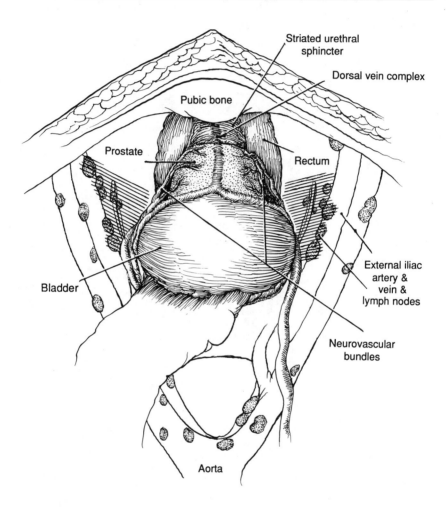

This is a schematic look at the prostate, bladder and lymph nodes. It's the view the surgeon has after the abdominal incision has been made. Inside the shaded area are the lymph nodes removed during a staging lymphadenectomy. You can see how easy it would be for cancer from the prostate to migrate toward these nodes.

Figure 5.3. *The radical retropubic prostatectomy* (continued)

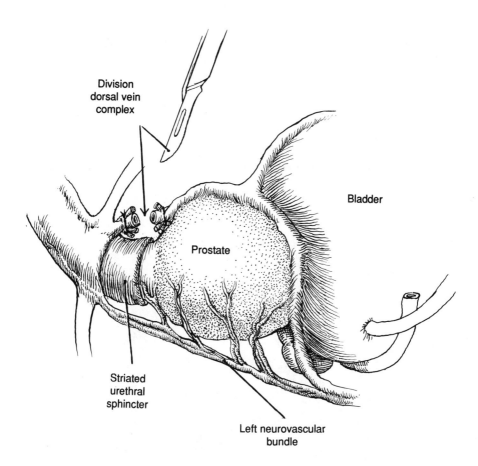

This is how the surgeon helps create the critical "bloodless field"—carefully cutting the dorsal vein complex, which travels over the urethra and prostate and carries a great deal of blood.

their prostate removed. And removing it now will help them avoid problems with urinary tract obstruction and bleeding later, when the cancer does return.)

If the cancer has spread massively to the lymph nodes, the surgeon will stop the operation at this point, because surgery won't help the situation. But if the lymph nodes are cancer-free—or nearly so (see above), and the cancer cells are not poorly differentiated—the operation continues.

Next, the major vein system that overlies the prostate and urethra (this is called the dorsal vein complex) is cut (Fig. 5.3). Blood loss must be kept to a minimum so that the operation can be performed in a "bloodless field." This is a crucial step; control of these veins makes a huge difference in the surgeon's ability to see what's happening, and it's particularly significant for what happens next—cutting through the urethra (Fig. 5.4). If the urethra is cut too

Figure 5.4. *The radical retropubic prostatectomy* (continued)

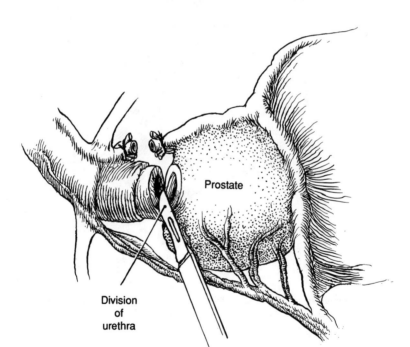

Prostate

Division
of
urethra

The surgeon now is cutting the urethra, which runs through the prostate. This is another delicate procedure—cutting the urethra too close to the prostate might mean some cancer is left behind; but cutting it too far from the prostate might mean damaging the urethral sphincter, which helps control urine. Bit by bit, the prostate is separated from all the tissue and blood vessels that are connected to it.

Figure 5.5. *The radical retropubic prostatectomy* (continued)

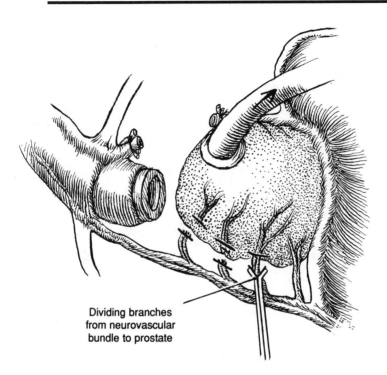

Dividing branches
from neurovascular
bundle to prostate

If it's possible—if the cancer has not penetrated the prostate wall—the surgeon can preserve the neurovascular bundles on either side of the prostate. To do that, the surgeon carefully separates each branch of these nerves and vessels from the prostate.

close to the prostate, some cancer might be left behind; but if it's cut too far away from the prostate, the urethral sphincter might be damaged—and such an injury can make a man incontinent.

Next, depending on the degree of cancer, the surgeon must make a decision that will affect the patient's potency—to leave intact the neurovascular bundles, the wafer-thin packets of nerves that sit on either side of the prostate, or to remove one or both along with the prostate (Fig. 5.5). These are the nerve bundles responsible for erection.

If we were to offer some friendly advice to men who are focusing on this aspect of the surgery, it would be this: *Think about what's really important!* The

Figure 5.6. *The radical retropubic prostatectomy* (continued)

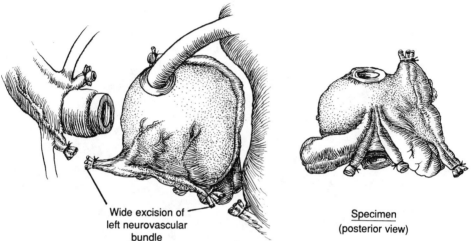

Wide excision of
left neurovascular
bundle

Specimen
(posterior view)

If it's not possible to preserve these nerve bundles—if they have been reached by the cancer—then the surgeon removes them along with the prostate; this is called "wide excision." The surgeon cuts out as much tissue as possible surrounding the prostate in an aggressive attempt to get every last bit of cancer.

primary goal here *isn't* to preserve potency, but to get rid of the cancer in a careful but thorough way. Please keep that in mind. Men can remain potent even if one bundle is removed, and can still have normal sensation, sex drive, and orgasm even if both bundles are removed.

There is no way for the surgeon to know for certain beforehand whether or not the bundles can be spared; only during surgery is it truly possible to see where the cancer is. If the surgeon decides to preserve the nerve bundles, the tiny branches that connect the nerves to the prostate are divided carefully. If, however, one or both bundles must be widely excised, the nerve bundles are cut near the urethra and beside the rectum.

Next, the surgeon goes to work on the prostate, making a cut to separate it at the bladder neck, which links the bladder to the prostate (Fig. 5.7 shows what the urethral sphincter looks like). The seminal vesicles and vas deferens on both sides are also removed (for more on the anatomy, see Chapter 1). The goal here

Figure 5.7. *The radical retropubic prostatectomy* (continued)

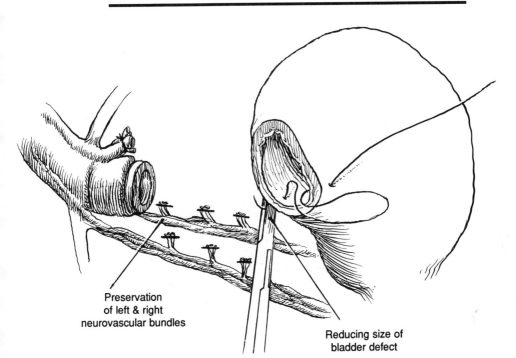

Preservation
of left & right
neurovascular bundles

Reducing size of
bladder defect

This shows the situation after the prostate has been removed. Note how big the bladder is in comparison to the urethra. The bladder opening must now be narrowed in size, so the two can be connected. This is done using sutures, or stitches.

is to remove as much surrounding tissue as possible along with the prostate. Finally, the surgeon must carefully rebuild the urinary tract, hooking up the bladder once again to the urethra and urethral sphincter, which is responsible for urinary control (this reconnection is called an anastomosis). The surgeon uses sutures, or stitches, to narrow the bladder neck so it matches the size of the urethra (Fig. 5.8). The Foley catheter is left in place after the operation.

After Surgery

Drains, exiting the abdomen (or perineum, in the radical perineal approach), will be left in place for about three to five days, and the Foley catheter, inserted

Figure 5.8. *The radical retropubic prostatectomy* (continued)

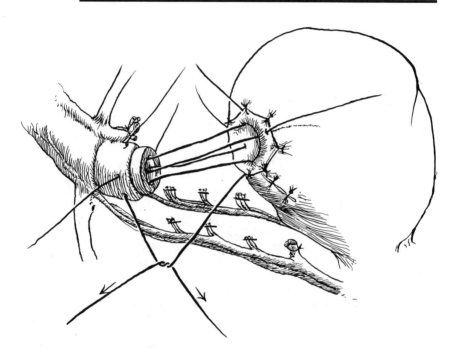

The operation's almost over now. Here, the surgeon will bridge this space by rebuilding the urinary tract—reconstructing the now-missing bladder neck, reconnecting the urethra and striated urethral sphincter, so urine can once again find its way out of the body.

in the penis and anchored by a tiny balloon in the bladder during surgery, will remain in place for two or three weeks. The main reason for the catheter is that it allows the anastomosis, the reconstructed urinary tract, a chance to heal. The drains are there to evacuate any urine that might leak from the anastomosis as it's healing; they stay in place until nothing more flows through them. *It is critical that the Foley catheter stay in place.* If it is inadvertently pulled out or removed too soon after surgery, this can be disastrous, and may lead to permanent incontinence. Your catheter should be securely taped to your thigh, and you should examine its mooring often. The catheter may take some getting used to, but remember—it's only temporary, and its presence is helping the body heal. While you're at home, keep the catheter connected to a large drainage bag most of the time, and use the leg bag only if you plan to go out of the house. The reason many doctors suggest this is that the leg bag doesn't hold as much urine, and if the bag becomes full and the patient doesn't realize what's happening, the urine can "back up" into him because it has no place else to go.

You'll be dealing with the catheter mostly at home; the economic trend these days is for patients to leave the hospital as soon as possible after any procedure, and prostate surgery is no exception. Fortunately, radical pros-tatectomy patients are actually *able* to go home and generally be more active sooner than ever before, and this is due largely to a new pain medication called ketorolac. As it turns out, one factor that kept men in the hospital was their inability to eat or to keep down oral painkillers after surgery. We always blamed this on the operation, but now we know what really happened—it was the pain medications they received after surgery that made them nauseated. Ketorolac belongs to a group of drugs called nonsteroidal anti-inflammatory agents (NSAIDs; these drugs include the over-the-counter painkillers Motrin or Nuprin). Patients on ketorolac usually are able to eat on the day after surgery— and for many men, this often is the first hurdle back toward normal life, even if it is bland hospital food!

Another hurdle is the crucial but often-dreaded first bowel movement after surgery. This is another item in the category of things men would rather not think about, but it has to happen sometime, and the sooner the better. Re-member, the prostate sits on top of the rectum; when it's removed, this part of the rectum is thin, fragile and particularly vulnerable to injury for the first three months after surgery. Therefore, it is critical that you don't have an enema or have your temperature taken rectally any time soon. And, it's absolutely essential that you have a bowel movement every day. For many men, this is easier said than done; pain medications, inactivity, slight dehydration (from not getting enough fluids before or after surgery)—all can add up to constipa-tion. To help keep things moving, you'll probably be given stool softeners or laxatives for several days. If you do become constipated, take mineral oil and milk of magnesia (but again, do not use an enema—you could perforate your rectum).

Other things you should do, or not do: Avoid lifting anything over ten pounds for six weeks from the day of surgery—and this includes grandchildren and the family pet! This is because, for the first six weeks, only sutures— stitches—are holding your incision together. After this time, the body's own mending device, firm scar tissue, will protect the incision. Heavy lifting can cause a hernia to develop in the incision; also, lifting or other strenuous activity may hurt the anastomosis connecting your bladder and urethra—and this could lead to long-term problems with urinary control. Keep telling yourself that this isn't forever—after six weeks, you can do anything you want.

And even during this healing time, you can eat and drink whatever you want, take long walks, and make as many trips as you'd like to up and down stairs. Also, you can drive a car five weeks after the surgery.

Expect to have some incontinence. This is normal, and it, too, is not permanent. It will go away soon—don't be discouraged. Also, expect to have some trouble with erections.

Finally, you'll be encouraged to sit in certain positions and to walk around almost immediately. This also is crucial—among other things, it can help reduce your risk of developing blood clots.

Results

Cancer Control

The bottom line, based on studies of hundreds of men who have had this procedure, is that radical prostatectomy *cures the vast majority of men with cancer confined to the prostate*. It also cures most men *even if cancer has reached or penetrated the prostate wall*, if—and this is a big if—two crucial conditions are met: If the tumor cells are pretty well differentiated (a Gleason score of 6 or lower), and if surgeons are able to cut out all the cancer. In surgical terms, this is called getting a "clear surgical margin." On the other hand, when a high-grade tumor has penetrated the prostate wall, or when the cancer has reached the seminal vesicles, the chances for a cure are not as certain.

One long-term study at Johns Hopkins, of 955 men with clinical stage T1 and T2 (A and B) cancer, found these results ten years after surgery: Only 4 percent had local recurrence of cancer, and 7 percent had distant metastases. And, using the PSA test, which is a highly sensitive measure for cancer recurrence, they found that 70 percent of the patients were cancer-free at ten years.

This study underlined the importance of the pathologic stage (the extent of cancer, determined at the time of surgery; see Chapter 3). At 10 years, the odds of being cancer-free, as measured by PSA levels, were 85 percent for men with disease confined to the prostate or who had very limited "capsular penetration," or cancer that has just barely penetrated the prostate wall.

At eight years after surgery, *all* patients with capsular penetration but "negative surgical margins"—this means the doctors were able to cut out all the cancer—and a Gleason score of 6 or less had an undetectable PSA. Fifty percent of men with capsular penetration and "positive surgical margins"—which means the surgeon's ability to cut out all the cancer is uncertain—and a Gleason score of 6 or less had an undetectable PSA at eight years. So did 50 percent of men with capsular penetration, negative surgical margins and a Gleason score of 7 or higher. And 25 percent of men with capsular penetration, positive surgical margins and a Gleason score of 7 or higher had an undetectable PSA eight years after surgery. (For more on positive surgical margins, see "Radiation after Prostatectomy," in Chapter 6.)

Some of the men who had an elevated PSA score went ahead and had radiation treatment; in 10 percent of these men, the radiation seemed to work—PSA plummeted to the undetectable range and stayed there for at least two years.

Why doesn't radical prostatectomy cure every man? Because the cancer has escaped the prostate before surgery, either locally, to the point where surgeons can't remove it all, or through impossible-to-detect, distant metastases. This is why many urologists make such a painstaking effort to figure out the exact stage of a man's cancer before surgery. They believe it's important to operate only on the patients who are going to benefit most and have the greatest long-term survival.

Urinary Continence

Incontinence is probably the most dreaded ramification of radical prostatectomy. But fortunately, when the operation is performed by an experienced surgeon, it's also among the rarest. In one Johns Hopkins study of 593 consecutive patients, 92 percent had complete urinary control after surgery. The remaining 8 percent had some stress incontinence (urine leakage at certain activities, such as running or playing golf). Of these men, 6 percent wore one or fewer pads a day. Only two men had stress incontinence serious enough to warrant placement of an artificial sphincter (see below), and no man was totally incontinent. In the next Johns Hopkins study, of 600 patients, no patient had stress incontinence severe enough to warrant placement of an artificial sphincter.

Of men over age 70, 86 percent were completely continent after surgery, as were 94 percent of the men who had both neurovascular bundles (clusters of nerves on either side of the prostate) preserved, 92 percent of the men who had one bundle removed, and 81 percent of the men who lost both nerve bundles. Also, there did not seem to be a link between potency and continence; 94

percent of potent men and 90 percent of impotent men remained totally continent.

What determines whether or not a man will remain continent? Most important is whether he has a strong sphincter to begin with. Some men have a poorly developed urinary sphincter—and it's almost impossible to determine this before the operation, because for men, the bladder neck and prostate are effective means of controlling urine. Also important is the skill of the surgeon in preserving the urinary sphincter and carefully rebuilding the urinary tract. But there are other factors, including the patient's age and whether both neurovascular bundles were removed. It's fairly clear, from studies at medical centers where radical prostatectomies are performed on older men, that men over 70 seem to have more problems with urinary control than younger men. It's not entirely clear whether preserving the nerve bundles improves urinary control: Men who had both nerve bundles removed appear to have a slightly higher rate of incontinence than men in whom both nerve bundles were preserved. However, it's possible that the urinary sphincter is sometimes damaged in the process of making a wide excision—cutting the bundles and as much tissue surrounding the prostate as possible.

What to Do about Incontinence.   Most men experience temporary urgency and stress incontinence after the catheter is removed—in fact, it would be remarkable if they didn't. Think about it: The urethra has been stretched and possibly irritated for three weeks by the catheter; it's probably going to take hours to days for it to recover from this insult.

Urinary control generally returns in three phases . Phase One—you're dry when lying down at night. Phase Two—you're dry when walking around. And Phase Three—you're dry when you stand up after sitting. Persistent stress incontinence (leaking urine when you stand up or exercise) is rare, and total incontinence is even more rare.

There's also something you can do to control stress incontinence—special exercises, called Kegel exercises, that strengthen the external sphincter. To help speed up your recovery, practice starting and stopping your urinary stream every time you go to the bathroom. The best way to do this is when standing to urinate: Try to shut off your urinary stream by contracting the muscles in your buttocks tightly. (There are other methods of performing these exercises, but by doing them this way you can be sure you're exercising the right muscles.) Only perform these exercises when you urinate—don't do them at other times, because you will tire out the sphincter muscle.

Until your urinary control returns completely, wear a pad, such as a Serenity pad, or disposable diaper, such as Depends. You can get these at the pharmacy or grocery store. Some men prefer using a special kind of padded underwear called Confidens Brief; your doctor should have good suggestions and perhaps even some samples for you to try. Whatever you do, *do not wear an incontinence device with an attached bag, a condom catheter or clamp!* If you use these devices, you won't develop the muscle control you need to be continent. Also, until your urinary control has returned, avoid drinking excessive amounts of fluids, and limit alcohol and caffeine—both can make the problem worse. Again, remember: You will get through this.

In extremely rare cases, when incontinence does not get better over time, your doctor may do cystometry to determine the state of the bladder. If you have urgency incontinence, anticholinergic drugs can dampen the involuntary bladder contractions. If you have stress incontinence, drugs that cause smooth muscle contractions, including decongestants or antidepressants (imiprimine, for instance, is an antidepressant drug that also inhibits urination), may be helpful. If incontinence persists for more than a year, or is severe, your doctor may suggest further treatment, possibly placement of an artificial sphincter. In this procedure, a rubbery cuff is positioned around the urethra and connected by tubing to a reservoir for fluid that's installed in the abdomen, and to a small pump, placed in the scrotum. The pump transfers fluid from the reservoir to inflate the cuff (and block the urethra), and a valve next to the pump can be released to deflate the cuff and allow urine to pass through the urethra.

The artificial sphincter is an elaborate device, but there are several simpler solutions that involve the injection of material (collagen) into the urethra or bladder neck. It's possible that with further refinements, these techniques will be sufficient for managing incontinence in almost all men who develop it.

Sexual Potency

After incontinence, impotence ranks right up there on the "most feared complications" list. But let's make sure we're all talking about the same thing: First of all, what is potency? The medical definition is simple—"an erection sufficient for vaginal penetration and orgasm." Having said that, it's worth repeating that men who are impotent after radical prostatectomy have *normal sensation, normal sex drive and can achieve a normal orgasm.* Their only problem may be in achieving or maintaining an erection. (For a more specific discussion of impotence after radical prostatectomy, and for suggestions on dealing with this problem, see Chapter 8.)

In a Johns Hopkins analysis of 503 potent men, 34 to 72 years old, 68 percent remained potent after radical prostatectomy. Age and the stage of cancer as well as surgical technique—the surgeon's skill, and whether or not one or both neurovascular bundles were removed during the operation—all can affect potency. The breakdown, by age: Potency was preserved in 91 percent of men younger than 50, in 75 percent of men aged 50 to 60, in 58 percent of men aged 60 to 70, and 25 percent of men over 70.

In men younger than 50, the potency rate is similar (about 90 percent) in men who kept both neurovascular bundles intact, and in men who had one nerve bundle removed. This suggests that all that's needed for men to achieve erection is one of these nerve bundles, and that nature has provided a spare.

In men older than 50, however, the sexual potency rate was higher in men who had both neurovascular bundles preserved than in men who lost one bundle. When the relative likelihood of impotence after surgery is adjusted for age, the risk is *twice as high* if the cancer has penetrated the prostate wall; if it has invaded the seminal vesicles; or if one neurovascular bundle has been removed.

To sum up: The men most likely to remain potent are younger, with disease confined to the prostate. These also are the men who will benefit most from surgery.

Complications

Like all surgery involving anesthesia, radical prostatectomy carries the risk of death, but *this is extremely rare.* In one hospital's study of 1,000 patients, there were two deaths—one man died three weeks after surgery, from a blood clot in his lung (for important tips on how to recognize symptoms of this, see below). The other man had a heart attack before surgery, as the anesthesia was beginning.

The most common complication during surgery is excess bleeding, usually a result of a blood vessel being injured during the operation. *That's why it is absolutely critical that your surgeon has mastered the techniques for ensuring a "bloodless field"* (see "An Anatomical Approach to Surgery," and "Are You in Good Hands? What to Look for in a Surgeon," in this chapter).

Less common complications include injuring the rectum or ureters; such injuries can be repaired during surgery, and extra surgical precautions can be taken to avoid permanent damage.

Other complications include blood clots and bladder neck contracture.

Blood Clots. These are among the most common, and potentially most serious, complications of radical prostatectomy. Blood clots that form in the legs' deep veins (this is called deep venous thrombosis) can be, at best, painful. At worst they can be fatal. The leg veins are, as one doctor describes it, "a straight shot to the lungs"; the worst-case scenario here is for a chunk of a blood clot in the leg to break free and shoot up to the lungs.

Blood clots in the legs can occur in as many as 12 percent of men after radical prostatectomy, and pulmonary embolisms, or blood clots in the lungs, occur in an estimated 2 percent to 5 percent of these men. (In one Johns Hopkins study of 1,300 radical prostatectomy patients, fewer than 2 percent had a blood clot, and two men died of a blood clot.)

Clearly, the best way to deal with this problem is *to prevent it from ever happening.* Some doctors do this by administering blood-thinning medications such as mini-dose heparin before surgery. Some doctors also give their patients compression devices—various forms of heavy-duty support hose—for the legs. One of these looks like a pair of "long johns," and is designed to force all blood into the deep veins, and keep the flow powerful and continuous. (Sluggish blood flow leads to clot formation.) Other hose have special compression chambers that control blood flow, and are designed to "milk" blood up the leg.

Important: If you have ever before had a blood clot, make sure your doctor knows about it. This could influence the way your anesthesia is administered. Also, men considered at higher risk of developing a blood clot may have a stronger blood-thinning medication administered by IV throughout their stay in the hospital. These preventive treatments are highly successful in preventing a blood clot from forming in the lungs.

Exercise is another crucial factor in helping to avert blood clots. Walking is good; it pumps blood back to the heart. Walk as soon as you're allowed to after surgery. Your doctor probably will encourage you to do dorsiflexion exercises —pumping your feet up and down to exercise the calf muscles. Do them often, about 100 times an hour in between naps. Also, it's a good idea not to sit upright in a firm chair (with your legs hanging down) for more than an hour at a time during the first four weeks. Try to sit with your legs elevated on a sofa, reclining chair, or comfortable chair with a footstool, as much as possible. This accomplishes two goals: One, because it raises your feet, it improves the blood flow from the veins in your legs. Two, it protects the area of surgery from bearing your full weight.

Note: Because patients are in and out of the hospital so fast these days, it's likely that any post-surgical trouble you experience will occur when you're at home. That's why it's essential that you and your family be aware of the warning signs of a clot in the leg or a clot that has gone to the lung. You may have a clot if you have swelling or tenderness in the leg, especially in the calf. Signs of a clot in the lungs include sudden chest pain—especially pain that gets worse when you take a deep breath—and coughing up blood. *If you have any of these signs, call your doctor immediately! Don't wait for your doctor's office hours if this happens in the middle of the night!* If you can't get to your doctor, go to an emergency room and tell the doctor there that you need to be evaluated for deep venous thrombosis or pulmonary embolism. Early treatment with anticoagulant medications generally takes care of the problem with excellent results. But if diagnosis—and therefore, treatment—is delayed, it's possible that a large clot to the lungs could be fatal.

Bladder Neck Contracture.   Often called constriction of the bladder neck and usually a result of scar tissue around the bladder neck, this complication has been reported in between 3 percent and 12 percent of men after surgery. Its symptoms are a dribbling urinary stream, but it can be difficult to distinguish this from the temporary incontinence that often occurs after radical prostatectomy. The contracture can be re-opened in outpatient surgery by a urologist, using a cystoscope, who makes a few tiny cuts to relax the tight scar tissue.

THE RADICAL PERINEAL APPROACH

Similar to the retropubic procedure in terms of before-surgery preparation and recovery, the radical perineal approach offers some advantages over that technique: There's less bleeding, because the major vein system that overlies the prostate (the dorsal vein complex) is not removed with the prostate. However, this also means that surgeons aren't able to cut out as much tissue as in the retropubic approach—so if the cancer has penetrated the prostate wall, "positive surgical margins" may be more likely here than in the retropubic approach. If the likelihood of cancer appearing in the pelvic lymph nodes is low (see table 3.3), there's no need for an abdominal incision. Many men, however, do have a laparoscopic lymph node dissection before getting a perineal prostatectomy just to be sure cancer hasn't reached the lymph nodes; see Chapter 3.

Call your doctor! Particularly if you have any of the warning signs of a blood clot

This is all part of being your own advocate. It doesn't mean that you have to be militant, or obnoxious, or that you should call your doctor in the middle of the night just to chat (please don't!).

What it *does* mean, however, is that you have certain rights. If you have a question or problem during office hours, by all means, go ahead and call; you may not always get the doctor, but you'll get somebody who can help.

And if you have a problem that you don't think can wait until morning, call at night. Most doctors have 24-hour answering services; many doctors have partners who share "on-call" time—they split it up, each taking a certain number of nights, weekends and holidays a year. They do this because they expect to get some calls at night, because they know from years of training and experience that medical emergencies don't always happen during office hours.

This won't be the first phone call your doctor gets in the middle of the night, and it certainly won't be the last. What would you rather do—wind up in the hospital as a result of a serious complication that should have been treated hours ago, or "bother your doctor?"

Another drawback to the perineal approach is that it's more difficult for surgeons to see—and thus protect—the neurovascular bundles, the thin packets of nerves that sit on either side of the prostate and are essential for erections. Therefore, preserving potency is not as certain. Also, the operation is not ideal for heavyset men, particularly men with what one doctor describes as a "large-barrel abdomen."

During Surgery: What Happens

You will be given general anesthesia, which means you'll be unconscious during the procedure. To reach the prostate, surgeons make an incision just above the rectum. The prostate is gradually separated from the rectum, bladder, urethra and vas deferens. The seminal vesicles are removed along with the prostate, and then the bladder is linked once again with the urethra.

WHAT HAPPENS IF MY
PSA GOES UP AFTER SURGERY?

If a man's PSA level goes up after a radical prostatectomy, this is an indication that there is prostate cancer somewhere. Maybe it's a local recurrence, in the area where the prostate used to be, or perhaps it's a distant metastasis—a tiny seed of cancer that got scattered long before the cancer was ever diagnosed.

How to tell which? Recently, Johns Hopkins investigators studied rising PSA levels in fifty-one men after radical prostatectomy. In 30 percent of these men, cancer returned locally; in 70 percent, the cancer showed up as distant metastases. Based on this study, the scientists found they can estimate which course the cancer will take using the *Gleason score* of the prostate specimen removed in surgery, the *pathologic stage* (which is based on study of the actual prostate—not just tissue samples, as in biopsy), and *timing*—when the PSA starts to rise.

Men most prone to distant metastases will have one or more of these conditions: Gleason scores of 8 or higher, cancer found in their seminal vesicles and lymph nodes during surgery, or a rise in PSA within a year after their surgery. Conversely, men with Gleason scores of 7 or lower, low pathologic stage, and/or increases in PSA several years after surgery most likely will have only a local recurrence of cancer. For these men, the good news is that this cancer may still be cured with external-beam radiation treatment to the prostate bed (the area where the prostate used to be. For more on an elevated PSA after radiation treatment, see Chapter 6).

RADICAL PROSTATECTOMY:
ONE MAN'S STORY

It was just a routine physical—until Peter Weaver's* doctor found a lump in his prostate.

*Weaver has allowed us to use his name in this book.

"I went in to the doctor's office sort of full of myself," recalls Weaver, who was 63 at the time. "I felt in great shape, I was jogging every day, doing some weights, eating well and having a good married life." He was stunned when his doctor found the lump. "I was sort of insulted, like, 'Me? This can't happen to *me*!' I had absolutely ZERO symptoms—no urinary problems, no aches, no pains, no sign of anything. It was a hidden time bomb, ticking away." The nodule was tiny, but a needle biopsy and transrectal ultrasound confirmed that it was cancerous—and "very operable."

Weaver, a syndicated financial columnist living in Washington, D.C., is a reporter, and he explored his treatment options just as he would research a story—chasing leads, talking to experts, putting himself in charge of getting the facts. After exploring every option, he decided to undergo surgery. His next step was to ask around until he was confident he'd found the best surgeon.

"It's a major operation," Weaver says. "I was in the hospital nine or ten days. (Today, most patients stay in the hospital only four or five days.) I went home with a catheter for urine for another two to three weeks." He had some trouble with incontinence for several months, and his sex life was disrupted for a few weeks. After about a year, he was back to normal.

That was five years ago. Now, he says proudly, his PSA tests have been "absolutely, totally normal." Several times a week, he runs three miles and works out with weights. He joined an athletic club. "My cholesterol's 155. The HDL (high-density lipoproteins) cholesterol is 45–50. The combination, my doctor says, is just perfect. I have a pulse of 60–64, a blood pressure of 120 over 80. I feel great."

For the last several years, Weaver has become involved in a prostate cancer support group. He has spoken and written about his experiences, and he has some advice for men in his situation.

First, he says, get a second opinion, and even a third. If you don't like what a doctor has to say—the doctor's success rate with impotence and incontinence, for example—"scratch his name off your list."

Ask your doctor as many questions as you need to, so you'll be prepared for the complications of surgery that will surely come. Because soon after surgery—if you're not expecting these complications—they can be overwhelming, he says: "You can't get an erection, you're leaking urine in your pants. From youth onward, you're made to feel that these are some of the worst possible things that can happen to a man." Even though the impotence and incontinence were only temporary for Weaver, they still affected his quality of life for months.

And know, too, that if impotence and incontinence don't go away, there *is* help, he says: "They've got medications, injections and devices available now that are incredible—that could give a cigar store Indian an erection!"

Weaver's last bit of advice for men? "Have a checkup every year, with the most experienced urologist you can find. Get a PSA test and digital exam. Take charge—be responsible for your own health." After all, "it's your body. You've got to look after it."

THE SHORT STORY

Radical prostatectomy is certainly not a new cure for prostate cancer; it's been around since 1904. There are two versions of this operation—the perineal approach, and the retropubic approach. The radical retropubic prostatectomy used to be notorious among surgeons for the extreme bleeding that went along with it, and both of these procedures used to have two devastating side effects—impotence and incontinence.

That picture has changed. The last fifteen years have seen dramatic improvements to the retropubic approach, based on new understanding of the prostate's anatomy. The development of new techniques has lessened the awful blood loss, and the operation has become far safer for patients. And, with what surgeons call "a bloodless field," it's now possible for them actually to see what they're doing—a major improvement! In the process, critical structures can be looked for and saved that previously were unrecognized and damaged as surgeons blindly felt their way. More precise techniques have reduced the likelihood of troublesome urinary incontinence to about 2 percent (and even those 2 percent aren't incontinent all the time). New anatomical discoveries also have made it possible for surgeons to preserve potency in the majority of men.

And perhaps most exciting, better understanding of the anatomical terrain means surgeons can now remove more tissue along with the prostate than anyone ever thought possible—which improves the operation's chances of cutting out all the cancer.

There are three goals to surgery: Removing all of the tumor, preserving urinary control, and preserving sexual function. Sexual function is number three because first, in order of importance, it is number three, and second, if it is lost, there are many ways to restore it to normal. Men who are impotent after radical prostatectomy have normal sensation, normal sex drive, and can achieve a normal orgasm. The one element they may be lacking is the ability to have an erection sufficient for intercourse, and this is a problem that can be fixed.

With the reduction in side effects, and with better screening techniques to identify men with localized prostate cancer, radical prostatectomies are now performed more often than ever before. Because of this, there's a wealth of information about long-term results, and the news is good: At ten years after surgery, 70 percent of patients have undetectable levels of PSA; only 4 percent develop local recurrence of cancer, and only 7 percent have distant metastases. Overall, 92 percent of men have complete urinary control, and only 2 percent of men have long-term, troublesome problems (wearing more than one pad a day). Total urinary incontinence is rare (and, as in impotence, there are several ways to improve this).

Recovery of sexual function is related to the age of the patient, and to surgical technique. Ninety percent of men younger than 50 remain potent after surgery; 75 percent of men in their fifties; 60 percent of men in their sixties, and 25 percent of men in their seventies remain potent.

There are two tiny bundles of nerves, one on either side of the prostate, that are essential for erection. Sometimes, depending on the extent to which the cancer has spread, one or both of these bundles must be removed. Men can still be potent even if one—but not both—of these bundles is removed. In men over 50, sexual potency is better in men who have both of these bundles preserved than in men who lose one bundle during surgery.

The men most likely to remain potent are younger, with disease confined to the prostate. These are also the men who are most likely to benefit from surgery.

Both the retropubic and perineal approaches are discussed in this chapter, as are all the possible complications and aftereffects you can expect, and ways to help you deal with them.

6

Other Treatments

Radiation and Cryoablation

RADIATION THERAPY FOR
PROSTATE CANCER: A LITTLE HISTORY

Like radical prostatectomy, radiation treatment for prostate cancer is not a new idea. In fact, it wasn't too long after urologist Hugh Hampton Young did that first radical prostatectomy (see Chapter 5) that he and another colleague at Johns Hopkins pioneered radiation therapy in this country (it had been developed a few years earlier in Europe). The treatment was primitive by today's standards, involving special radium applicators placed in tissue surrounding the prostate—the urethra, bladder and rectum.

But the next few decades laid the groundwork for some of today's radiation therapies: X-ray treatments were introduced, followed by radon "seeds" that could be inserted in the prostate tumor.

These fledgling attempts at curing prostate cancer, however, were not distinguished by astounding success. Compared to today's high-powered technology, the low-energy X-ray beams produced throughout the 1930s were lackluster, and their ability to penetrate the prostate was mediocre and imprecise. Radiation treatment, therefore, was only palliative—it could relieve pain and symptoms, but it did not eradicate the cancer.

In the 1940s, the impact of hormones on the prostate was discovered, and radiation was all but abandoned in favor of castration and hormonal drugs. But radiation's exile was not long, thanks largely to scientists who revolutionized the field, using an exciting new machine called a linear accelerator. They produced penetrating, high-powered beams that could target radiation doses to a specific site without harming surrounding tissue. And suddenly, radiation was off the bench and back in the ballgame as a major player—*a treatment that could actually cure localized cancer, not just relieve the symptoms of advanced disease.*

In the decades since then, radiation therapy has been refined and made even more powerful. There are two standard approaches—sending radiation into the tumor from the outside, with external-beam therapy, and implanting radioactive seeds directly into the tumor (this is called interstitial brachytherapy). Also, within the last few years, a new technique called three-dimensional conformal therapy has come on the scene. It increases external-beam therapy's potential by maximizing the dose of radiation to the prostate tumor while keeping the risk of damaging nearby tissue to a minimum.

External-Beam Therapy

How does an X-ray machine work? The simplest way to think of it is to imagine yourself getting a suntan. The difference here is that you can't feel or see the X-ray energy hitting your body, and the "tan" occurs internally. (What happens is that the radiation particles destroy DNA, causing targeted cells to die.) The best way to get a good, even tan is in increments, not all at once. Similarly, the most effective radiation doses are spread out over several weeks, with each treatment lasting only a few minutes at a time. (The goal here, besides killing the prostate cancer, is to do as little harm as possible to the surrounding tissue—the rectum, bowel, bladder, bone, and skin.)

To help your radiation oncologists get a good picture of the terrain of the targeted area—the prostate and surrounding organs—you will probably be given a "treatment-planning" CT scan. Some doctors also use computer simulators to fine-tune the dose of radiation and fields of treatment for you—these can vary, depending on factors such as the stage and grade of your tumor, the contour of your pelvis, and your size (for some large or heavyset men, a different degree of energy works better).

For high-grade tumors (Gleason score 7 or higher) or malignancies greater than clinical stage T2b (B1), doctors make sure the field of treatment covers the prostate, seminal vesicles and surrounding tissue, including nearby lymph

Figure 6.1. *External-beam radiation treatment*

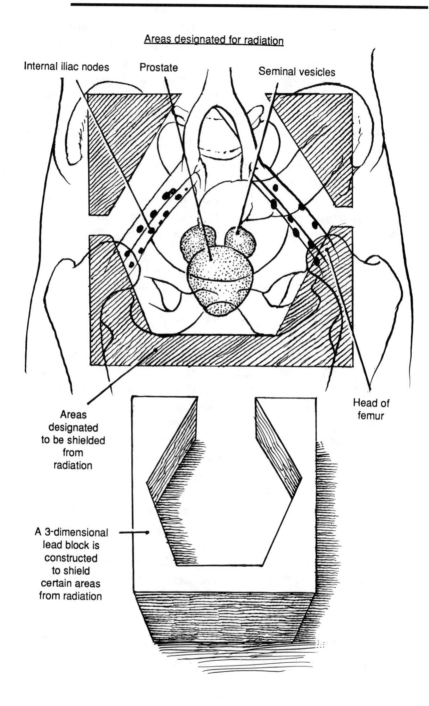

Areas designated for radiation

Internal iliac nodes   Prostate   Seminal vesicles

Areas designated to be shielded from radiation

A 3-dimensional lead block is constructed to shield certain areas from radiation

Head of femur

nodes, where the cancer may have spread after penetrating the prostate wall. Radiation is delivered to the front, back and each side of the patient. (The specific map of treatment can vary from man to man.) A major goal here is to safeguard as much of the surrounding territory—the cancer-free organs and tissue—as possible. Doctors particularly want to shield bone from radiation, to avoid harming key blood-forming cells that reside in the bone marrow. One way to protect cancer-free areas is to shield them with blocks of lead, which the radiation can't penetrate. Other steps can also be taken—one way to protect the bowel, for instance, is for the patient to have a full bladder during treatment; this pushes the bowel away from the pelvis. Another technique is to have the patient lie on a hard pillow that pushes the bowel out of the way, into the upper abdomen.

To make treatment easier to tolerate (and thus minimize side effects), a "sandwich" approach—in which the radiation dose is split in two, with a break in between—may become more common. The purpose of this technique is to give the bowel and part of the bladder a "breather," a window of opportunity to recover from the shock of the treatment. In men who have small (stage T1 or T2, or A and B), low-grade tumors—where the risk of cancer having spread beyond the prostate is minuscule—radiation is limited to the prostate alone.

What Happens

Radiation treatment means going to the hospital on a daily or near-daily basis and lying flat on your back or stomach on a table for a few minutes as a big X-ray machine (similar to, but larger than, ones you've seen at the dentist's office) moves in an arc or circle over the targeted fields. That's it. Then you go home. Most radiation treatment takes seven to eight weeks and is done during weekdays, leaving weekends free.

What If I've Had a TUR Procedure for BPH?

Your predicament is just the same as that of men who have a radical prostatectomy—you've got to wait for the swelling and inflammation to go

Opposite: Here we see the regions targeted for external-beam radiation treatment: the prostate, the seminal vesicles, and the lymph nodes. There are two goals here: to eradicate the cancer, and, equally important, to minimize harm to surrounding tissue. (Here, for example, we can see that the portion of the rectum immediately behind the prostate and seminal vesicles is unavoidably in the radiation field.) Doctors particularly want to shield bone from radiation, to avoid harming key blood-forming cells that reside in the bone marrow. One way to protect these cancer-free areas is to shield them with blocks of lead, which the radiation can't penetrate.

down, generally about eight to twelve weeks, before you can undergo any new treatment. This waiting period, though it may seem agonizingly slow, is critical—it helps minimize your risk of becoming incontinent or developing scar tissue around the urethra from radiation damage to not-yet-healed tissue. (Some men who have undergone a TUR procedure may be more likely to develop a urethral stricture, which is easily treatable; see "Complications," below.)

Complications

For the first few days or even the first couple of weeks of external-beam radiation therapy, you may feel nothing out of the ordinary; it takes a while for the cumulative doses of radiation to build up and have an effect. But by the third to fifth week, many men react with symptoms that can range from mild to severe; in most cases, these generally go away within days to weeks after the course of treatment is over. Sometimes, men develop these symptoms six months or more after treatment.

Most common complications are bowel problems (diarrhea, rectal itching or burning, urgency to have a bowel movement, painful cramps) and urinary trouble (feelings of urgency, painful or difficult urination, stress incontinence, and the need to urinate frequently, especially at night). For as many as 85 percent of men, these symptoms become acute enough to require medication.

In one analysis of 1,020 men treated in two large studies, about 7 percent of men needed to go to the hospital for treatment of more severe urinary problems. These included blood in the urine, bladder inflammation, and urethral stricture or bladder neck contracture—both caused when scar tissue develops and impedes urine's progress out of the body. Urethral strictures accounted for more than half of these problems, and they seemed to develop mostly in men who had undergone a TUR procedure for BPH. Fewer than one percent of the men needed surgery to fix these problems. (A bladder neck contracture can be re-opened in outpatient surgery by a urologist, using a cystoscope, who makes a few tiny cuts to relax the tight scar tissue. Most urethral strictures respond well to dilation—stretching the urethra, in one or two sessions. Stubborn strictures may also be treated with tiny incisions, like those done to ease bladder neck contractures.)

Just a little over 3 percent of the men in this study experienced chronic

Opposite: The lateral (side) radiation field, again with the prostate and seminal vesicles. From this side, much of the rectum is shielded from the radiation.

Figure 6.2. *External-beam radiation treatment*

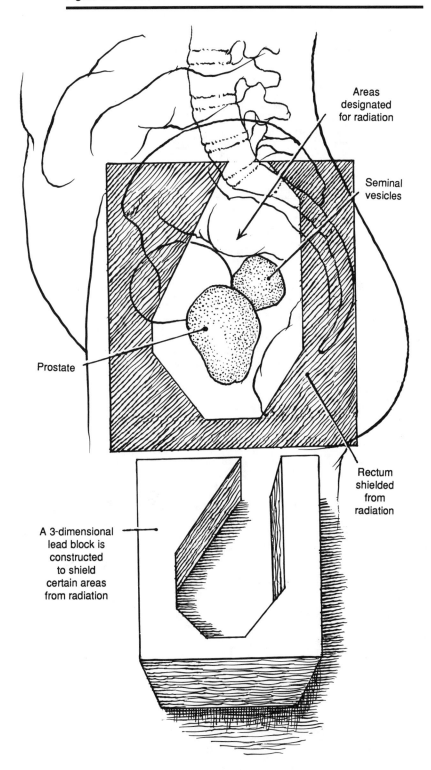

Areas
designated
for radiation

Seminal
vesicles

Prostate

Rectum
shielded
from
radiation

A 3-dimensional
lead block is
constructed
to shield
certain areas
from radiation

Figure 6.3. *External-beam radiation treatment*

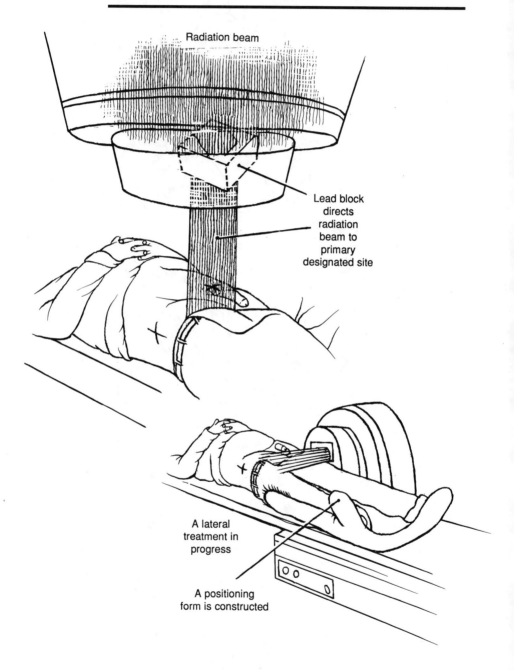

intestinal problems, including rectal inflammation, diarrhea, rectal bleeding, an intestinal ulcer or development of an anal stricture (tight scar tissue that can interfere with bowel movement); fewer than one percent experienced bowel obstruction or perforation. And complications that proved fatal were extremely rare—0.2 percent.

Sexual Function

Sexual potency after external-beam therapy is reported to remain in between 54 percent and 86 percent of men. There is a range here because sexual potency is difficult to measure: Age, stage of disease, and a man's sex life before treatment all play a role in his ability to have an erection afterward. Men younger than 60, who are sexually active and who are treated when the cancer is in the earlier stages (confined to the prostate) are most likely to remain potent after radiation treatment. However, many men treated with radiation are older, and more likely to have problems with impotence anyway—either because they're taking medications that can interfere with sexual function, or simply because of their age.

One fact you should know about radiation therapy is that its effect on potency is slower and much more insidious than radical prostatectomy's more immediate impact. Radiation seems to cause a man's ability to have an erection to diminish over time (months to years); about half the men who receive it are impotent at seven years after radiation treatment. (For more on impotence, see Chapter 8.) This is probably because radiation acts on the blood vessels, causing an eventual decrease in blood flow to the penis.

Results

It's difficult to show any real differences between the results of radiation and radical prostatectomy, if you look at overall fifteen-year survival rates of men with prostate cancer after both treatments. A large study from Stanford report-

Opposite: The simplest way to think of radiation therapy is to imagine yourself getting a suntan. The difference here is that you can't feel or see the X-ray energy hitting your body, and the "tan" occurs internally. (What happens is that the radiation particles destroy DNA, causing targeted cells to die.) The best way to get a good, even tan is in increments, not all at once. That's why the radiation doses are spread out over several weeks, with each treatment lasting only a few minutes at a time.

Here we can see the lead block, which protects cancer-free areas, in the machine. Note the marks on this man's skin that align the machine with his body before each session. A positioning form ensures that the radiation always targets the same area.

ed an overall survival of 50 percent, fifteen years after treatment, for men with stages T1a and T1b (A1 and A2) disease. From these statistics, radiation therapy looks highly promising. However, most of the patients who are initially diagnosed with localized prostate cancer who die during the first fifteen years after *any* form of treatment die from other causes—so studies of overall survival don't always reveal the whole story.

Other studies of radiation therapy use different measuring sticks—prostate biopsies and PSA tests. Depending on how many biopsies are taken, anywhere from 30 percent to 90 percent of men who have received external-beam radiation therapy can have a positive biopsy two years or more after treatment. Although this does not mean that *all* of these men will have treatment failure— that their cancer will come back—long-term follow-up studies have found that many patients do. At five years after treatment, only 25 percent of patients will have low or undetectable levels of PSA. At ten years, only 10 percent will. However, despite the fact that PSA may be measurable, many of these men have not yet demonstrated any clinical signs of treatment failure (urinary tract obstruction, for example); *these findings suggest that radiation therapy can effectively control local symptoms from prostate cancer in many patients.* And frankly, for many older men—a 75-year-old man who gets radiation today, for example—it isn't going to matter too much if PSA rises slightly ten years from now, if the therapy has controlled the cancer.

The bottom line is that the standard radiation therapy administered over the last decade does not always eradicate prostate cancer, and in many men, PSA levels will rise over time. Because of this, doctors are working to improve radiation techniques—among other things, to give the prostate more radiation while minimizing side effects to surrounding tissue. But there has been a decrease in doctors' enthusiasm for using radiation therapy as curative treatment in *young men who have the potential to live for many years*—and who could be cured with surgery.

Studies of radiation therapy in locally advanced disease (stages T3 and T4, or C disease) have shown less promising results. The problem is that often, by the time cancer in these stages is even diagnosed, it's too late—it has already scattered offshoots in microscopic amounts to the pelvic lymph nodes. And when this is the case, irradiating the pelvis doesn't seem to help prevent distant metastases. Radiation doesn't seem to help stop local spread of cancer in all of these patients, either. Ten years after treatment, as many as 40 percent of these men will have a recurrence of cancer locally, in the prostate and surrounding tissue. (Three-dimensional conformal therapy, however—discussed later in this chapter—may improve local control of prostate cancer.)

To boost the odds for survival in these men, some doctors are trying a combined approach—giving patients hormonal therapy two months before and during radiation treatment. Early results of these trials are encouraging, but long-term studies are needed to know the true difference this double-barrelled approach will make.

One Note about Evaluating Radiation Treatment (or Any Treatment): Many studies of radiation and prostate cancer have been published in the medical literature, and they're not standardized—their definitions of success vary. In measuring local control of prostate cancer, for example, some studies base their results on a normal digital rectal examination, or a normal PSA score, or a negative prostate biopsy at eighteen to twenty-four months after radiation (this seems to be the most accurate approach). So in weighing the results of *any* studies, look at the criteria the investigators use, the boundaries they draw (for example, a six-month study probably isn't going to be very helpful), and the endpoints they use to measure their results (a normal digital rectal exam, for instance, may not tell the whole story—cancer could be there, even if doctors can't feel it).

What Happens If My PSA Goes Up after Radiation Treatment?

The purpose of radiation treatment is to disable the prostate, to stop cancer there from continuing to grow. Because the prostate is the source of PSA, it's pretty obvious that something is wrong if PSA is still being made, and there are two possibilities here: Either the cancer has returned locally, to the prostate or surrounding tissue, or a distant metastasis—a tiny bit of cancer that probably escaped the prostate before treatment began—has started causing trouble.

Some doctors advocate "salvage" procedures—additional treatments, such as radical prostatectomy or cryotherapy. Radical prostatectomy is generally not a good idea; the risk of complications after the prostate has been irradiated is so high that many surgeons have a hard time justifying the procedure. Also, by the time most men who initially had radiation treatment seek surgery, it may be too late for surgery to cure the cancer; it has already spread outside the prostate. (This includes men who originally had clinical stage T3 or C disease. Remember, men with cancer that has spread beyond the prostate aren't considered good candidates for surgery in the first place; having had radiation therapy is just another strike against the odds of cure. Also, surgery is not advisable for patients who have advanced, palpable cancer after radiation therapy, for men with PSA levels greater than 10 or 20, or with poorly differentiated cancer—a Gleason score of 8 or higher.)

Radical prostatectomy may be considered in the small subset of men who initially had cancer confined to the prostate, if the local recurrence of cancer appears to be well- to moderately well-differentiated (a Gleason score of 7 or lower) and still confined within the prostate, and if the PSA level is less than 10. But even in these, the best possible candidates for prostate surgery after radiation treatment, the complications are much higher than for men who have surgery first. The risk of incontinence is as high as 25 percent, and other injuries—to delicate rectal tissue made even more fragile by radiation, for example—also are much more common.

Recently cryotherapy—freezing the prostate—has been considered as a "Plan B" for radiation with a rising PSA. But at the writing of this book, there is only preliminary information available on how often this affects the tumor, and on the complications that might accompany cryotherapy after the prostate has been irradiated. (Cryotherapy is discussed later in this chapter.)

The bottom line, for most patients who have a progressive increase in PSA after radiation therapy, is that it's unlikely that any form of additional treatment will cure the cancer. One option is that these patients begin hormone therapy in an attempt to shrink the tumor (for a discussion of hormone therapy, see Chapter 7). Another is that they be followed closely with watchful waiting, and that they receive additional treatment only if or when they have symptoms of metastatic disease (for a discussion of when to begin treatment, see Chapter 7).

Radiation after Prostatectomy

PSA is a good litmus test for the success of prostate cancer treatment: Soon after radical prostatectomy, a man's PSA level should plummet—ideally, into oblivion. If it doesn't drop that far, or if it goes away and comes back, some patients move to Plan B—external-beam radiation treatment. (This is the opposite of the situation described above, and the long-term prognosis is often different for these men.)

Radiation after prostatectomy is also used in some men who have "positive surgical margins"—if the edges of the removed tissue show cancer cells. However, there are several considerations here: One is that *just because the surgical margins are positive does not necessarily mean that cancer is left behind.* How can this be? When cancer reaches beyond the prostate to invade nearby tissue, it produces a dense scar tissue that acts, as one surgeon describes it, "like Super Glue." As a surgeon removes the prostate, this thick scar tissue sticks to the surrounding cancer cells—picking them up like a lint brush. So in some cases, although the pathologist may see cancer cells at the margin—and make a judgment of "positive surgical margins"—there are no cancer cells left inside the patient; the sticky scar tissue took them all away.

A study at Johns Hopkins involved such instances, when a surgeon removed the prostate, looked at it, suspected that some cancer cells were present, went back and cut out more of the surrounding tissue. Even when the pathologist believed there was a positive surgical margin at the edge of the prostate, in 40 percent of these patients there turned out to be no cancer left behind in that adjacent tissue.

Another factor to consider here is that in patients with cancer that has extended beyond the prostate to the point where it is not possible for surgeons to remove it all, it's a pretty likely bet that there are other cancer cells floating around elsewhere—that cancer has already escaped from this tissue near the prostate, that it has already metastasized. And that any attempts at local treatment (such as radiation to this area) will not be able to reach all the cancer. Finally, radiation after radical prostatectomy can make a man more prone to problems with urinary control and sexual function; the radiation may damage tissue already made vulnerable by the surgery.

As a general rule, men with organ-confined cancer or men with cancer that has penetrated the prostate but still was removed in its entirety (men who had "negative surgical margins") and Gleason scores of 6 or less should not receive radiation therapy after radical prostatectomy.

The best candidates for radiation after radical prostatectomy are men who have positive surgical margins—but cancer that has not yet reached the pelvic lymph nodes and seminal vesicles. However, even this is not a crystal-clear decision; not all of these men are going to need radiation. For many of these men, the radical prostatectomy will be enough to control the cancer. One option is for men to have regular PSA tests and begin radiation treatment *only* if the PSA starts going up.

And there's yet another consideration: Not all of these men with rising PSAs are going to be helped by the radiation, because of the problem with distant metastases we mentioned above. So what you and your doctor need to determine is, why is the PSA going up? Is it local recurrence of cancer, or the presentation of distant metastases?

Recently, investigators at Johns Hopkins studied 51 radical prostatectomy patients who experienced a rise in PSA after surgery. These men were followed until the location of the recurrent cancer could be identified; 30 percent of these men developed palpable local recurrence of cancer that was confirmed by biopsy; 70 percent showed signs of distant metastases with positive bone scans.

In this study, distant metastases were present in nearly all men who had early elevations of PSA during the first year after radical prostatectomy, men whose tumors had a high Gleason score (8 or higher), and men with cancer in the seminal vesicles or lymph nodes. Therefore, radiation therapy to the prostate bed (the area where the prostate used to be) probably isn't going to get all the cancer in these men.

However, men in this study who had a late rise in PSA, men with low-grade disease (Gleason 7 or lower), and men with cancer-free seminal vesicles and pelvic lymph nodes were more likely to have local recurrence of cancer—cancer that has not yet metastasized. These men, then, would be more likely to benefit from radiation therapy to the prostate bed.

Should a man have radiation therapy immediately after surgery? No. It should be delayed at least three months, to give the body a chance to heal—and particularly to give the urinary tract a chance to recover. Irradiating a tender, sewn-together urinary tract is not the best way to encourage this inflamed tissue to heal.

Interstitial Brachytherapy (Implanting Radioactive Seeds)

This is basically hand-to-hand combat, instead of missiles launched from far away. The idea here is that the farther away energy gets from its source—the more tissue a radiation beam has to pass through to reach its target—the less effective it will be in killing cancer. And that implanting tiny sources of radiation *directly in the cancerous tissue* (*brachy* comes from the Greek word meaning "short," as in "a short distance away from the malignancy") will really blast the tumor—and, as an added bonus, minimize the risk of harming innocent civilians, the cancer-free cells nearby.

The concept is not new. Pierre Curie thought of it nearly a century ago—even before external-beam radiation treatment came on the scene—and doctors in New York tried it several years later; they inserted thin glass tubes with a radioactive substance called radon directly into tumors. The treatment killed tissue, all right, but the results were uneven; some of the targeted tissue was devastated while other tissue remained unscathed. In the next decades, scientists improved the technique, but its popularity waned as hormonal treatment developed and as external-beam radiation therapy got better (see above). In the 1950s and 1960s, however, improvements in dosages and radioactive materials helped foster a comeback for interstitial therapy: Doctors implanted radio-active gold "seeds," or tiny chunks of radioactive material, in men with pros-tate cancer; this was combined with external-beam radiation therapy. A few years later, doctors began using radioactive iodine seeds to fight prostate cancer.

Over the years, several other radioactive materials, including palladium, have been tested, and the means of implanting them have evolved from a subjective, free-hand technique (which requires surgery to give the doctor access to the prostate) to state-of-the-art, ultrasound- and CT-guided systems involving templates. (Some of these techniques mean open surgery is not necessary, although laparoscopic surgery may still be used to see whether cancer is in the pelvic lymph nodes—see Chapter 3.)

So, doctors have become highly sophisticated in targeting and placing these radioactive seeds. But do they work? The bottom line is: *Not as well as radical prostatectomy or external-beam radiation therapy.* And who should get this treatment? It's not ideally suited for men with a large, bulky tumor, a high-grade (Gleason score 7 or above) tumor, or lymph node metastases. Most implantation regimens don't include the seminal vesicles or tissue outside the prostate—so if there's the slightest risk that cancer has spread to these areas, implanting radiation seeds *within* the prostate won't do anything to fight the cancer *outside* it. And implanting foreign particles—no matter how tiny—into the body may cause infection over time as the body moves to fight these invaders. (To avoid this risk, some implants are removed after several days.)

Radiation seeds are not recommended for men who have had a previous TUR procedure; for one thing, because they've had significant amounts of tissue around the urethra removed to alleviate their BPH symptoms, there's not a lot left to hold the seeds in place. Perhaps because of this, men who have had a TUR are much more likely to develop urinary problems from this therapy.

The ideal patient for radioactive seeds is a man who is *also* ideally suited for external-beam radiation therapy and radical prostatectomy—and both of these treatments can cure prostate cancer in men with localized disease. So the question is, *is interstitial brachytherapy equally good or better?* And the answer for now is, probably not, although the treatment is continually improving. Before the development of sophisticated guidance systems, major problems arose from seeds being either too far apart or too close together, resulting in an uneven distribution of radiation throughout the prostate—some cancer cells were killed, but some weren't. In many cases, the cancer returned, or never completely went away in the first place. Better placement may change this picture.

Basic Approaches

There are many variations, but the basic means of access is the transperineal approach, reaching the prostate through the perineum, the area between the scrotum and rectum. Before beginning interstitial brachytherapy, you should undergo an extensive physical examination and a cystoscopy (see Chapter 9) to evaluate your particular anatomy and make sure the cancer is contained within the prostate. You should also have a CT scan, so your doctors can get a closer look at the prostate and plan the way the treatment will be administered.

One transperineal approach involves open surgery and begins much like the radical prostatectomy—with a Foley catheter, an abdominal incision and a staging lymph node dissection (see Chapter 3) to make sure the cancer has not spread to the pelvic lymph nodes. If the lymph nodes are cancer-free, the procedure continues. When doctors reach the prostate and can see the tumor, they draw an outline by implanting tiny bits of material, which can be seen on an X-ray, around its edges—like dotted lines or stakes marking a boundary. Then the doctor inserts a long needle through the perineum into the prostate, far enough so that its tip sticks out of the bladder neck. This is called a stabilizing needle, and it becomes an axis that helps hold a template in place. The result is a highly sophisticated kind of "paint-by-numbers" map of the prostate that helps doctors know exactly where to insert the other needles. The doctor's finger, inserted in the patient's rectum, helps guide placement and depth of the needles. With this approach, it's also possible for doctors to place seeds in the seminal vesicles (however, this may cause severe rectal complications—see below).

Now, instead of simply inserting the radioactive seeds, the doctors send the patient out of the operating room and to the hospital's radiation oncology department. "Dummy" (not radioactive) seeds are implanted, and then photographed by an X-ray machine. These fake seeds make possible ultra-precise, three-dimensional placement of each of the real radioactive seeds, which are implanted next. Also, the amount of radioactive material can be fine-tuned from seed to seed to ensure an even distribution of radiation. Now comes a little help from outside—external-beam radiation therapy. The radiation zeroes in on the implants and turns them into little antennae, which help focus and amplify the radiation. The seeds are removed—which should minimize the risk of infection—and a course of external-beam radiation therapy will begin two to four weeks later.

Avoiding Open Surgery

Several transperineal procedures don't require open surgery at all. One is done just with fluoroscopy (an X-ray image that appears live on a TV screen instead of as a still photograph). Another involves a perineal template like the one described above, and uses CT scanning for extra precision in placing the needles. Over the course of several CT scans, doctors are able to create a three-dimensional image of the prostate. A computerized guidance system helps determine where the seeds should go, how deeply they should be inserted, and how strong their radiation should be.

Many doctors are encouraged by new techniques that use transrectal ultrasound and a sophisticated grid to guide placement of the implants. Like the CT scanner, the transrectal ultrasound enables doctors to develop beforehand a three-dimensional map of the prostate; this guarantees a much more even distribution of radiation throughout the gland. During the procedure, a Foley catheter is inserted through the urethra into the bladder, an ultrasound probe is inserted in the rectum, and needles are placed according to the electronic grid. In this approach, long stabilizing needles are used that don't have anything to do with placement of the seeds. Because there's no abdominal incision here, and therefore doctors don't have full access to all sides of the prostate, they use these needles basically to skewer the prostate and move it around so the seeds can be placed in the appropriate spots. Doctors also use fluoroscopy and ultrasound to double-check the position of the seeds. In some studies, this has been shown to ensure a more accurate, even distribution of the seeds.

Complications

Evaluating the complications of interstitial brachytherapy is confusing for doctors as well as patients—mainly because there are many studies out there whose results and criteria vary widely. Some reasons for this are that different surgeons have different techniques and, frankly, levels of expertise; that some doctors implant seeds in patients who would be ruled out for this treatment by other doctors; and that some doctors leading various studies may not specify, may lump in different categories, or may not even be aware of all the complications their patients have had. Any time you see gaping holes in percentages (like, "From 5 percent to 85 percent of men had . . ."), it's probably safe to assume that truly accurate results are hard to come by.

Having said this, we can also say that there are some complications you can expect from implantation of radioactive seeds. They include the following.

The incidence of death from any of the procedures is extremely low. There is a huge fluctuation in the incidence of late (not immediately after surgery) complications—ranging from zero to 72 percent—depending on which study one chooses to quote; the most common range is from 10 percent to 25 percent.

Rectal Problems.   Several studies report that from 20 percent to 25 percent of men suffered rectal complications, such as diarrhea, cramps or bleeding; most of these problems were not severe. Men who were treated more aggressively (in one study, men with larger, stage T3 or T4, or C, tumors got radioactive iodine seeds plus external-beam radiation) or men who had larger tumors (and therefore got more seeds or a higher dose of radiation) tended to develop more severe rectal problems, such as ulcers. Stool softeners, steroid enemas and anti-inflammatory drugs may help mild rectal ulcers go away, but more serious ulcers that eat away tissue may require reconstructive surgery.

Prostatitis.   In one study of 115 patients who had radioactive iodine seeds implanted, five men developed prostatitis (for a discussion of prostatitis, see Chapter 11) and reported severe irritative urinary symptoms. "Three of these patients were essentially 'prostate cripples,' who were truly disabled by their frequent and painful voiding," wrote two of the investigators. Symptoms in the other two men got better after a TUR procedure (in which many of the radioactive seeds were removed) and long-term regimens of antibiotics. The investigators suspect that in these men, the seeds had become infected.

Urinary Problems.   From 10 percent to 37 percent of men in several studies had urinary problems—including urethral stricture, bladder neck contracture, and damage to the urethra—that caused irritative urinary symptoms. Most of these occurred in men who had already experienced such problems (from BPH, for example) or who had undergone a TUR procedure. For example, incontinence, which occurred in 5 percent of men, was not a problem for men who had not had the TUR procedure. Another factor in the development of urinary problems seems to be placement of the seeds—trouble seems much more likely to develop when seeds are planted too close to the urethra. Some doctors are now hoping to avoid this problem by leaving a larger cushion of seed-free tissue around the urethra. However, in sparing the urethra, will they also be sparing some cancer? This is not certain.

Sexual Problems.   These can include impotence, ejaculatory pain, pain in the testicles, and blood in the semen. The incidence of impotence seems to have a lot to do with a man's potency before the procedure. One study, for example, found that only 7 percent of men reported impotence. In other studies, impotence is much more common. Note: In men who have radioactive seeds implanted, a man's ability to have an erection appears to diminish over time, just as it does in men who get external-beam radiation treatment.

Results

Results, too, vary widely, depending on such factors as the stage and grade of tumors, the length of time after treatment a patient is followed, and the criteria used to define cancer control. Many studies just look at results of prostate biopsies—not incorporating other important signs that something is wrong with the prostate, like a lump that can be felt in a digital rectal exam, or symptoms of urinary obstruction (from a tumor that is large enough to disrupt urinary flow), or changes in PSA or acid phosphatase levels. It's significant that the best results for cancer control—a zero percent failure rate in some cases— generally come from the studies with the shortest follow-up time. How can an eighteen-month study possibly be as thorough, or ultimately helpful, as a ten-year study?

One long-term study predicted a local relapse rate (where cancer returns to the prostate or surrounding tissue) of 52 percent at fifteen years, with a failure rate during this time of about 11 percent a year. The average time it took for local recurrence to be diagnosed was nine years.

With external-beam radiation treatment, the five-year mark after treatment is a big milestone; in most cases, if cancer's going to come back, it happens before then. But with interstitial brachytherapy, in a significant number of men cancer comes back after five years. In one study, for instance, only 57 percent of the men who ultimately would have a relapse were diagnosed within five years. In another study, it took at least six to eight years before half of the men experienced local relapse.

Other studies have found that men with higher tumor stage and grade were more likely not to be cured by radiation seeds (which makes sense, considering that most implantation programs don't do anything to fight cancer outside the prostate). Also, some studies have found that a significant number of men—20 percent in one study—who got radioactive iodine implants required radical prostatectomy to help fight cancer that had returned. With external-beam radiation therapy, this number is much lower, about 8 percent. (Note: Many urologists feel that radical prostatectomy after *any* radiation treatment is not going to be very successful and will not perform the operation on these men.)

And in studies comparing seed implantation's results in controlling cancer to other therapies, the seeds have come in a distinct third to radical prostatectomy and external-beam radiation therapy. In no major study has interstitial brachytherapy ever proved a *better* method than the other two main forms of treatment for prostate cancer. However, many studies looking at "relapse-free survival" have shown, at ten years after seed implantation, that 58 percent or more of men are still alive and cancer-free, and one study found that 53 percent of men who didn't have cancer in the lymph nodes were alive and cancer-free after fifteen years. The bottom line from a host of studies seems to be that seed implantation—if it doesn't ultimately cure prostate cancer—can at least delay it significantly, for years.

"Salvage" Therapy

There are many medical centers in this country trying all manner of techniques, sometimes one after another, in a desperate attempt to buy time or cure prostate cancer that has come back after treatment. Some men whose prostate cancer returns after getting radioactive seeds go on to have what's called "salvage" therapy. This can include having a radical prostatectomy and orchiectomy (castration, removal of the testes), or undergoing other radiation treatment—getting more seeds, or having external-beam therapy.

These men are more likely to have complications. Understandably, operating on a prostate whose tissue has been damaged by radiation seeds is going to be more difficult than operating on an otherwise healthy prostate with just a bit of cancer. And in the medical literature there is no good evidence that salvage radical prostatectomy is actually curing many patients.

Three-Dimensional Conformal Therapy

This approach has great potential to sharpen the cancer-fighting ability of external-beam radiation while reducing the damage to nearby tissue. In fact, some doctors believe three-dimensional conformal therapy will eclipse other radiation treatments for prostate cancer before the end of the century.

Little more than a decade ago, the idea here—zeroing in on the prostate more accurately and completely, but leaving surrounding tissue little the worse for wear—would have seemed like a nice daydream to most radiation oncologists. But over the last several years, great technological strides have made 3-D conformal therapy seem, suddenly, not only achievable but highly promising.

This therapy developed because scientists looked at what was *not* happening with radiation treatment: Conventional approaches, studies found, weren't precise enough. For one thing, they weren't accurately estimating the volume of their target; and because of this, they often didn't supply enough radiation to kill the whole tumor. What was happening in some men, researchers have learned, was like what happens when a speaker with an inadequate microphone tries to make himself understood to an audience of a hundred thousand people in a vast amphitheater—some, maybe even most of the crowd can hear him, but that still leaves hundreds or even thousands who aren't getting his message. In traditional radiation treatment for prostate cancer, this inadequate coverage meant that *many men who suffered local relapses of prostate cancer did so because they were underdosed.*

In other research studies, something else was becoming clear: *The dose of radiation received has a lot to do with who gets cured and who doesn't.* In other words, men who receive *higher* doses of radiation have lower relapse rates than men who receive lower radiation doses. However, *in traditional radiation treatment, higher dosage almost always means more, and worse, side effects* (the nearby bladder and rectum are particularly susceptible to injury).

Enter the high-tech advances: Intricate software and imaging systems that allow 3-D treatment planning and computer-controlled radiation delivery systems; elaborate computer programs that can zip through sophisticated mathematical calculations of prostate volume and radiation dose per millimeter (or even smaller) of tissue; amazing technological advances that make it possible for doctors to custom-design a 3-D model and treatment plan, so each patient's prostate tumor can get the most precise and thorough radiation coverage possible.

Treatment planning begins with a series of CT images that give enough cross-section views of the prostate, seminal vesicles, and surrounding terrain (including the bladder wall, rectal wall, small bowel, bony structures and skin) to create a three-dimensional reconstruction. Dosage, and the area over which it will be distributed, can be calculated plane by plane, millimeter by millimeter. Each radiation beam—the 3-D approach allows more segments of treatment than traditional therapy—is automatically shaped by the computer so the energy focuses on the tumor *alone* (in the prostate as well as in tissue outside the gland where cancer has spread), rather than its entire neighborhood. A special body cast is custom-built for each patient to minimize movement during a treatment session, and also to make sure that a man's exact position can be reproduced every time. Several quality-control mechanisms are built into this approach; after-the-fact or instantaneous means of verifying that the radiation went to the right spot for the right length of time help guarantee the most successful treatment possible.

Right now, it's impossible to predict how well these techniques will work. There's just not enough information yet to give meaningful results on PSA levels after treatment or to predict long-term survival rates; however, this information should be available within a few years. At eighteen months after treatment in one study, only 3 percent of the men had a local recurrence of cancer (two of these were men with stage T2c, or B2, cancer; and five had stage T3 or T4, or C, disease. The best we can say right now is that early results suggest an excellent potential for 3-D conformal therapy.

Radiation Treatment: One Man's Story

Craig, a retired internist, was 78 years old when his prostate cancer was diagnosed. He had recently undergone a TUR procedure to alleviate symptoms of BPH; no cancer was found at that time, when a pathologist examined the chips of tissue taken from his prostate. But within a year, Craig's urologist found a nodule during a routine digital rectal exam, which turned out to be cancer localized to the prostate, with a Gleason score of 6.

Because of his age, Craig agreed with his doctors that external-beam radiation therapy was his best option. (Also, because of his age, he received treatment only in the prostate and seminal vesicles.) Craig began receiving doses of radiation every day. After a few days of treatment he began experiencing severe bowel problems, including debilitating diarrhea. These symptoms got better after Craig's radiation oncologist changed his treatments to four times a week, which gave his lower gastrointestinal tract a chance to recover. The new treatment schedule helped considerably, he recalls, and "things subsided fairly well."

That was twelve years ago. The radiation treatment worked, and he has been cancer-free ever since. "I went to see my urologist last year, and he joked with me, 'I don't know why you're coming back, because your ten-year warranty is up!'" Since his treatment, Craig has traveled extensively with his family.

They've been, among other places, to London, Copenhagen, Prague, and Vienna; they've taken ocean cruises and flown to South America.

This is particularly remarkable because a few years after his treatment Craig began to be plagued with episodes of severe diarrhea, infection, and bowel problems that his doctors have been largely at a loss to explain. "I've had cultures, searches for parasites, everything you can think of, and they can't find any explanation." (One set of problems, including blood in his bowel movements, was attributed to some large polyps in his intestinal tract; these were removed several years ago, however, and the episodes of diarrhea have continued.)

The conclusion reached by a number of doctors, including a urologist, a radiation oncologist, an internist, and a gastroenterologist, is that Craig has what's called an "irritable bowel" (a spastic, overly reactive colon prone to diarrhea) and that it is "secondary to"—a delayed effect of—his radiation treatment.

This is not uncommon; many men have delayed effects of radiation treatment, but these usually begin within a few months of treatment. In Craig's case, his bowel problems may have been made worse by some of the antibiotics he's been given over the years to combat infection. Craig's self-diagnosis? "I think very probably the radiation made the colon irritable, and then the prolonged treatment with the mycins (antibiotics) might have been a contributing factor."

Despite the episodes of bowel problems over the years, Craig does not seem to have slowed down too much over the last decade. In between their globe-trotting expeditions, he and his wife are restoring an old family home on Maryland's Eastern Shore. For Craig, radiation treatments have meant a gift of time and—bowel problems aside—good health. He has made the most of both.

CRYOABLATION
(FREEZING THE PROSTATE)

This technique sounds great: For starters, it involves no surgery. Instead, extremely cold liquid nitrogen is used to freeze the entire prostate, causing cancer cells within the gland to rupture as they begin to thaw.

The idea itself is not new. Many years ago, when the technique was first introduced, the freezing was accomplished through the urethra. Today, using ultrasound to guide them, doctors circulate the freezing liquid nitrogen through five metallic probes, which are placed in the prostate gland through the perineum. The freezing continues until the ultrasound shows that an "iceball" has been created. The procedure can take longer than an hour, and the hospital stay is generally one or two days.

Doctors who perform cryoablation (also called cryotherapy) must be well-acquainted with transrectal ultrasound, so they can be sure that the prostate is frozen completely. During the procedure, the tissue around the urethra is heated so it won't be destroyed along with the rest of the prostate.

The advantages of cryoablation include a short hospital stay and the absence of serious problems with urinary control. Fans of this procedure emphasize cryoablation's ease of treatment and freedom from early side effects.

However, only about one-third of men appear to be potent afterward; this may be because, in an attempt to destroy all the cancer, many doctors who perform this procedure deliberately attempt to freeze the nerve bundles that are essential for erection.

The big unknown here is whether cryoablation actually cures prostate cancer. Prostate cancer begins as a "multifocal" disease—many bits of cancer cells sprouting up in many sites within the prostate. *So to cure it, it's necessary to eliminate the entire prostate.* But that doesn't happen with cryoablation. During the procedure, the tissue around the urethra is protected by heat. Does the heat that preserves the urethra also spare a few scattered cancer cells? This is not clear.

Another concern is that, unlike most treatments for prostate cancer—or for any disease, for that matter—cryoablation is not backed up by years of solid, careful laboratory research. In this country, by the time almost any procedure is tried on humans, it's been thoroughly tested, sometimes for decades, in laboratory studies and in animals to see if it even works, and to make sure it's safe. There was little laboratory testing of this technique before doctors began using it in men. It has not been proven that cryoablation can completely destroy the prostate in a dog, much less a man.

There are no long-term studies on how well cryoablation works. But we do know that at two years after treatment, 20 percent of men have positive biopsies, and a large percentage of patients have elevated levels of PSA.

Currently, cryoablation is used to treat men with localized prostate cancer as well as men who have undergone unsuccessful radiation treatment. Again, we come back to the critical question: Does it work? As more men opt for this therapy, this question is becoming increasingly important. To answer it, we need thoughtful studies that not only determine the risks of late complications, but that demonstrate cryoablation's long-term success in controlling cancer.

THE SHORT STORY

External-beam radiation therapy is an excellent treatment option for many men with prostate cancer. First and foremost, it requires no surgery—this is a key advantage for older men, as well as for men with other health problems that might preclude major surgery. Also, it can be used in men with prostate tumors that are too far advanced to be cured by surgery.

There are two standard approaches to radiation treatment for prostate cancer—sending radiation into the tumor from the outside, with external-beam radiation therapy, and implanting radioactive seeds directly into the tumor; this is called interstitial brachytherapy.

Currently, the "gold standard" for radiation is external-beam radiation therapy. Sophisticated refinements have transformed it from the imprecise, mostly palliative treatment it was just decades ago into a powerful treatment that can cure localized cancer—not just relieve the symptoms of advanced disease.

How does an X-ray machine work? The simplest way to think of it is to imagine yourself getting a suntan. The difference here is that you can't feel or see the X-ray energy hitting your body, and the "tan" occurs internally, as the radiation particles destroy DNA, causing targeted cells to die. The best way to get a good, even tan is in increments, not all at once. Therefore, radiation doses are spread out over several weeks, with each treatment lasting only minutes at a time. The goal here, besides killing the cancer, is to do as little harm as possible to the surrounding tissue—the rectum, bowel, bladder, bone and skin.

External-beam radiation therapy's effects may not be as durable in the long run as those of radical prostatectomy; it is often associated with positive biopsies and, over time, with increases in PSA. This is why external-beam radiation therapy is an ideal option for older patients. However, within the last few years, an exciting new technique called 3-D conformal radiation therapy has come on the scene. It increases external-beam therapy's potential by maximizing the dose of radiation to the prostate tumor, while keeping the risk of damaging nearby tissue to a minimum—and it may improve long-term results.

Interstitial brachytherapy is basically hand-to-hand combat, instead of missiles launched from far away. The idea here is that the farther energy gets from its source—the more tissue a radiation beam has to pass through to reach its target—the less effective it will be in killing cancer. And that implanting tiny sources of radiation directly in the cancerous tissue (*brachy* comes from the Greek word meaning "short," as in "a short distance away from the malignancy") will really blast the tumor—and, as an added bonus, minimize the risk of harming innocent civilians, the cancer-free cells nearby.

In the past, interstitial brachytherapy has not been as successful in controlling prostate cancer as external-beam radiation therapy. However, the development of advanced guidance ultrasound systems, three-dimensional treatment planning and templates to ensure an even distribution of radiation throughout the prostate may improve this technique's results.

Recently, cryotherapy—killing prostate cells by freezing them—has become increasingly popular as a less-invasive form of treatment for localized prostate cancer. Although it appears to be well tolerated, and involves only a short hospital stay, it remains to be determined whether it will be as effective as external-beam radiation or radical prostatectomy in curing prostate cancer.

7

Treating Advanced Prostate Cancer

READ THIS FIRST

One day, as new and better drug therapies and combinations are developed, it may be possible to cure prostate cancer at any stage—or at least to restrain it, to make sure that it never leaves the prostate, or that it stays well-differentiated and slow-growing rather than becoming an aggressive, lethal invader of tissue and bone.

But that day is not here yet.

This is the part of the book we wish we didn't have to write, and that nobody would ever have to read. When prostate cancer is advanced, when it has swept through the prostate to the lymph nodes or bone, the options for treating it are limited. Cure is no longer possible. Instead, your doctor's goal is to stave off the cancer—to buy more time, to alleviate symptoms and, finally, to ease debilitating pain.

There are many schools of thought on treating prostate cancer that has spread beyond the prostate to the lymph nodes or bone (stage N+, M+, D1, or D2). All of them involve hormone therapy—shutting down the hormones that feed the prostate and nourish the cancer. (This is also called "hormone deprivation" therapy.) But there are huge differences in medical opinion: Should hormone therapy begin while a man still feels fine, or should it wait until symptoms begin? Should it target the hormones that most directly involve the prostate, or should it try to smother *all* the body's androgen (male hormone) activity? This idea of turning off all androgens is called total androgen blockade (or total androgen ablation), and many doctors believe in it. But is this total shutdown necessary?

And what's the best method of stopping these hormones? Think of a car going through a series of checkpoints—points A, B, C and D—to cross over a border into another country. You want to stop this car from reaching the other side. At what point do you stop it? Do you set up a roadblock at Point A, the first stop along the way? Or do you simply wall off the border at Point D, so the car can never cross over? Or do you divert the car at some point in between?

The androgens that affect the prostate reach their destination through a process, involving several steps, that begins in the brain. Medical roadblocks are now available to stop or detour this process at Point A (the brain), Point D (the prostate), or at several spots in between. Some of them work better than others, and some are more expensive. But ultimately, all of these means of hormone therapy will fail to control the cancer. This treatment failure may take years if a man is lucky and has a tumor that's particularly responsive to hormone therapy. It may only take months if he's not—if he has a faster-growing tumor that doesn't respond well to hormone therapy because many of its cells are indifferent to it.

Ultimately, what kills men with advanced prostate cancer are these malignant hormone-insensitive, or androgen-insensitive, cells. And right now, we don't have any way to stop them. Standard chemotherapy—a host of drugs that work so well in treating other kinds of cancer—doesn't help, mainly because it's designed to target cells that are dividing much faster than those in prostate cancer. (Newer chemotherapeutic drugs that target growth factors may produce better results.)

Which leaves us, finally, with palliative treatment—easing symptoms and pain, and keeping up nutrition in men who don't feel like eating. In this stage of treatment, thankfully, there *is* much that can be done, and *you have a right to demand everything possible*—medication or a procedure to ease pain or symptoms of urinary obstruction—to make the situation better.

A final note, before we begin to discuss each of these issues in detail: There are a lot of treatments out there. We are going to tell you what we think of them. The opinions here—like those throughout the book—are based on decades of clinical experience and research, and they bear the perspectives of physician and patient. Your doctor may disagree, or may prescribe a medication that this book will say is not effective.

One reason for these differences of opinion is that doctors treating men with end-stage cancer are desperate. Most of them—the best of them—care deeply about their patients, and are willing to try every last-ditch measure they can think of to help them. Say a study trumpets the benefits of the latest drug—one drug, for example, created a stir in the medical community because it was said (with debatable accuracy) to prolong life for several months. Many caring physicians will go ahead and prescribe such a medication, *even though, deep down, they realize it probably won't help.* They figure that there's a race against time, and they're losing it. And that any effort is better than none.

Ultimately, what you decide to do, what drugs and treatments you decide to try, is up to you—as it should be. Read this material, plus any other information you can get your hands on (for some suggestions on where else to look for answers, see page 289). Talk to your doctor, and get a second opinion; talk to your family, to any other prostate cancer patients you can find, and make the best, most informed decisions you can.

HORMONES AND PROSTATE CANCER: AN OVERVIEW

Doctors have long known that hormones play a major role in the life of the prostate. In 1786, an English surgeon named John Hunter became the first to demonstrate in animals that a radical operation, castration, caused the sex accessory tissues, including the prostate, to shrink.

But it wasn't until the 1930s that anyone discovered why this happened. At the University of Chicago, a trio of investigators discovered that removing the testes *shut down production of testosterone.* And, when shots of testosterone were injected back into castrated animals, these tissues were restored to normal size and function. This Nobel Prize–winning research included another valuable finding—that castration also could shrink prostate cancer.

The researchers were able to achieve the same effect chemically; they found they could shut down testosterone with doses of female hormones called estrogens. Estrogens blocked a signal, transmitted in the brain by the pituitary gland, called *luteinizing hormone* (LH), which stimulates testosterone. The oral estrogen, called DES (diethylstilbestrol), is what's known as a chemical castrator; it causes impotence.

For now, hormonal therapy means one of two main choices: Surgical castration, a "one-shot effect"; or chemical castration, a lifetime of medication.

Impotence is likely with almost every kind of hormone therapy; 90 percent of men on hormone therapy lose sexual drive and the ability to have an erection. In the future, however, new hormone treatments (discussed later in this chapter) may prove effective without causing impotence.

For a time, hormone therapy *does* control prostate cancer. But what some doctors used to believe—that prostate tumors are nourished *only* by hormones, that hormone starvation will stop the cancer from spreading—is, unfortunately, not the whole story. Ultimately, hormone therapy will not stop the disease's progression.

Why Hormones Don't Cure

Why not? Because prostate cancer, scientists have learned, is "heterogeneous," a cellular melting pot. It's a bunch of different cells mixed up together—so a drug or hormone treatment that targets *one* kind of cell, for instance, won't have any effect against another variety. The cancer is made up of many different kinds of cells, and some of them have learned to be resistant, to grow in the absence of androgens, or male hormones. These are called *androgen-independent, or -insensitive* cells.

For years, scientists have been working to understand why hormonal treatment eventually fails—why some cancer cells seem to kick in and grow with such vengeance. "There's probably no area of cancer therapy where we've got as many good options as we do for treating the hormonally responsive element of prostate cancer," says a Johns Hopkins cancer researcher. "In sharp contrast, we have almost nothing that has proved very useful in managing the hormonally *independent* portion of the cancer."

When a man starts hormone therapy, the early results are successful and highly encouraging: The tumor shrinks, PSA levels drop in the blood, and the patient feels better. But in the prostate, only the hormone-*dependent* cancer cells have been affected. The rest, the cancer cells that have nothing to do with hormones, go on about their merry, proliferative business, oblivious to the hormonal war being fought just cells away.

Scientists believe that these androgen-independent cells probably inhabit the prostate for years; they don't just suddenly appear one day after the cancer is diagnosed. And so to do battle with them, many scientists feel, in the future hormone therapy must be combined with something else—chemotherapy, drugs targeted specifically at these androgen-independent cells. Today, however, effective treatment along these lines is not yet possible in men, and is only under experimental study.

Cell Birth and Cell Death

There are several ways to treat a cancer. "One," explains a Johns Hopkins cancer researcher, "is to slow down or prevent the growth. Essentially, the cancer is producing problems because it's continually growing." In cancer, cells simply can't stop dividing—new cells are continually churned out, eventually overrunning other tissue as they fill up their initial location. This is rampant population explosion.

In prostate cancer, the rate of cell division, or *birth* of new cells, is relatively low. Cancer begins amassing—cells begin building up and spreading to invade new tissue—because something happens to throw off the normal process of cell *death*. So if scientists can't stop new cells from being born, maybe they can help other cells to die at a faster rate. This treatment idea is being explored aggressively.

Telling Cancer Cells When to Die

Scientists know that all cells, cancerous and normal, have a genetic pathway called programmed cell death. The problem is, cells often ignore this pathway. In the normal prostate, androgens keep androgen-dependent cells alive; these cells become relatively immortal (it's like pumping air to a deep-sea diver). But when this life-giving supply of hormones is shut off—by physical or chemical castration—the picture changes. The change in hormones triggers a series of events in which certain genes are expressed, and new proteins are made. Some scientists believe these new proteins prompt a buildup of free calcium in the cells. And the prolonged increase in calcium activates what one Johns Hopkins scientist describes as a "suicide enzyme." This "suicide" enzyme, something called a calcium-magnesium-dependent endonuclease, functions as a sort of wrecking ball. It breaks down the DNA in the nucleus, and wipes out the cell's genetic memory bank. The cell no longer replicates, but dies. Over time, it begins to fragment; tiny chunks are later recycled as building materials by other cells. "This is an active process," the scientist explains, "in which the cell that is destined to die is actively involved in its own death."

This process happens all the time, particularly during fetal development, "or we wouldn't be able to develop as people who have arms and legs and appendages," the scientist continues. "When you're developing, you have limb buds.

In order to develop digits—our fingers, for example—the cells that are in between the fingers literally have to die. And that's a particularly tricky, coordinated process. You can imagine—you've got to make some cells die and other cells have to live, right next to them."

Androgen-independent cells, while all this is going on, experience no such increase in calcium. Although they possess a similar suicide pathway, it is not activated.

This is an area of intensive work for prostate cancer researchers—figuring out how to kill these cells, or better yet, how to get them to kill themselves.

For several years, scientists have been able to kill these cells in the laboratory. "Experimentally," says the scientist, "we've been able to demonstrate that if we take the most poorly differentiated, metastatic, fast-growing, androgen-independent cell lines available, and we use agents that can elevate the intracellular calcium, the cells will then undergo programmed cell death and die." What's happening to these androgen-independent cells involves the same pathway that's activated in the hormonally dependent prostate cells after castration. "Which suggests to us that the pathway is fundamentally retained in the androgen-independent cancer cells," the scientist adds. "This gives us a target." In other words, one day chemotherapeutic drugs may be able to trigger the elusive suicide pathway in the hard-to-kill, androgen-independent cells.

"The big problem with chemotherapy is how to get the cancer cells to die without killing normal cells. We're at that very difficult crossroads now," says the scientist. The standard cancer-fighting arsenal includes chemotherapeutic agents that can lead to cell death—drugs such as cytoxan. But unfortunately, such drugs seem most effective in treating leukemia and other rapidly dividing cancers. Prostate cancer cells, in comparison, are sluggish, and often have time to repair damage caused by chemotherapy before they divide again—it's as if the damage never occurred.

So scientists are trying to figure out how to kill cells without depending on cell division. Programmed cell death—triggered by the suicide pathway—does not require cell division.

"What we need to do," the scientist concludes, "is get the proliferation rate below the death rate." Simply *slowing* cancer growth won't help a man with a metastatic tumor who's losing weight and has bone pain. It won't shrink his tumor or relieve his symptoms; it will just slow down the progression of his disease.

What is needed, urgently, is a way to reduce the tumor—in other words, a form of therapy that can stimulate programmed cell death.

WHERE TO BREAK THE CHAIN?
SPECIFIC WAYS TO
CONTROL HORMONES

Remember the car trying to cross the border, and all the roadblocks set up to stop it at various points along the way? This is the key to how hormone therapy works. Each therapy targets a different link in the chain of hormonal interactions that affect the prostate.

This is a long and complicated chain; put together on paper, it's a confusing jumble of letters, mostly consonants, that looks like alphabet soup. And if you're like most men, just thinking about this muddle will make your eyes glaze over. But, stripped down to its essential steps, this code is not so tough to crack—you can do it! (And, you need to master this information, so you can not only understand what your doctor's talking about, but help choose the treatment option that's best for you.)

To understand this hormonal chain, let's start at the beginning—the brain, where the hypothalamus makes, among other things, a substance called *LHRH* (luteinizing hormone-releasing hormone), which acts as a chemical signal. It's dispatched in pulses, like Morse code or flashes of light, to the nearby pituitary gland. Its message? "Make *LH* and *FSH*," it tells the pituitary.

LH (luteinizing hormone) and FSH (follicle-stimulating hormone) are other chemical signals, and they bring us to the testicles, or testes, where LH motivates certain cells (called testicular Leydig cells) to make *testosterone*. (FSH has its major effect on sperm production.)

And testosterone brings us to the prostate. Testosterone circulates in the blood and enters the prostate by diffusion, like water through a tea bag. Soon it undergoes a metamorphosis: Testosterone is transformed, by an enzyme called 5-alpha-reductase, into a hormone called *DHT* (dihydrotestosterone)—which is more than twice as powerful as testosterone. Several studies have shown that the prostate contains less 5-alpha-reductase when it is cancerous; therefore, DHT is not believed to be as important in prostate cancer as it is in the normal prostate or in BPH. Both testosterone and DHT can bind to the same receptor in the prostate cell—like two different keys fitting the same lock. (DHT *really*

Figure 7.1. *Sources of male hormone production and the "chain of command," and where key hormone therapies actually work*

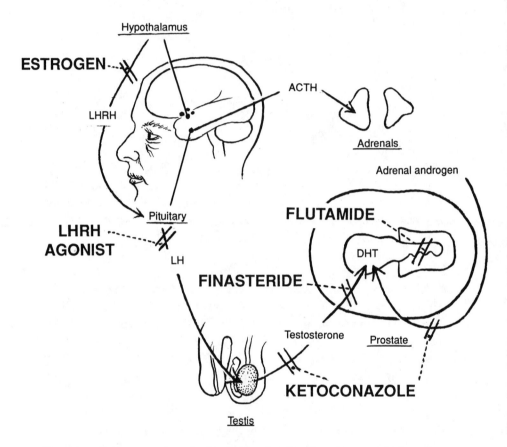

Shown in capital letters are drugs that block either the *effect* of testosterone and other androgens (flutamide and finasteride) or the *production* of testosterone itself (LHRH agonists, estrogens, ketoconazole).

binds to it, with great affinity; testosterone does not cling as strongly to the receptor.) When DHT and testosterone hook up to the receptor, it attaches itself to DNA, which then activates certain genes.

Testosterone in the blood circulates back to square one, the hypothalamus, which acts as a thermostat. It measures the level of testosterone and decides whether to boost or cut back on its LHRH production, and the cycle begins all over again (scientists call this a "feedback loop").

Also, the adrenal glands, which sit on top of the kidneys, make weak male hormones called "adrenal androgens," including androstenedione, dehydro-epiandrosterone (DHEA), and dehydroepiandrosterone sulfate (DHEAS), plus small amounts of testosterone. These are minor players, believed to make up only 5 percent or less of the total androgen stimulation to the prostate. Their total effect on the prostate is a controversial issue (discussed in this chapter).

So there are several potential checkpoints in this chain of events. Currently, hormone therapy can target the hypothalamus (LHRH), the pituitary (LH, FSH), the adrenal gland (adrenal androgens), the testes (testosterone) and the prostate (DHT). They can be used individually or in combination.

Men on hormonal therapy should go back to their doctor every three to six months for a digital rectal exam, a PSA test, and a creatinine test, which tests for impaired kidney function. They also should get a bone scan once or twice a year if the PSA begins to rise.

SURGICAL CASTRATION

Surgical removal of a man's testicles (also called an orchiectomy) is the easiest and least expensive way to control testosterone. As surgical procedures go, it's simple. The operation can be performed under spinal anesthesia or, if the patient is not strong enough to tolerate this, even a local anesthetic. This is what happens: A surgeon makes a small incision in the scrotum, and brings out each testicle individually through this opening. Then the surgeon cuts the vas deferens and blood vessels that supply each testicle, and the testicles are removed. Some surgeons perform what's called "subcapsular orchiectomy." In this operation, the surgeon opens the lining to the testicles and empties the contents of each testicle. The lining is closed again, and this empty shell is placed back inside the scrotum—so nothing looks different; in other words, no one can tell from outward appearance that there's nothing inside the scrotum. The basic differences here are cosmetic—and therefore psychological—and for some men, this makes the thought of castration easier to accept. However, some surgeons don't like to perform this operation because they worry that some testosterone-producing cells may be left behind.

After surgery, patients usually can go home from the hospital the same day—or, at the very latest, the next day. The only major complication to worry

A word on castration and impotence:
What's really important here?

Castration—chemical or otherwise—is an awful thought, one that makes most men shudder. Loss of sexual function or sense of identity is not a pleasant concept; it can be even worse when combined with the fear and uncertainty that are part of having cancer. This is a scary time, but you are not alone. It might help to talk to your doctor, or family, or men who are going through this, too—see the "Where to Get Help" section at the back of this book.

For many men with prostate cancer, when it comes down to choosing between sexual potency and death, the sex life takes a back seat to survival. When hormonal therapy can truly mean the difference between life and death and you're preoccupied with sexual potency, you're missing the bigger point.

It's time for plain speaking again: Get over it. Now is the time to cherish life: Treasure every extra, precious moment you get to spend with your loved ones. Make the most of every day. Now is the time, while you still can, to do the things you've always wanted to do—take that trip you've always dreamed of, for instance. Take your wife out dancing. Learn to sail. Teach your grandchild how to fish. Realize there is so much more to living than sexual potency.

about with surgical castration is bleeding. However, this shouldn't be a problem if the surgeon makes a point of checking that all bleeding is stopped before the scrotum is closed, and that a compression dressing is left in place to control the smaller, harder-to-see blood vessels.

Castration works fast; it reduces the body's amount of testosterone by 95 percent almost immediately, and permanently. Boom—within about three hours after surgery, testosterone levels begin to plummet to a level called the "castrate range." This is considered the gold standard, an important point of comparison in monitoring hormone therapy—as certain drugs are judged by their ability to reduce testosterone to this range.

Some doctors used to believe that several months after castration, the body began producing more testosterone at other sites—and that this was the reason prostate cancer continued to grow. This is not true. There is no delayed increase in testosterone and anyway, that's not why prostate tumors keep growing—they continue to spread because of the cancer cells that are *not* affected by hormone therapy.

What happens to the prostate tumor after castration? It begins to shrink, and men with symptoms of obstruction or pain caused by the cancer begin to feel better right away.

Castration's advantages are that it's effective almost immediately and that its results are permanent—there's no need to take daily medication. And, because it is a "one-shot" treatment, it's relatively inexpensive.

Side Effects

Its disadvantages are certainly psychological (this can vary depending on a man's age and stage of illness)—and cosmetic. (To help alleviate the stigma of castration, some surgeons perform what's called a "subcapsular technique"— see above—in which *only* the testosterone-producing parts of the testicles are removed, and the outer shell remains. Also, testicular implants—which make the testicles appear normal—are available for some men.)

Castration is irreversible, and for many men, this is too final a treatment. In one 1989 survey, only 22 percent of prostate cancer patients opted for surgical castration; 78 percent of these men chose alternative hormonal therapy (they picked LHRH analogs, discussed in this chapter).

Testosterone is the hormone that makes men feel "manly." When it is missing, some of the characteristics associated with being male vanish along with it. Side effects of castration—surgical or medical—can include tenderness, pain or swelling of the breasts (this is called gynecomastia), and loss of sex drive. Impotence is not an absolute certainty; 10 percent of men do remain potent. However, they are rare exceptions to the rule. (Impotence here, unlike impotence in other situations, means loss of libido as well as the ability to achieve an erection.)

Hot Flashes

The other major side effect is hot flashes, and these are like the hot flashes experienced by women during menopause—a sudden rush of warmth in the face, neck, upper chest and back, lasting from a few seconds to an hour. Although they aren't harmful to a man's health, they can be bothersome. They probably occur because the change in hormones affects the hypothalamus, the brain's "thermostat" for regulating body temperature, and the brain's response to this makes the body feel out of kilter. The blast of heat happens because blood vessels underneath the skin are dilating; this causes sweating, which helps bring the body back to normal.

Hot flashes are unpredictable; no one knows what sets them off, or what makes them go away. Some men don't have any; other men are plagued by them. There is some evidence that outside triggers such as radiant heaters, eating hot food, drinking alcohol or taking certain medications can bring them on. However, there is help: Hot flashes can be treated with low doses of oral estrogen (one milligram of DES a day) or with progestational drugs such as medroxyprogesterone (Provera), or megestrol acetate (Megace). Some doctors also believe that clonidine, a blood pressure drug, can reduce the number and duration of hot flashes.

Other Changes

Finally, many men who have been castrated report that they don't feel "normal"; they may also feel irritable and less aggressive. Weight gain, loss of muscle mass and subtle changes in physical appearance—differences in skin tone and hair growth—also are common. However, contrary to popular belief, there is no change in the pitch of the voice—nor, unfortunately, do balding men regrow a full head of hair. The long-term effects can include osteoporosis—loss of bone density, in which bones become thinner, more brittle and easier to break.

Who should not undergo this procedure? First of all, if you're not prepared to accept the physical and psychological ramifications of castration, it's not for you. Choose another form of treatment. Also, this procedure may not be best for men who are on anticoagulant medications that might cause excessive bleeding.

MEDICAL CASTRATION

Medical castration can be accomplished in three ways: By shutting down the hypothalamic-pituitary connection (discussed earlier in this chapter); by directly blocking the ability of the testicles to make testosterone; or by blocking the effects of testosterone at the target organ—the prostate.

Drugs That Shut Down the Hypothalamic-Pituitary Connection

Estrogens

Many men, for many reasons, don't want to undergo surgical castration, so they opt for chemical castration—taking drugs that accomplish the same result without the cosmetic change.

DES, the main oral estrogen, targets a different checkpoint—the hypothalamus and pituitary connection, instead of the testicles. It works by blocking the release of LHRH, which in turn blocks the release of LH and FSH, virtually shutting down the Leydig cells, the testicles' testosterone-making factories. So testosterone drops to the castrate range.

The effect is not as speedy as with surgical castration; it generally takes ten to fourteen days for testosterone to fall to the castrate range. And, it's not permanent—in most cases, the testicles start making testosterone again soon after a man stops taking DES.

We talk about DES here because it's the most widely used oral estrogen, and it's the gold standard of estrogen therapy for prostate cancer. Other drugs, such as Premarin and ethinyl estradiol (both medications used by women during menopause) are considered as effective as DES; neither is better. Another drug, called cholotriansene (TACE), is a synthetic estrogen that lowers testosterone but doesn't completely shut down its production; it also permits the body to make a little bit of LH. (It has proven to be ineffective, and is no longer used in attempts to lower testosterone levels to the castrate range.) A drug called polyestradiol phosphate (Esradurin), injected once a month, may be easier to tolerate for men with gastrointestinal problems. And for men with advanced prostate cancer who haven't responded to other estrogen drugs, diethylstilbestrol diphosphate (Stilphostrol) may bring relief of symptoms. It is administered intravenously, at 500 to 2,000 milligrams a day.

Several years ago, an estrogen-related drug called estramustine phosphate (EMCYT) generated some enthusiasm among doctors in Europe for its ability to diminish testosterone and to kill some cancer cells. (This drug is related to the chemical weapon mustard gas used in World War I.) But more recent studies have shown that, although it uses different mechanisms to achieve its effects, it doesn't prolong survival any longer than DES. And it can have side effects including nausea.

Therefore, we believe that *among oral estrogens,* DES is the way to go. It's relatively inexpensive (far cheaper than some LHRH analogs, for instance) and it accomplishes the same goal as surgery—reducing testosterone to the castrate range.

Now, what's the right dosage? How much DES do you need to take? This has been a source of great controversy in the medical community. Decades ago, doctors gave high-powered doses of DES—ten to twenty milligrams a day—thinking that this would not only eliminate testosterone, it might also kill cancer cells. This didn't happen; testosterone was lowered, but that was it. Then, studies by the Veterans Administration showed that lower doses could achieve the same results. But even five milligrams a day proved to be too much. One study found that, over time, men on five milligrams of DES a day died—from heart disease caused by the estrogen, not from prostate cancer! Then doctors tried three milligrams, and then one milligram a day. *And one milligram of DES a day proved sufficient to suppress testosterone without endangering the heart.* A large study in Europe found that men on one milligram of DES a day showed no signs of *irreversible* damage to the cardiovascular system.

Other studies have proved that there is no statistical difference between the lifespans of men who were castrated and those who took one milligram of DES a day. (Some doctors argue that it takes three milligrams of DES a day to lower testosterone to the castrate range. This is true. However, if there's no difference in the length of survival, and the heart-related side effects are fewer with one milligram than with three milligrams, what's to be gained by taking the higher dose?)

Other Side Effects.   The main side effect is enlargement of the breasts. This problem can be eliminated, however, with three low-dose treatments of radiation, given directly to the breast *before* estrogen is started. In high doses, DES can cause dangerous cardiovascular problems. However, when it's taken in doses of one milligram a day, side effects such as edema (water retention, which causes swelling in the ankles) can be managed effectively with diuretics. Some physicians recommend that their patients on DES take an aspirin every day to avoid other cardiovascular side effects such as thrombophlebitis (blood clots in the legs), and also to lower the risk of a heart attack. Because of the risk of cardiovascular problems, men with a history of heart disease or thrombophlebitis should not use estrogen as their main form of treatment.

Estrogen does not cause hot flashes, although patients do develop the same problems with sexual function as men who are castrated (see "Surgical Castration," above).

Conclusion: One milligram of DES a day is just as effective as higher doses, and one milligram of DES is just as effective as surgical castration in prolonging life.

LHRH Agonists

LHRH agonists shut down production of LH and FSH. Here's how they work: LHRH is a small protein, built of ten blocks of amino acid. A synthetic substance called an LHRH-analog, or agonist, made by changing one of the ten blocks, works by inhibiting LH (the hormone that tells the pituitary gland to make testosterone). The hypothalamus acts like a lighthouse, sending out LHRH in signal pulses—like Morse code in flashes of light—to the pituitary gland. LHRH agonists work by providing prolonged signals—by turning on the light and keeping it on, instead of just sending flashes. So these drugs trick the pituitary; because the pituitary receives no flashes, or pulses, it thinks no signal is being sent—and it doesn't make LH.

These drugs don't work right away. In fact, for about a week after a man begins taking an LHRH agonist, his testosterone level kicks into overdrive. This is called a "flare," and it happens because the constant LHRH signal initially stimulates LH production. But by about ten days, testosterone falls into the castrate range. For the first few weeks, doctors often prescribe another drug, such as flutamide, to block this surge.

The most commonly prescribed LHRH agonists are leuprolide (Lupron) and goserelin (Zoladex). In large studies, researchers have found that these LHRH agonists are equivalent to treatment with DES or surgical castration in their ability to lengthen the time until the cancer progresses, and to prolong survival. These drugs are given in monthly injections.

To sum up: LHRH agonists are basically equivalent in testosterone-lowering and lifespan-lengthening results to DES, which is basically equivalent to surgical castration.

The chief advantages of LHRH agonists are that they avoid the need for surgery, and that they don't cause breast swelling as often as treatment with estrogen. Also, they don't have the risk of cardiovascular complications that can accompany estrogen treatment.

Side Effects. Like surgical castration, however, LHRH agonist treatment does cause hot flashes, loss of sex drive, and impotence. Other disadvantages include the need to get monthly shots, and the tremendous expense—LHRH agonists cost hundreds of dollars a month.

Drugs That Inhibit Production of Testosterone

Ketoconazole

This drug got its start as an antifungal agent. Then doctors noticed that men taking it developed breast enlargement—clearly, more than fungal problems were being treated here! Doctors learned that ketoconazole blocks production of testosterone by the testicles as well as androgens made by the adrenal gland. It works quickly; taking 400 milligrams of ketoconazole every eight hours reduces testosterone to the castrate range within twenty-four hours. The drug's effects are reversible, and testosterone goes back up again as soon as a man stops taking ketoconazole. It's debatable whether the drug is as effective as other hormonal treatments for long-term use; ketoconazole causes a surge in production of LH that might, over time, overpower the drug's tight clamp on testosterone. Therefore, *ketoconazole generally is used in short-term situations where fast action is needed*—in a man with acute spinal pain, for example, or in a man with DIC (disseminated intravascular coagulation, a blood-clotting disorder that develops in some men with advanced prostate cancer). In addition to the hormonal effects, some derivatives of ketoconazole have also been shown to have some effect in directly blocking the growth of cancer cells; this potential is undergoing intense investigation. One technicality: The drug is not approved by the FDA for use in the treatment of prostate cancer. It can have adverse effects on the liver. Because it can also suppress the production of steroids normally produced by the adrenal gland, ketoconazole should be prescribed along with a corticosteroid such as prednisone (five milligrams a day), to compensate for this loss.

Conclusion: Ketoconazole is not a drug for the long haul, but it is helpful in some situations.

Drugs That Block the Effects of Hormones at the Prostate

Antiandrogens

These drugs don't care how much LHRH, LH, FSH, testosterone, or DHT you make; it doesn't matter to them. (Actually, antiandrogens cause testosterone levels to go *up* because of an increase in LH.) All they do is make sure testosterone and DHT don't reach their targets—the receptors. In other words, antiandrogens act as dummy keys in the "locks," or receptors. When testosterone and DHT reach the receptors, there's already a key sitting in the lock—so they can't enter the lock and activate the receptors. Therefore, the tumor doesn't get the hormones it needs to nourish its androgen-dependent cells.

Flutamide is the most widely used anti-androgen. Casodex, a new, not-yet-approved drug, is another; so is cyproterone acetate, an antiandrogen that's used in Europe but is not yet approved in this country.

Their potential advantage is that, because testosterone is not suppressed, they preserve potency. In men taking flutamide, for example, 87 percent remain potent. (This is not true, however, for cyproterone acetate. This drug, like estrogen, also suppresses the hypothalamus-pituitary connection—so it lowers LH, which affects testosterone production. Thus, it does produce impotence.)

But do antiandrogens work? The answer, for now, is probably not enough *when they're used by themselves.* They also produce breast enlargement in 74 percent of the men who take them.

In total androgen blockade (see below), flutamide is given along with an LHRH agonist. In new research, scientists are looking into combining flutamide with something else—perhaps finasteride (discussed later in this chapter) to increase its effectiveness.

Side effects: Flutamide's major side effect is diarrhea. Also, it can cause significant liver damage in some men; therefore, it's a good idea for men taking flutamide to have their liver function checked after the first few months of treatment.

5-alpha Reductase Inhibitors

In prostate cells, testosterone is converted by an enzyme called 5-alpha reductase into a more potent hormone, DHT; 5-alpha reductase inhibitors—drugs such as finasteride (Proscar)—block this enzyme. Finasteride's big advantage is that it preserves potency because testosterone levels in the blood remain unchanged (for more on finasteride and prostate cancer, see Chapter 10).

Finasteride works well in shrinking benign enlargement of the prostate, where DHT plays a major role. But in prostate cancer, testosterone is more of a villain than DHT, and finasteride does little to stop it. So by itself, finasteride is not enough. However, finasteride may prove more effective when combined with flutamide (discussed later in this chapter).

"Total" Androgen Ablation, or Blockade

This idea is not new. Investigators have been pursuing this concept since the 1930s, when scientists first began to understand the ramifications of shutting down every single hormone that could possibly affect the prostate. Some approaches have been more drastic than others—surgical removal of the adrenal glands or the pituitary, for instance.

The theory here is that even low levels of testosterone and DHT—produced by the adrenal androgens—can stimulate cancer in the prostate, and that they must be stopped. This can be accomplished by combining whatever achieves a castrate level of testosterone—surgical castration, estrogen or an LHRH agonist—with flutamide.

Total androgen blockade became a hot concept in the medical community about a decade ago, due largely to the work of one scientist. This scientist reported that combining an LHRH agonist with an anti-androgen was far more successful than using either approach alone. But there are a few things you should know about this research: One is that *no other scientist has ever reproduced this man's spectacular results.* In his study, 97 percent of men with advanced cancers who were treated with an LHRH agonist plus flutamide were still alive eighteen months later.

The sad truth is that in nearly every other doctor's experience, only half of patients diagnosed with metastatic prostate cancer are alive two or three years later, and no treatment, so far, has made a real difference in those numbers. The survival rates for men with *advanced* prostate cancer in 1995 are not much different from the rates in 1965.

Most studies since then have shown either no difference in survival or an overall survival time lengthened by only a few months. One study, however, has produced results that suggest that patients with *only minimally advanced disease*—men with just a few metastases—have the most potential to benefit from the combined therapy of castration or an LHRH agonist plus flutamide. For men with minimal disease, total androgen blockade might be a reasonable option; it might prolong life. (This currently is being tested in a large study in the United States. In the next few years, we should know much more about the true benefits of this form of treatment.) However, for most men, and particularly for men with widely metastasized disease, it probably will not be of great benefit.

The big advantage of the combined therapy is that it seems to stretch out the time that hormones work—the time to progression of cancer is lengthened by several months. However, overall survival is not significantly better for the men on the combined treatment. In a huge analysis of about five thousand prostate cancer patients in Europe and America, doctors studied overall survival and found, at five years after treatment, a 3 percent difference between the men on total androgen blockade and the men who underwent castration or took LHRH agonists alone. This is not a stunning display of the success of total androgen blockade.

And, after a certain point, some patients actually benefit from *stopping* flutamide. For example, when a man taking flutamide in combined therapy begins to relapse—when his prostate cancer begins growing again, and his PSA level goes up—one step his doctors should take right away is to *stop* the flutamide. In from 40 to 75 percent of these men, PSA levels drop when flutamide is stopped. Paradoxically, flutamide can make some patients—who initially were helped by it—worse. Exactly why this happens is not clear. In certain prostate cancers, over time, the androgen receptors (the part of the cell responsive to hormones) undergo a mutation—and all of a sudden, flutamide *stimulates* the cancer. Remember, flutamide normally acts like a dummy key in the "lock" (the receptor), whose purpose is to block testosterone and DHT from activating the receptor. With this mutation, however, the flutamide key actually works—it turns in the lock and activates the receptor.

Because of this odd twist in flutamide's effectiveness, some doctors have questioned the long-term value of taking the drug, and believe it should be used only for a few months by men taking LHRH agonists.

There is one crucial concept here that you need to understand: *Ultimately, total androgen blockade is going to stop working, just as every other kind of hormone therapy does.* Anyone who leads you to believe otherwise is not doing you a favor. And when hormone treatment stops working, it's not because of the tiny amounts of testosterone and DHT being made by the adrenal androgens—in other words, it's not the fault of some renegade hormones that are sneaking through the hormonal blockade. It's because of the hormonally *independent* portion of the cancer—the cells that couldn't care less what hormones its host is taking, because *hormones have no effect on this portion of the tumor.* Using hormones to fight these cells is like trying to kill a cockroach with hair spray instead of insecticide. The problem is, we haven't found the right "Raid" yet.

As one Johns Hopkins molecular biologist explains, "Cancer cells are very efficient. And as they keep dividing, they jettison some dead weight. One of the first pieces of unnecessary baggage to go may be the system of controls—the part of the cell that takes orders from hormones. Over time, the deadliest cancer cells survive because they become pure, stripped-down growing machines."

If adrenal androgens really were the key to fighting prostate cancer, flutamide should produce a dramatic improvement in men who were castrated, took estrogen or an LHRH agonist and then had a relapse. This just isn't the case. Sadly, what happens for these men is that beginning total androgen blockade has very little effect—again, suggesting that this approach is not the answer.

Finally, other studies have demonstrated that adrenal androgens have little effect on the prostate. In one investigation at Johns Hopkins, researchers studied four men who had their pituitary glands removed before they reached puberty—which means that *not only did their bodies fail to make LH, they failed to make a hormone that stimulates the adrenal gland, so it was virtually shut down; in other words, they had total androgen blockade.* They also studied three men who had a genetic disorder called Kallmann's syndrome (in which the hypothalamus doesn't make LHRH, and therefore, the pituitary glands don't make LH or FSH), and one unfortunate man who had been castrated at age seven, when a dog bit off his testicles. The average age of these men was about 65. Using age-matched "control" (normal) patients for comparison, the investigators showed *no disparity in prostate size* in men with both testosterone and the adrenal hormones out of commission and in men with only testosterone missing. (In all of these men, the prostate was tiny. In all, there were no Leydig cells, the tiny testosterone-making factories in the testicles.) In other words, *total androgen blockade made no difference.*

HOW LONG DO HORMONES WORK?

This varies from man to man. Ten percent of men with M+ (D2) disease—metastatic prostate cancer—live less than six months. Ten percent live longer than ten years. The rest fall somewhere in the middle; statistics show that half of these men live three years or less, and only 25 percent are alive after five years. What accounts for the extreme disparity in these numbers? *It all has to do with the ratio of hormone-sensitive cells to hormone-insensitive cells, and how fast the cancer grows.* In some men, nearly every cell is responsive to hormones; in other men, very few cells are hormone-sensitive. Some cancers take hundreds of days to double in size; others double every few weeks.

There is a mathematical model of how these cancer cells grow, called tumor kinetics. A tumor must double in size thirty times before a doctor can even feel it—before there's a centimeter of cancer. This growth is logarithmic—two cells, then four, then eight, etc. Say a tumor is at its tenth doubling; it has 1,024 cells. And say that three-fourths of these cells are responsive to hormones. The patient is castrated, and all the hormone-responsive cells drop out of the picture, leaving only 256 cells. What happens? These cells aren't affected by the hormones; they continue to grow. The now-smaller tumor doubles. There are 512 cells. It doubles again—1,024 cells. It's back to where it started. And when it doubles again, there will be twice as many cells as before.

Now say only 1 percent of this cancer is not responsive to hormones. It's going to take many more doublings before this tumor becomes dangerous. So how long hormones work depends on two things: The ratio of hormone-resistant cells to hormone-dependent cells, and how long it takes for the cancer to double in size. Relapse will come a lot sooner in a man whose cancer doubles every 30 days, for example, than in a man whose cancer takes 100 days to double.

WHEN TO BEGIN HORMONE THERAPY? EARLY VERSUS LATE TREATMENT: MORE CONTROVERSY

Should a man with stage T3, T4, or N+ (C or D1) cancer—*but no symptoms*—begin hormone therapy? Many doctors believe he should, the sooner the better. "Treat the tumor while a greater percentage of cells are responsive to hormones, and the patient should do better," says one oncologist.

That is certainly one option, but we doubt that ultimately it will make a difference in prolonging life. Hormone therapy never cures; at best, it palliates cancer. An excellent example of this is a study done by the Veterans Administration Cooperative Urological Research Group, in which 1,764 men received either a placebo, surgical castration, 5 milligrams of DES a day, or the DES plus surgical castration. When prostate cancer began to progress in the men on the

I have cancer in my lymph nodes. What do I do now?

There is cancer in your lymph nodes. Maybe you learned about this before surgery—maybe your surgeon looked at the lymph nodes, found cancer there, and decided not to remove your prostate. Maybe this has come about after surgery—perhaps you have already undergone a radical prostatectomy, and a pathologist has found some cancer in the lymph tissue that was removed during the operation.

What should you do now?

Every man, at every stage of prostate cancer, needs a course of action, a plan for the future. And right now, more than anything, you need answers.

Your doctor may draw up an immediate plan of attack: Radiation therapy, hormone therapy, chemotherapy, or even all of the above. Many well-meaning doctors suggest one or more of these options because they want to do something—anything—right away, to hold off the cancer for as long as possible.

But let's wait a minute. Now, before you embrace any of these approaches, is the time for us to examine some hard facts together:

The first fact is that once prostate cancer has established itself in the lymph nodes, it has almost certainly set up shop at other sites as well, most commonly in bone. The second is that to cure the disease—to get rid of all the cancer—it would be necessary to find and eliminate cancer cells at all of these sites throughout the body.

Radiation to the prostate is aimed at a specific, limited area—the prostate and surrounding tissue. Therefore, frankly, radiation isn't going to have any effect on the cancer cells growing outside this targeted area. Nor will hormone therapy cure this advanced prostate cancer; at this point, it simply isn't good enough to eliminate ▶

▶ all the cancer cells growing outside the prostate. Also, unfortunately, at present there is no effective form of chemotherapy able to achieve this vital goal, either.

At the writing of this book, there is not any form of treatment that will eliminate all the cancerous cells once the cancer has reached the lymph nodes.

And so, again, the big, tough question: What should you do? Although all these forms of treatment may be necessary someday, we believe that taking any of these steps *now* will not prolong your life. (And conversely, *not* taking them now *will not shorten* your life.) All that will happen, if you begin these forms of treatment now, is that your quality of life will be disrupted.

For these reasons, we believe that men in this situation should opt for watchful waiting now. This decision of watchful waiting may be one of the hardest you'll ever have to make, but remember: Watchful waiting doesn't mean being passive. It means treating specific symptoms *if and when* they arise. In this case, watchful waiting should also mean that your doctor will monitor your health very carefully and that you will have a physical examination, including a digital rectal exam, PSA, and serum creatinine tests, every three to six months, as well as a bone scan every six to twelve months.

The very understandable problem most people have in accepting this approach is the uncertainty associated with it. What is my cancer going to do? Will it just sit there for years, or will it begin to spread quickly? And, the biggest worry of all, how long have I got to live? Am I going to die soon?

No doctor can answer these questions, because in every man, prostate cancer is different. However, although we don't know the absolute answers for your specific cancer, we do know some things, and they are reassuring. ▶

▶ We know what generally happens to men in your situation who are followed carefully with watchful waiting: Gradually, over time, the PSA level will go up. At some point, the bone scan will become positive. This is the time to begin hormone therapy. Once hormone treatment is under way, the PSA level almost always falls dramatically and stays low indefinitely—for some men, this can mean *many years.* However, at some point down the road, if the patient lives long enough, the PSA will begin to rise again, as the hormone-resistant cells start to multiply. This is when both patients and their physicians begin to worry, because if these cells cannot be stopped, a man's lifespan is generally only one or two years from this point.

Now, having said this, we also add that for men facing this today, there is great hope. Within the next five to ten years, we expect major new advances that will make it possible for us to control these hormone-resistant cells. Monumental research efforts are being focused on finding new and better ways to treat advanced prostate cancer. And it is entirely possible, if and when you ever reach the point where the hormonal therapy is no longer working, that more effective treatments will be there waiting for you.

Therefore, it is impossible to tell any man with prostate cancer how long he will live today because there is great and reasonable hope that he will have a much brighter outlook tomorrow.

So, to sum up: All of this means that if you have positive lymph nodes and embark on a plan of watchful waiting, you will be avoiding unnecessary side effects today from treatments that will not prolong your life; that these treatments will be there tomorrow, if you develop symptoms and need them. And that, in the future, there is a strong likelihood that we will have new treatments available for you that will do a better job of controlling this cancer.

There is great hope that, one day soon, we will rewrite the textbooks on advanced prostate cancer.

placebos—this happened to 70 percent of the men with stage T3 or T4 (C), and to all of the men with stage N+ and M+ (D) cancer—they began hormone therapy. The study, though not originally intended for this purpose, turned into a comparison of early hormone therapy versus delayed treatment. *There was no difference in survival between the men who started hormone therapy late and the men who had been on it all along.*

So what this means is that whether we treat a man with castration immediately—as soon as the diagnosis of advanced disease is made—or we wait until he has symptoms and then perform the castration, the survival is exactly the same. There is no evidence that any kind of hormone therapy works better earlier than later, when a man begins experiencing symptoms such as urinary obstruction or bone pain. We don't believe that *any* man who is asymptomatic—feeling no symptoms—is going to feel any better once he has been deprived of his normal hormones. To repeat a point: The cancer cells that ultimately prove fatal in prostate cancer are the hormone-insensitive cells. They keep right on growing, unfazed by hormone therapy. To these cells, whether hormone therapy comes earlier or later does not matter.

For an asymptomatic man, early hormonal therapy means going from feeling fine and "normal" to experiencing hot flashes, loss of libido and the ability to have an erection, weight gain, changes in muscle mass, skin and hair growth and the subtle changes in personality that accompany the loss of male hormones. The long-term effects of hormone therapy can include osteoporosis—loss of bone density, which leaves bones more brittle and easy to break.

What's the point of going through this early, when ultimately it's not going to work any better than if a man waits to start hormone therapy until he develops symptoms of advanced disease?

HORMONE THERAPY: CONCLUSIONS AND A LOOK INTO THE FUTURE

This is not to say that hormone therapy does not work. It does work. It does prolong life, and it does ease many symptoms of advanced prostate cancer. The take-home message here is this: There's no evidence that giving a man early hormone therapy, or giving more hormone therapy than is necessary, works any better than giving adequate hormone therapy if and when a patient needs it.

The other truth we have to face is that hormone therapy does not cure prostate cancer. And if a man lives long enough, this cancer will progress. Despite so many refinements in hormone therapy, the death rate for advanced prostate cancer is about the same as it has always been. And the reason these men are dying has nothing to do with the hormone-responsive cells; we can control those cells. It's the hormone-insensitive cells we can't seem to kill. So what we need, urgently, is a better way to target this group of cells.

But until we have such a treatment, perhaps the best strategy with hormone therapy is to find ways of lowering its costs or minimizing its side effects. Are the most expensive hormone treatments necessarily the best? Probably not. Surgical castration and one milligram a day of DES are equally effective. Even though one milligram does not lower testosterone dependably to the castrate range—as three milligrams a day does—this might not be necessary, since castration and one milligram of DES seem to be equal in terms of survival. DES is a lot cheaper than LHRH agonists, which can cost several hundred dollars a month. And DES's biggest side effect, painful breast swelling, can be taken care of relatively cheaply with radiation treatment. However, men with a history of heart disease or thrombophlebitis should not use DES as their main form of treatment.

Another way to improve hormone therapy would be to diminish its side effects—particularly impotence. One hope in this area may be flutamide, perhaps combined with finasteride—both preserve potency in most men. The theory here is the "one-two punch." Flutamide blocks the binding of testosterone and DHT to receptors in the prostate (the "keys-in-the-lock" idea). With help from finasteride, which decreases the amount of DHT floating around inside the prostate, only testosterone is left to bind to the receptor. Therefore, because testosterone's link to the receptor is relatively weak, it becomes easier for flutamide to jolt testosterone out of the way—to knock the key out of the lock.

Will this work? It needs further investigation, but laboratory studies are promising. The result would be hormonal treatment that doesn't make men impotent and doesn't leave them feeling "unmanly," or suffering any of the other side effects from conventional hormone therapy. This should be a major focus of research in the near future—developing effective hormone therapy with fewer side effects.

WHAT HAPPENS WHEN HORMONE THERAPY DOESN'T SEEM TO BE WORKING?

What should you do? First, let's make sure that you're receiving the maximum benefit from hormone therapy—that it's doing the job it's supposed to do, and that it's not making things worse.

If you've been castrated, make sure that all the tissue was taken out. This is easier than it sounds; all you need is a blood test to measure your testosterone level. Similarly, if you're taking estrogen or an LHRH agonist, make sure you're getting the recommended dosage and taking your pills regularly—taking a pill at six one morning and at midnight the next night, for example, might mean the level of hormones is fluctuating. Again, a blood test can confirm whether your testosterone level is at the crucial castrate range. In either case, if there's too much testosterone in the blood, dosage regularity is probably the problem, and it can be fixed.

If your testosterone is in the castrate range and you're not on flutamide, you could try taking it to see whether this makes your PSA levels fall. Some men are helped by this. If, however, you already are taking flutamide in addition to castration, estrogen or an LHRH agonist, try stopping the flutamide.

In a few men, prostate cancer comes back as a kind of tumor called a small-cell carcinoma. This may be the case if there is a large recurrence of cancer in the pelvis or liver—especially if your PSA level is low. A biopsy should find this out. It's an important fact to know because small-cell prostate cancers have a make-up similar to other small-cell cancers (of the lung, for example), and they respond to the same kinds of chemotherapy drugs used to treat these other small-cell tumors.

If all of these options for hormone therapy have been tried, and the cancer is not a small-cell carcinoma, the next step may be to try and control the cancer and its symptoms with other kinds of drugs—chemotherapy. However, this option is recommended only for men who are strong enough to withstand chemotherapy's side effects. The other option is to treat specific symptoms as the cancer progresses.

Chemotherapy

This is going to be an extremely short discussion—mainly because *standard chemotherapy doesn't work in fighting prostate cancer.* Unfortunately, it's a waste of money and the time it takes to get over the side effects, which can be debilitating for some men. Not only does it fail to cure the cancer, it doesn't even prolong survival to any significant degree, and its side effects only add to the unpleasantness of having prostate cancer—which can be awful enough without any additional help.

That's it.

"Conventional chemotherapy drugs have not shown a lot of benefit to patients," says one Johns Hopkins oncologist, "and there's no evidence that they have an impact on survival." (The one exception may be men with a kind of cancer called small-cell carcinoma; see above.)

Suramin

But then there's suramin. Suramin is not a standard chemotherapeutic drug—actually, it was originally used to eradicate internal parasites more than fifty years ago. Decades later, in the early 1980s, this synthetic compound was investigated as a potential treatment for AIDS. Doctors had discovered that suramin had a unique ability to invade cells and disturb their most basic elements. Suramin, they found, could hook itself up to various substances called growth factors—which serve as switches to activate processes that promote cell division—and upset their normal activities with the effect of a bull in a china shop.

Then doctors at the National Cancer Institute began wondering whether suramin could cause the same chaos in prostate cancer. They knew suramin was capable of thwarting the activity of such growth factors as basic fibroblast growth factor and epidermal growth factor—both believed to be important to sustaining and promoting the growth of prostate cancer cells. Spurred by such growth factors, these cancer cells somehow revert to a more primitive state, which encourages them to mass-produce.

The scientists also knew that suramin could inhibit growth in specific varieties of prostate cancer cells. And finally—a bonus—suramin also seemed to lower the level of adrenal androgens.

So suramin looked highly promising as the first drug with the potential not only to lower the adrenal androgens but to target the hormone-resistant cells that, so far, have successfully eluded every other attempt to kill them. Could suramin perform as expected—could it interrupt factors that feed cancer cells and make them grow? In other words, could it slow down the proliferation of cancer cells?

The jury is still out on suramin. The bottom line is that it has helped some men; it has not helped other men, and its effects don't seem to be long-lasting. In one study, suramin caused reduction or "complete disappearance" of cancer metastases in soft tissue—masses in the pelvis, lymph nodes, and even nodules under the skin. However, in only a few men did the improvements last longer than three months. Only a few men showed an improvement in metastases to the bone, and these gains were slow in coming—it took about nine months or longer. In some men, bone metastases got better; in others, they got worse. Some men showed no change at all, and in other men, the cancer continued to progress. PSA levels dropped in some men, but in only a few of these men did this improvement last longer than three months.

A majority of the men in this study who had experienced severe bone pain found significant relief. However, this often happened within the first weeks of treatment and wasn't accompanied by an obvious shrinking of the cancer. In fact, the doctors weren't sure this was even due to suramin—it could have been the result of corticosteroid treatments, which are known to ease terrible bone pain.

Side Effects

In addition to inhibiting growth of cancer, suramin can also suppress the body's immune system. Its side effects can include infection, particularly in the urinary tract; a reversible drop in the number of platelets in the blood; fatigue, decreased appetite; rash; and pain and weakness in the hands and feet.

Why One Drug Probably Isn't Enough

Currently, researchers are working hard to develop analogs, or "cousins" of suramin—to make it more powerful, with fewer side effects. And scientists are investigating whether suramin given in combination with another drug—EMCYT, perhaps—might be more effective.

"We're talking about the very end of a lifetime of a tumor here," says the Johns Hopkins oncologist. "By this point, tumors become resistant to drugs in many ways; they express different pathways of resistance. If you treat with

Drug A, for instance, this may be effective against a certain portion of the tumor, but probably not all of it—some part of that tumor is probably going to be resistant to that treatment. Therefore, because we're dealing with a heterogeneous disease, it's unlikely that any *one* drug is going to make a significant impact."

Timing of treatment also may make drugs such as suramin more effective. Some doctors are letting PSA be the guide to beginning additional treatment. "In following men on hormonal therapy," says the oncologist, "if we see that the PSA is rising—even before patients develop problems—that is probably a better time to start (with other drugs) because the disease is not as extensive as it becomes if you wait until pain, weight loss and other cancer-related symptoms begin."

HELP IF YOU'RE IN PAIN

"Pain is very closely associated with quality of life," says a Johns Hopkins oncologist. "People in pain have a reduced appetite; they lose weight. They're often depressed. Sometimes they're bedridden, the pain is so bad. If we control the pain aggressively, we often see patients getting stronger and eating better. Aggressive pain management is clearly to the patient's benefit."

It's not only beneficial, it's your *right* as a patient not to suffer. Far too many men with advanced prostate cancer endure excruciating pain in the course of their disease. Several studies have shown that an average of 72 percent of men with advanced prostate cancer are in pain. In one recent study of 201 men with prostate cancer, 47 percent reported feeling pain that ranged from "moderate to very bad"—*despite the use of painkillers.* This tells us several things. One is that, as diseases go, prostate cancer is more painful than most. Its particular patterns of spreading—metastases to bone, and particularly to the spine—make it second only to cervical cancer in terms of severe pain. But this study also shows us something else: These 201 men were on analgesics—painkillers —yet they still hurt. Some of them even felt miserable pain. *Does this mean that painkillers don't work? No. It means the doctors treating these men weren't giving them enough medication to make them comfortable.*

There is no excuse for that. And often, both sides—doctors as well as patients—are at fault. A recent article by University of Colorado scientists cited some reasons why prostate cancer patients often are under-medicated.

Here are some of the reasons why doctors may not give enough pain medication: One is that many doctors just don't learn enough about pain medication in medical school and in their subsequent professional training; they learn how to save or prolong lives, but not always how to make their patients comfortable. (This is improving as medical schools and continuing education courses are doing a better job teaching doctors how to manage patients' pain.)

But perhaps a bigger problem—and this also has to do with the way health care professionals are educated—is the very real fear that patients will get addicted. *This is hogwash.* The sole purpose of these drugs is to alleviate pain, and frankly, few patients need these medications more desperately than people with cancer—especially men with metastatic prostate cancer whose pain is extreme.

And yet every day all over this country, this study showed, some doctors prescribe painkillers at inadequate dosages; some nurses withhold doses of painkillers; and some pharmacists refuse to provide drugs.

In addition, some doctors worry about controlling the side effects of analgesics (see below). They worry about inadvertently precipitating a patient's death—or worse, being an unwitting part in a patient's suicide attempt—if he overdoses.

Other problems listed in this University of Colorado study come under the category of communication failure. Some guidelines for drug dosages (printed in medical reference books and other sources) are not appropriate for the particular intensity of cancer pain. And sometimes—this is increasingly common—if a patient is being looked after by a group of physicians, there may not be a clear understanding of who's responsible for pain management. The pain may "fall through the cracks."

You're a patient; what can you do? If you're suffering terrible pain, talk to your physician. If you're being treated by a group practice, demand that one doctor oversee your pain and other symptoms. If you're still not satisfied with the care you're getting, look for another doctor—preferably, someone who treats many cancer patients and is attuned to their particular, intense pain.

Another option is to contact the National Hospice Organization, a group whose goal is to "enable patients to carry on an alert, pain-free life and to manage other symptoms," so their days "may be spent with dignity and quality at home or in a home-like setting." (See "Where to Get Help," at the back of this book.)

Most hospice programs—and there are hundreds throughout the country—are directed by physicians, and care is administered by a spectrum of health-care professionals, including nurses, psychologists, members of the clergy, and social workers. Care is available twenty-four hours a day, every day, and it is centered around patients and their families.

There are also some regulatory issues, the University of Colorado study showed. When potentially addictive narcotics (strong painkillers like morphine) are involved, so is the government. That's why most of these drugs are called "controlled substances." Some governmental red tape can include limits on refills; however, this is not an insurmountable hassle—it just means patients need to get their doctors to write new prescriptions when their medication runs out.

But finally, the study showed a variety of reasons why the *patients themselves* didn't ask for adequate pain medication. Some men aren't very good at expressing their symptoms, or conveying the depth of their pain, the researchers found. Some men feel it isn't "macho" to admit that their pain is intolerable. (If you have a problem with this, it may help to take along a family member who feels no such hesitation when you go to see the doctor.) Other men are afraid of becoming addicted—and some of these men aren't helped any when zealous family members urge them to "just say no" to drugs!

Some men believe that the pain is just an inevitable part of having the cancer and that nothing can be done to help them. Others worry about the pain yet to come, and want to save the "big guns," the strongest medications, until the pain becomes intolerable. (Actually, with heavy-duty painkillers like morphine, relief *always* comes when doctors boost the dosage, so there is nothing to be gained by seeing how much pain you can stand.) Some men don't want to be labeled as "bad" patients because they complain about their pain. And finally, the study said, some men—ever the breadwinners—worry that costly pain medication will use up all their families' resources. For these men, methadone may be a good option—at around $30 a month, it's the cheapest narcotic.

The bottom line is that you—or a loved one with prostate cancer—do not need to suffer terrible pain. There is help available. Take it.

Drugs for Pain

It makes sense to treat each level and kind of pain differently. At the lowest level is mild pain that responds to aspirin, acetaminophen (Tylenol), or ibuprofen (Advil or Motrin). Next come low-powered opiates, drugs such as codeine. As opiates go, these drugs are considered weak. In terms of pain relief, they can't hold a candle to high-powered opiates such as morphine—the highest rung on the pain ladder. (However, these milder opiates generally are sufficient to ease moderate pain.) The biggest advantage to strong opiates is "their lack of ceiling effect," as one study puts it. "Increasing the dose always increases the pain relief," although it can also increase the side effects.

In addition, other drugs not generally classified as painkillers—particularly corticosteroids—have proved helpful in reducing inflammation and bringing relief from some spinal pain. Ask your doctor if one of these drugs might be right for you.

If you are elderly, have other health problems, or are taking other medications, certain painkillers may have a stronger effect in you than in other men. Be sure to discuss these factors, the side effects of various drugs, and the form in which you should take these drugs—a pill, or liquid, rectal suppository, skin patch, or shot—with your doctor. If you need additional information, your pharmacist may also be able to provide you with the package insert sheets for various drugs. These generally are impenetrable, written in tiny print, and confusing—they contain more information than most people want to know. They also tend to list every possible side effect, even the unlikely ones. However, some people find this information helpful. (For more sources of information, see "Where to Get Help," at the back of this book.)

Drugs for Milder Pain

Listed here are some nonsteroidal anti-inflammatory drugs (NSAIDs) and some of their brand names. (Just because we don't mention the brand name here doesn't mean it isn't a good drug.) Over-the-counter drugs include aspirin; acetaminophen (brand names include Tylenol and Datril); and ibuprofen (brand names include Motrin, Advil and Nuprin). Prescription drugs include diflunisal (Dolobid); choline magnesium trisalicylate (Trisilate); salsalate (Disalcid); naproxen (Naprosyn); naproxen sodium (Anaprox); indomethacin (Indocin); sulindac (Clinoril); and ketorolac (Toradol).

Drugs for Moderate to Severe Pain

Here are prescription drugs, and some of their brand names. (Again, not all brand names are mentioned here.) They include fenatyl (Duragesic); propoxyphene (Darvon, Darvocet); codeine (Tylenol with codeine); oxycodone (Tylox, Percocet, Percodan); meperidine (Demerol); methadone (Dolophine); hydromorphone (Dilaudid); and morphine (Roxanol).

Treating Specific Pain

Until recently, a widespread treatment called "hemi-body" irradiation was commonly used to ease pain in prostate cancer patients with metastases to bone in several places. Hemi-body irradiation involved what radiologists call "wide fields" of radiation—large expanses of the body, and comparatively high doses of radiation. The problem was that this often wiped out key blood-forming cells in the bone marrow and compromised the body's immune system, resulting in such complications as infections and the need for transfusions.

Now, for pain that is concentrated in one area—a portion of the spine, for instance—more specific pain treatment is a far better approach. Two good options are "spot" radiation and radioactive strontium-89.

"Spot" Radiation

This is localized external-beam radiation treatment, targeted at one or several painful bone metastases. It won't prevent new metastases from cropping up in bone, but it generally helps ease pain in the sites it does treat. Spot radiation often results in several months of dramatic relief from pain, and it helps prevent spinal cord compression (see below). In recent studies, 55 percent of patients received complete relief from pain, 33 percent had partial relief, and only 12 percent had little or no response.

Radioactive Strontium

A new approach to bone pain has arrived with the development of a compound called radioactive strontium-89—a radioactive isotope that is injected into the body as an outpatient procedure.

Strontium-89 is specially tailored for bone pain. Like calcium, it is taken up immediately by bone, as water is absorbed by a sponge—except this compound tends to zoom right past healthy bone and zero in on metastatic cancer. (Strontium-89 is soaked up by tumor in bone, instead of by bone marrow, at a ratio of ten to one.) Relief from pain has been reported in from half to 80 percent of patients.

Strontium-89 has a long half-life—fifty-one days—in the body; a single shot of the compound has proved effective at relieving pain for an average of six months. One advantage of this, as compared to spot radiation, is that it acts on *new sites of metastasis* that crop up while it stays in the body, as well as the older sites of cancer it originally was intended to treat.

And, strontium-89 can be used in combination with spot radiation. In one study, doctors found that this combined approach—strontium-89 plus spot radiation—delayed progression of pain seven months longer than radiation alone.

Side Effects. The few side effects associated with strontium-89 include the potential for bone marrow damage; this is characterized by a drop in platelets. Also, some men report a mild increase in pain for the first couple of days after receiving the injection; this can be controlled with other pain medication. And a safety note: Because this radioactive substance is excreted in the urine, for the first forty-eight hours after receiving the injection urine must be taken care of in a certain way; this means you must urinate into a special container—not into the toilet—and dispose of this as directed by your doctor.

WHEN ADDITIONAL TREATMENT MAY BE NEEDED

In addition to causing extreme pain, metastases of cancer to bone can cause two other catastrophic complications—spinal cord compression and pathologic fracture.

Spinal Cord Compression

About one-third of men with metastatic prostate cancer may be at risk for spinal cord compression—when proliferating cancer cells cause part of the spinal column to collapse, trapping and sometimes crushing nearby nerves. If you have severe pain in your back that accompanies leg weakness, loss of sensation (often beginning with numbness or tingling in the toes), trouble walking, constipation or urinary retention, you may be at risk, and you need an MRI scan right away. *An MRI scan is essential—it gives details of the spinal cord and can show early signs of compression.* If spinal cord compression is an immediate danger, the MRI will show the cancer invading the dura, the membrane surrounding the spinal cord; this is called extradural compression. If your hospital doesn't have an MRI machine, it's worth it to make arrangements to travel to another hospital. *This is a very serious problem—a true emergency—and it requires aggressive, immediate treatment.* It is far better to treat potential spinal cord compression early than to try and repair the damage after it happens.

Patients in imminent danger of spinal cord compression should be treated with large doses of corticosteroids (usually a drug called decadron) for forty-eight hours. Then, depending on how your body responds to this, your doctor will make a decision on what to do next—this could mean spot radiation treatment to the spine, or something called surgical decompression, an operation to ease the cancer's pressure on the spinal cord.

If you have not yet begun hormone therapy, now is an excellent time to begin—and fast—with immediate castration or treatment with flutamide (see above). Giving an LHRH agonist alone in this situation is not a good idea, because it can cause a surge in testosterone that could aggravate the cancer sitting so precariously in the spine.

Spinal cord compression is yet another blow in a series of unpleasant complications of prostate cancer, and it has the greatest potential to ruin quality of life—it can lead to paralysis, with an accompanying loss of bowel and bladder function. Most significantly, it can result in the loss of a patient's independence and feeling of dignity.

If you begin to feel any of the warning signs mentioned above, *call your doctor immediately; don't wait until your next scheduled appointment!* This may mean the difference between remaining able to walk and being bedridden.

Pathologic Fracture

When cancer invades bones, they become brittle. Brittle bones break. Therefore, men with metastatic prostate cancer are prone to broken bones (called pathologic fractures). Most susceptible are bones that bear much of the body's weight, in the hip and thigh. Sometimes, doctors can take steps to protect bones at risk—putting pins in the hip bone to strengthen it, for example. Such steps are a good idea when a bone has a large chunk of cancer (greater than three centimeters in diameter) that takes up at least half of the bone's outer shell.

Other Complications

Urinary Tract Obstruction

If you're having any of these symptoms—weak urine flow; hesitancy in starting urination; a need to push or strain to get urine to flow; intermittent urine stream (starts and stops several times); difficulty in stopping urination; "dribbling" after urination; a sense of not being able to empty the bladder completely; or not being able to urinate at all—it's probable that the cancer has become extensive enough to block your urinary tract. Several procedures are available to ease these symptoms, including a TUR procedure or the placement of stents. (For more procedures to relieve obstruction, see Chapter 10 and talk to your doctor.)

Weight Loss

What's wrong with losing weight—particularly if you've spent the better part of your life trying to do just that? The problem here is that people who have cancer need to eat. Losing weight means losing strength and the body's reserve for fighting off illness.

No appetite? Able to eat just a little at a time? The thought of vitamins makes you gag? Then do what pregnant women with bad morning sickness do: Eat less, more often. Have small, nutritious snacks throughout the day. Make every calorie count. Empty calories in sugared iced tea or soda won't do your body as much good as the calories in juice, for instance; the same goes for the empty calories in a doughnut versus the calories in a muffin or slice of banana bread. Finally, if you just can't force yourself to eat as much food as your body needs, you may want to try a calorie-packed liquid nutrition supplement like Ensure or Sustacal. Most hospitals have nutritionists available to help you solve dietary problems like these. That's what these people are there for—use them!

In severe cases of weight loss, doctors can insert a gastrostomy tube, which bypasses the upper digestive tract and allows patients to get much-needed nutrition in liquid form. This tube "really takes the burden from the patient's shoulders," says one Johns Hopkins gastroenterologist. This tube provides a painless route for food to get to your stomach. It's comfortable and discreet—hidden by clothes—and it can be removed when your appetite comes back and you don't need it anymore.

Constipation

This is another big problem for many men taking strong painkillers like morphine, which sedate the digestive tract as they relieve pain. Many doctors go ahead and prescribe mild laxatives or stool softeners at the same time they prescribe opiate analgesics. Another option is adding fiber supplements to your diet; these are available in a variety of forms, including mixtures you can add to fruit juice. You don't have to have a bowel movement every day, but you should be having one every two to three days—and when it does happen, it should not be uncomfortable.

SHOULD YOU BE IN A STUDY?

Clearly, this depends on the study and the medical institution that's taking part in it. One potential downside to participating in any study of a new drug or procedure is that the treatment you receive may be ineffective, or not as effective as treatment that's already available—particularly if it's a double-blind study and you get the placebo. Also, one reason scientists may be testing a drug is for any potential side effects.

However, there are many advantages to participating in a study. Medical studies are strictly controlled, with well-defined rules (participants can stop being in the study whenever they want) and review boards that include doctors, nurses, lawyers, scientists, clergy members, and laypeople. Often, people who take part in medical studies are followed more closely, and thus receive better medical care, than the general public—and usually at little or no cost. (Sometimes, if a medication proves helpful, participants are even given a free supply as a reward for their help!)

Participating in a study often means access to new drugs that aren't yet available to others; you may get first crack at a new breakthrough. And many people who volunteer for a medical study say that they feel that they are doing something important—that their contribution will advance medical science, and that it ultimately will help other people.

"If they're motivated and feel well, patients should always explore this option," says a Johns Hopkins oncologist. "They shouldn't give up. For many patients, being in a study gives them a new outlook and new hope."

THE SHORT STORY

When cancer spreads beyond the prostate, it cannot be cured—but it can be controlled. The main way to do this is by hormone therapy—shutting down the hormones that feed the prostate and nourish the cancer. There are several kinds of hormone therapy; each one targets a different link in the hormonal chain of events that affects the prostate.

Prostate growth is tightly controlled by a major hormone, testosterone, which is made by the testicles. Testosterone circulates in the blood and enters the prostate, where it's soon transformed into another powerful hormone called DHT, the active hormone within the prostate.

The amount of testosterone that circulates in the blood is carefully monitored by the brain, and this is where the whole hormone chain really begins. The hypothalamus makes a substance called LHRH, a chemical signal that's dispatched to the nearby pituitary gland. It tells the pituitary gland to make, among other things, a hormone called LH. LH, in turn, tells the testicles to make testosterone. Think of the domino effect—LHRH, LH, testosterone, DHT.

The major goal of hormone therapy is to reduce testosterone, which stimulates the prostate tumor. What's the best approach? There are several good places to break this hormone chain—drugs that can target the hypothalamus (LHRH), the pituitary (LH), the adrenal gland (adrenal androgens), the testicles (testosterone) or the prostate (DHT).

The cheapest and easiest way to control testosterone is by a simple surgical procedure, castration (also called an orchiectomy). Castration works fast; it reduces the body's amount of testosterone by 95 percent almost immediately, and permanently. Within about three hours after surgery, testosterone levels begin to plummet to a level called the "castrate range."

Many men, for many reasons, don't want to undergo surgical castration, so they opt for chemical castration—taking drugs that accomplish the same result. There are several options: One is a group of drugs called *estrogens*. DES, the main oral estrogen, targets the hypothalamus-pituitary connection, instead of the testicles. It works by blocking the release of LHRH—which, in turn, blocks LH and FSH, and this virtually shuts down the testosterone-making factories in the testicles. So testosterone drops to the castrate range. (Note: Men with a history of heart disease or thrombophlebitis should not use DES as their main form of treatment.)

LHRH agonists are another option. LHRH agonists shut down production of LH. The most commonly prescribed LHRH agonists are leuprolide and goserelin. These drugs are equivalent to treatment with DES or to surgical castration in their ability to lower testosterone and lengthen a man's lifespan.

A drug called *ketoconazole* blocks production of testosterone by targeting the testicles. Also, the effects of testosterone on the prostate itself can be blocked by interfering with testosterone's conversion to DHT—this is what a drug called *finasteride* does—or by blocking the effects of testosterone and DHT on the prostate cell by neutralizing their effect. This is what *flutamide,* an "anti-androgen" drug, does.

The standard forms of hormone therapy for men with prostate cancer are *castration, estrogens, and LHRH agonists.* All three achieve a similar effect—lowering testosterone to the crucial "castrate range." There is no good evidence that another approach, called total androgen ablation, makes any significant difference in lengthening life expectancy. (The theory behind this approach is that even low levels of testosterone and DHT, produced by the adrenal gland, can stimulate cancer in the prostate, and that they must be stopped. This is done by combining a standard hormone treatment, such as castration, with flutamide.)

Hormone therapy works in almost every man; it prolongs life and eases many symptoms of advanced prostate cancer. In some men, its effects last for years. Why doesn't it cure the disease? Because prostate cancer is "heterogeneous"—it's a bunch of different cells mixed up together. Some of these cells respond to hormones; some of them don't. This means that a hormone treatment which targets one kind of cell, the kind that responds to hormones, has absolutely no effect on the hormone-insensitive cells all around it. They keep right on growing, unfazed. Ultimately, if a man lives long enough, these cells eventually overtake the hormone-sensitive cells. And right now, we don't have any way to stop them.

This fact has two important implications for patients: One, there's no evidence that starting hormone therapy early in the course of prostate cancer is any more effective in prolonging survival than starting treatment *if and when a patient needs it*—when a man has bone pain from the cancer, for instance. Again, the cells that ultimately prove fatal are the hormone-insensitive cells—and to these cells, whether hormone therapy comes earlier or later does not matter one bit. Two, there is no good evidence that other forms of hormone manipulation—total androgen ablation, for instance—provide much benefit after hormone therapy has stopped working.

If hormones lose their effect on the tumor, there are several other options for treatment of the disease and specific symptoms, including new chemotherapy drugs, "spot" radiation to painful sites of metastases (chunks of cancer that have broken off from the main tumor and established themselves in new locations, such as the bone), a radioactive substance called strontium-89, which is specially tailored to treat bone pain, and a whole host of powerful pain medications. *There is no reason for any man with prostate cancer to live in excruciating pain.* Aggressive pain management is not only beneficial—it's been shown that men who aren't in terrible pain live longer—it's your right as a patient. Help is available; take it.

All of these options are discussed in detail in this chapter.

8

Help for Impotence after Prostate Treatment

Men who are impotent after prostatectomy or radiation therapy have normal sensation and normal sex drive, and they can achieve a normal orgasm. Their only trouble may be in achieving or maintaining an erection.

And this is a problem that can be fixed.

The purpose of this chapter is not to itemize every possible cause for impotence—there are many—or to discuss every treatment in detail, but to let you know two things: First, that you're not alone, and second, that help is available.

Here are some statistics: By age 65, about 25 percent of all men are impotent. In the United States, an estimated 10 million men are impotent.

Aging is one reason for impotence. But impotence can also result from medical conditions such as diabetes, hypertension, or multiple sclerosis; from certain medications; from overuse of alcohol, cigarettes or other drugs; even from emotional or psychological problems. For most men, impotence does not have to be a permanent situation. In other words: If there's a will, there's generally a way.

WHAT HAPPENS IN
NORMAL SEXUAL FUNCTION?

Normal erection in men can be reduced in medical terms to a "vascular event," but this seems too simple a description for the delicate, complex interplay between blood vessels (veins and arteries) and nerves. The penis itself is a remarkable structure, made up of nerves, smooth muscle tissue, and blood vessels. It has three cylindrical, spongy chambers that are essential to erection; one of these is called the corpus spongiosum, and the other two are called the corpora cavernosa.

When sexual function is normal, this is what happens: A man becomes sexually aroused. A substance called nitric oxide is released by the nerve endings, and the smooth muscle tissue in the penis begins to relax. The spongy chambers (also called sinusoids) within this smooth muscle tissue begin to dilate. Meanwhile, arteries continue to pump blood, as usual, into these spongy chambers of the penis. As the penis elongates, the veins are stretched; they clamp down against the thick tissue that surrounds the corpora cavernosa —shutting themselves off so the blood can't leave the penis. The chambers become engorged, and this keeps the penis "inflated" during sexual activity. An erection is born.

After ejaculation, nitric oxide stops being released; the smooth muscle tissue contracts and the blood flow to the penis is reduced—the veins ease their viselike grip. Once again, blood is allowed to leave the penis, and the erection goes away.

WHAT CAN GO WRONG?

There are four components to normal sexual function in men—*libido* (sex drive), *erection, emission of fluid* (ejaculation), and *orgasm*. All of these elements are regulated separately; there is no centralized "sex control center."

Libido

The sex drive is controlled by the male hormone, testosterone, which is produced almost exclusively by the testicles. (To get the "big picture," it may help to review the anatomy in Chapter 1.) One major cause for a diminished libido in men undergoing treatment for prostate diseases is a drop in testosterone. However, other factors—environmental as well as psychological—can have an impact on sex drive (see below).

Erection

Probably the most common sexual problem for men after prostate treatment is the inability to have an erection sufficient for sexual intercourse; this is called erectile dysfunction. The nerves that lead to and from the penis are extremely important to erection. Particularly essential are nerves in the two bundles that sit on either side of the prostate. Even if these nerve bundles are not removed during radical prostatectomy, they can still be damaged by the surgery. They also can be injured during other procedures including laser prostatectomy, if the laser's energy extends too far beyond the prostate, and, rarely, by the TUR procedure to treat BPH. *But remember, these nerves are only necessary for erection—not for sensation and not for orgasm.* Loss of erection after radical prostatectomy is what doctors call "multifactorial"—in other words, it's probably not caused by one single problem.

Even if both nerve bundles are preserved during surgery, some men still can be impotent afterward—and doctors don't always know why. For example, if both bundles are preserved, potency returns after surgery in about 90 percent of men in their forties, 80 percent of men in their fifties, and about 70 percent of men in their sixties. (Only about 25 percent of men over age 70 are potent.) If one bundle is removed, potency returns in about 90 percent of men in their forties, 60 percent of men in their fifties, and half of men in their sixties.

Let's look at the men in their forties—90 percent are potent with one or both bundles remaining after radical prostatectomy. *But 10 percent aren't.* These younger men have the best odds of potency of all patients, yet even some of these are impotent after surgery. What these figures show is that even when both bundles are preserved, recovery of the ability to have an erection is not certain, and that the older a man gets, the more uncertain this ability becomes. Why is this? No one knows for sure.

Erection problems can also result from vascular injury—damage to the blood vessels in the penis. The arteries that supply blood to the penis must be intact for a normal erection. This blood supply can suffer after radiation treatment; in fact, damage to these arteries is believed to be the main cause of impotence after radiation treatment. In a few men, this blood supply also can be reduced by radical prostatectomy—even though the major arteries that supply the penis do not normally travel next to the prostate. (In these men, for some reason the major blood supply to the penis runs *inside* the pelvis—instead of outside, as it does in most men. When this is the case, these arteries can be damaged inadvertently during radical prostatectomy.)

Another problem with erections in men after radical prostatectomy or radiation therapy results from a problem called "venous leak." What happens here is that, although the blood flows normally into the penis, it doesn't stay there; the veins can't keep it trapped inside. Exactly why this occurs is not clear.

Dry Ejaculation

In normal ejaculation, several events must take place. Sperm, which are made in the testicles, travel to the epididymis, a "greenhouse," in which they mature. During orgasm, sperm are rocketed from the epididymis through the vas deferens during a series of powerful muscle contractions. They shoot through the ejaculatory ducts and mix with fluid produced by the prostate and the seminal vesicles. Simultaneously, a muscular valve in the bladder neck slams shut, forcing this fluid out the only possible exit—through the urethra and penis to the outside world, rather than backward into the bladder.

In most men who have undergone a TUR procedure for BPH, this valve is damaged; and therefore, because there's no barrier to keep sperm from going back into the bladder, it isn't forced out the urethra (this is called "dry," or retrograde ejaculation).

After radical prostatectomy, there is usually no emission of fluid because the prostate and seminal vesicles, which produce the vast majority of this fluid, are gone and the vas deferens has been shut off. (A few men, however, do continue to produce a small amount of ejaculate. This fluid comes from the nearby Cowper's glands; like the prostate and seminal vesicles, these are known as "sex accessory" tissues.)

After radiation therapy, many men also have a loss of ejaculate fluid because the glands responsible for making this fluid are "dried up." In any event—no matter what causes "dry" ejaculation—the lack of fluid should not interfere with orgasm. The reason is that *orgasm doesn't really have much to do with the prostate.* Think about it—women don't have prostates, yet they do have orgasms. Why? Because . . .

Orgasm

Orgasm happens primarily in the brain. For orgasm to take place, there must be sensation and stimulation. In men who are impotent after radical prostatectomy, TUR or radiation therapy, sensation is not interrupted; therefore, orgasm should always be possible and it should be no different from the way it was before treatment. (Except for men receiving hormonal therapy. For them, orgasm is not an issue—even though a few can still have erections—because the hormone treatment causes a loss of libido, a lack of interest in sexual activity.)

WHAT CAN YOU DO ABOUT IMPOTENCE?

Talk to your doctor. The first thing you can expect is to have a detailed history and physical taken. The doctor is going to try to pinpoint the exact problem, and figure out what's causing it. Is it trouble with libido, erection, ejaculation, or orgasm? Even though it may seem pretty obvious—you were potent before prostate surgery and impotent afterward—the doctor needs to rule out the possibility that any other medical or psychological problem is causing this.

You may be asked to fill out a questionnaire so you don't have to discuss details face to face, or your doctor may ask you some very specific questions. You'll probably be embarrassed; most men would rather be almost anywhere else, discussing almost any other topic, than in a doctor's office talking about impotence. But you shouldn't be embarrassed. This is private, sensitive, confidential information. Everything you discuss in the doctor's office will remain there. Remember: This certainly won't be the first time that your doctor has heard about such problems, and it won't be the last—remember the 10 million men! And finally, remind yourself that this discussion is the first step to solving the problem.

Probably one of the first questions your doctor will ask is whether you ever wake up at night with an erection. Most men have several erections while they're asleep; these are usually associated with dreaming, and they happen during a particular phase of sleep called REM, for rapid eye movement sleep. (Because men tend to wake up in the morning with these erections, they often connect them with having a full bladder; this is just coincidence.) The idea behind this question is to make sure there's no mental or emotional problem causing the impotence. In other words, if a man can't produce an erection during sexual activity but has several a night while he sleeps, this is a clue that the nature of the problem is not physiological, but psychological. This type of erection problem is called "psychogenic," and it's often treated successfully with counseling.

Your doctor will also ask whether you have a history of cardiovascular disease. Men who have had a heart attack, men who have coronary artery disease, hypertension, elevated blood lipids, or who smoke have a greater chance of having vascular problems. (Aside from the obvious health risks, smoking causes arteries to contract. What's one of the first steps involved in erection? The arteries dilate; they fill up the penis with blood. If they're contracted, they won't be able to dilate very well. Smoking is an easily reversible cause of impotence. Any man who smokes should quit!)

A history of neurological disease—diabetes, for example—may be a cause of impotence. Also, certain drugs may contribute to sexual problems, and combined with prostate treatment, they may result in impotence. Cimetidine, for example, is a drug used to treat ulcer disease; but it's also an antiandrogen; it blocks the action of testosterone. Other medications that can cause impotence include drugs to treat high blood pressure such as beta blockers and thiazides, medications to treat depression such as monoamine oxidase inhibitors and tricyclic antidepressants, antipsychotic drugs, sedatives, drugs to treat anxiety, and drugs of abuse such as opiates. And don't forget alcohol and cigarettes—they're drugs, too. Basically, it's a good idea if you're on *any* medication to check with your doctor and make sure the side effects don't include impotence. Switching from one drug to another may make a big difference.

Diagnostic Tests

Your doctor may want you to undergo further evaluation, which may include something called a "nocturnal penile tumescence test." This is to see whether you have erections during your sleep (see above). If your doctor suspects a problem with penile blood flow, you may need to undergo pulsed Doppler evaluation. This test uses high-resolution ultrasound to evaluate the arteries' blood supply to the penis. Another test involves the injection of smooth muscle relaxants through a small needle directly into the penis; the idea here is to see whether an erection can be produced. If this shot doesn't cause an erection, this is a good hint that there's a vascular problem—trouble with arterial blood flow. Sometimes during this test a man develops an erection but gradually loses it; this usually signifies that there's a problem with the veins—they're not shutting off the blood supply, so the blood is escaping from the penis, and thus the erection is failing.

RECOVERY OF POTENCY
AFTER RADICAL PROSTATECTOMY

You've had a radical prostatectomy, and one or both bundles were preserved. Which means that the potential for erection is there. So what's the problem? Why isn't it happening?

The first bit of advice your doctor should give you here is, "Be patient." Erections return gradually. Your body has been through a trauma; it needs time to recover. This doesn't mean you should give up on sexual relations until the day you wake up with a full erection. Also, know that the erection you have two months after surgery is not necessarily the same one you'll have two years from now. *Most patients experience an improvement in their erections over time; the quality improves month by month.*

Normally, men become sexually aroused, have an erection and then pursue sexual activity. But after radical prostatectomy, the stimuli that cause an erection are different; visual stimulation is not nearly as important as tactile sensation—what the penis can feel directly. In other words, soon after surgery, the only way a man can achieve an erection is with direct sexual stimulation. This changes the sequence of events. Now, men need sexual stimulation to produce an erection sufficient for intercourse. For this reason, don't be afraid to experiment with sexual activity—you can do no harm!

Also, if you have a partial erection, go ahead and attempt intercourse— vaginal stimulation will be the major factor that encourages further erections. So don't wait until you have the "perfect erection." (If you do, you could be waiting a long time and missing out on this important aspect of your life.) Use of lubrications such as K-Y jelly also will help tremendously.

At first, sexual stimulation is the major thing that produces erections in men recovering from radical prostatectomy, and because the best stimulation is vaginal stimulation, we encourage patients to use whatever erection they have to get vaginal penetration. Often they'll notice that the erection soon becomes much firmer.

Early on, however, erections are not sufficient for traditional vaginal penetration. One common reason for this is the venous leak—even though the arteries are doing their job and filling the penis with blood, producing a partial erection, the veins aren't keeping the blood trapped inside the penis. To improve this situation, many men find that if they attempt sexual activity standing up, they'll be able to achieve a much firmer erection. (The blood has to travel all the way back up to the heart, and this takes longer if a man is standing up than if he's lying down.) Sexual activity can continue either while a man remains standing, or while he's kneeling. Also, it may help to attempt entry from behind; the vagina opens more easily if a woman is bending forward.

Another way to combat venous leak is for men to place a soft tourniquet at the base of the penis *before* they begin foreplay or sexual stimulation. The purpose of the tourniquet is to *keep blood in the penis,* once the stimulation causes the arteries to dilate and penile blood flow to increase. The tourniquet doesn't impede blood flow *into* the penis; it just keeps it from going back out. (A material called Coban works well for many patients. This is a transparent tape that can be cut into strips one-half inch to three-quarters of an inch wide. It does not stick to hair, and it can be bought in most drugstores.)

The return of sexual potency has a lot to do with the patient's age and stage of the tumor. For some men, it can take as long as four years for full potency to return. For others, intercourse is possible just a few weeks after surgery. In any case, you don't have to wait for the penis to become erect on its own. If you are not having erections yet, you may wish to try a vacuum erection device (see below).

Finally, it's worth repeating that almost all men who can't obtain an erection after radical prostatectomy still have normal penile sensation and are able to achieve a normal orgasm. Therefore, even if your body can't produce an erection, it will still be possible for you to restore sexual function. There are three basic approaches, discussed below.

Solutions to the Problem

Our hope is that you will use this chapter as a starting point. Think about the nitty-gritty aspects of each of these options; imagine yourself using each one. Some men, for example, reject the option of penile injections because they are squeamish, or they don't want to associate the minor pain of a needle stick with having sexual intercourse; other men hate the idea of using a pump; still other men don't want to undergo the surgery needed to have a penile implant.

Talk to your sexual partner, and talk to your doctor. Talk to men who have—and men who used to have—this problem, and see what solutions they recommend. Read all you can on the subject of impotence (some suggestions of where to look are in the "Where to Get Help" list at the end of this book) and then make the best, most informed decision possible about the option that's best for you.

Vacuum Devices

The idea here is to create suction using an airtight tube that is placed temporarily around the penis. An attached pump withdraws air, creating a reduced atmospheric pressure—a vacuum—around the penis, causing it to become engorged with blood. The penis becomes erect. Then a constricting ring, like a rubber band around the neck of a balloon, keeps the blood trapped in the penis, so the erection can be sustained. (This imitates the clamping action of the veins in normal erection.) It usually takes about five minutes to produce the erection, and this generally lasts for about half an hour. (The erection probably shouldn't last much longer than that; leaving the constricting band on too long can cause distention or swelling due to fluid retention in the penis.)

This erection is not quite the same as a normal erection—it begins only above the constricting band. But it is sufficient for successful intercourse. Vacuum devices have few complications; these can include trouble with ejaculation, pain in the penis, and tiny, pinpoint-sized bruises. (Men taking aspirin or other blood-thinning medications may be more likely to experience such complications.) Some men are highly satisfied with the result of vacuum devices; others are not.

Penile Injections

To recap: The keys to a normal erection are for the arteries to open and fill the penis with blood, and for the veins to close, so the blood can't escape the penis; the smooth muscle tissue also needs to relax. Several drugs can produce erections by making these events happen. They are vasodilators; they open up blood vessels, making a wider channel for blood to go through. They also cause the smooth muscle tissue to relax and the veins to close. The main advantage here is that these drugs produce an absolutely normal erection. Some of these erection-producing drugs include papaverine, phentolamine, and prostaglandin E-1.

It usually takes less than five minutes for one of these drugs to work, and the erection can last as long as a couple of hours. It will be important for your doctor to determine the *lowest possible dose* you need to achieve an erection; this will help reduce the risk of side effects. Other ways to help lessen side effects include limiting injections to no more than once a day, and using an insulin syringe (which has a smaller needle than many syringes) to minimize pain and bleeding from the injection. Also, men should compress the site where the needle went in for three minutes after the injection; this also helps reduce bleeding and tissue damage.

Penile injection is not for everybody. These erection-producing agents won't help men with vascular problems. However, they do work in most patients. Because of the nature of this therapy—giving the penis a shot—it obviously is not ideal for men who can't see well, men with poor hand-eye coordination, or men who are very overweight. Also, because many erection-producing drugs reduce blood pressure, this can cause problems for some men with heart disease.

One side effect is that if the injection is too strong, it can produce a prolonged erection that may require some medical therapy to relieve it. Some doctors ask patients who opt for penile injections to sign a consent form because of some other side effects—some of them long-term—associated with the injections. These can include tiny blood clots, burning pain after injection, damage to the urethra, or minor infection. But the worst is that in some men, over time, painless, fibrous knots of tissue build up in the corpora cavernosa, and this can cause the penis to become curved. Doctors aren't entirely sure why this happens; it may be related to the frequency of injection, strength or dosage of the drug used, and the amount of bleeding resulting from the shots. Some doctors believe compressing the site at the time of injection may be critical to minimizing this risk; also, keeping the dosage to a minimum, or using a blend of several drugs may help.

The future looks much more promising, however: On the horizon are better drug-delivery systems that may render the syringe—and its worst side effects—obsolete. New approaches include a salve to rub on the penis and erection-producing suppositories to place inside the urethra.

Penile Implants

Penile implants, or prostheses, are available in several varieties; the simplest are bendable, and the more complicated ones are inflatable or mechanical. The implants are not a new idea, but they have improved considerably since they were first introduced about twenty years ago. The bendable prostheses, for example, were exactly the same size *all the time*—whether or not the penis was in the erect position—which, as you can imagine, often proved awkward in social settings. Earlier models of the inflatable prostheses that did allow for a "non-erect" size sometimes failed to work and needed to be replaced.

If these relatively clumsy but functional early designs were the prosthetic equivalent of the typewriter, then the latest models are more like a Macintosh computer—sleek, sophisticated and user-friendly. They are more reliable, easier for surgeons to implant, and are designed to look more natural in the "non-erect" phase—even the bendable prostheses, which are more malleable than before. *And they can restore sexual function entirely to normal.*

Now, most prostheses are implanted into the penis through an incision in the scrotum. Some of the more complicated devices involve a pump and a reservoir for fluid, housed in the abdomen or scrotum, and inflatable chambers, which are placed in the corpora cavernosa. (Fluid is pumped into the penis to create an erection and is then held there by a valve. Afterward, the valve is released, and the fluid returns to the reservoir.)

Penile prostheses used to be offered routinely to most impotent men. Now, with other good treatments available, many urologists have come to regard penile prostheses as a last resort because they do involve surgery—and thus, they carry the risk of complications. These can include infection, scarring, damage within the corpora cavernosa, or a problem with any part of the prosthesis. However, these side effects are relatively rare. Most men who have penile prostheses are satisfied with the result and have a normal sex life.

THE SHORT STORY

Men who are impotent after prostatectomy or radiation therapy have normal sensation, normal sex drive and can achieve a normal orgasm. Their only trouble may be in achieving or maintaining an erection—that's the bad news. The good news is that this is a problem that can always be treated.

Why does impotence occur? There are many possible reasons, in addition to the fact that a man has had prostate treatment. Aging is one reason for impotence. But impotence can also result from medical conditions such as diabetes or hypertension, from certain medications, from overuse of alcohol, cigarettes or other drugs, even from emotional or psychological problems.

The bottom line is that for most men, impotence does not have to be a permanent situation. If there's a will, there's generally a way.

What can go wrong? Normal sexual function in men has four components—libido (sex drive), erection, emission of fluid (ejaculation), and orgasm.

Libido is stimulated by the male hormone, testosterone, which is produced mainly by the testicles. When testosterone levels drop, the sex drive is diminished.

Erections are controlled by nerves that lead to and from the penis; particularly important are the nerves in two bundles that sit on either side of the prostate. In normal erection, sexual stimulation causes these nerves to release chemicals that increase blood flow into the penis. As the penis becomes engorged with blood, veins clamp down—shutting themselves off, so the blood can't leave the penis. This keeps the penis erect during sexual activity. But sometimes these nerves are damaged—during a surgical procedure, for instance. Sometimes the arteries that pump blood into the penis are injured—after radiation therapy, perhaps. Or sometimes, for various reasons, the veins that are supposed to keep blood trapped inside the penis just don't do their job. When a man has trouble with an erection, doctors call this "erectile dysfunction."

Ejaculation involves powerful muscle contractions in the epididymis, vas deferens, prostate and seminal vesicles. During orgasm, a muscular valve in the bladder neck slams shut, forcing semen out the only possible exit—through the urethra and penis to the outside world, rather than backward into the bladder. But certain prostate treatments can result in the loss of this fluid. In a TUR procedure to treat BPH, for instance, the valve in the bladder neck is sometimes destroyed—so, because there's no barrier to keep sperm from going back into the bladder, it isn't forced out the urethra. After radical prostatectomy, there's usually no emission of fluid because the prostate and seminal vesicles, which make most of it, are gone and the vas deferens has been shut off. After radiation therapy, many men also have a loss of ejaculate fluid because the glands responsible for making it are "dried up."

Orgasm doesn't really have much to do with the prostate. Orgasm happens primarily in the brain; as long as sensation is intact, orgasm can occur even in the absence of an erection and ejaculation. *This is the key reason why normal sexual function can be restored to most men who are impotent after prostate treatment.* (The one exception here is men receiving hormone therapy; because this causes a loss of libido, there is a general lack of interest in sexual activity.)

The most common sexual problem that troubles men after prostate treatment is the loss of erection, and there are several good ways to restore this, including vacuum erection devices, penile injections (injecting tiny amounts of erection-producing drugs into the penis), and penile prostheses.

The take-home message here is that after treatment for prostate disease (except for men treated with hormone therapy), recovery of sexual function is almost certain. Take heart!

Part II

Enlargement of the Prostate and Prostatitis

9

Understanding BPH and How It's Diagnosed

Benjamin Franklin reportedly suffered from it; so did Thomas Jefferson. So will most men, if they live long enough. This almost inevitable condition, called *benign prostatic hyperplasia* (BPH), is the enlargement of the prostate.

BPH is not prostate cancer, and having it doesn't mean a man is more likely to get prostate cancer. Unlike prostate cancer, which grows outward and invades surrounding tissue, the cell growth in benign enlargement is inward, involving the prostate's innermost core. The key word here is *benign.* (In this case, *hyperplasia* means an increase in the number of cells in the prostate, which causes it to become enlarged.) By itself, an enlarged prostate causes no symptoms and does no harm. If it weren't for the fact that the prostate encircles the urethra (the tube that carries urine from the bladder through the prostate to the penis), BPH might never require treatment. It takes years to develop; in fact, most men don't realize they have BPH until the prostate begins to tighten around the urethra and hinder urine flow.

Like wrinkles and gray hair, BPH seems to come with the territory of aging. One exception to this rule seems to be men in Asia; however, BPH—as well as prostate cancer, both of which were once rare in China and Japan—is becoming increasingly common in the Far East. Some scientists believe this is related to increased "Westernization" of the traditional diet, which is low in fat and animal protein.

In this country, studies have found that the incidence of BPH increases every year after age 40; it's present in 50 percent of men aged 51 to 60, and 80 percent of men who reach age 80. Twenty-five percent of these men—more than 350 thousand a year in this country alone—eventually will require surgery (some of them more than once) to relieve the urinary obstruction BPH causes, making BPH the most common cause of surgery in American men over age 55. The yearly cost of BPH surgery in the United States is well over $3 billion. Clearly, BPH is a significant medical problem in this country, and the numbers will only increase as our lifespans continue to lengthen.

But if BPH is almost a certainty for most men, its annoying symptoms don't have to be. Never before have so many good treatment options—medical and surgical—been available for BPH, and never before have so many men sought, and found, relief from their symptoms.

WHAT MAKES THE PROSTATE GROW?

From birth to the age of puberty, a boy's prostate is tiny. But with the onset of puberty, something happens: There is a surge in the production of the male hormone testosterone, and the prostate begins to grow, doubling again and again until it reaches, at about age 20, the size of a walnut. Then the rate of growth slows down, although the prostate continues to grow for the rest of a man's life. With age, the prostate also gets heavier; this corresponds with the development of obstructive urinary symptoms in BPH.

Where Growth Begins: Location, Location, Location

The prostate has five distinct zones. For this chapter, only one of these—the tiniest, an area known as the transition zone—is important. The transition zone makes up *only about 5 percent* of the normal prostate gland in young men. Yet this tiny ring of tissue is the source of all the trouble in BPH. It's located right in the center of the prostate, and it makes a natural circle around the urethra. Several things happen here, which in combination produce BPH: Beginning at age 30 or 40, tissue in the transition zone begins to expand; bulbous, glandular nodules begin to spring up like mushrooms among the prostate cells lining the urethra. Over time, as this growth continues, the landscape of the transition zone changes dramatically. As they emerge, the nodules tend to form clusters, or lobes, at certain characteristic sites (see figure 9.1).

Figure 9.1. *The many shapes of BPH*

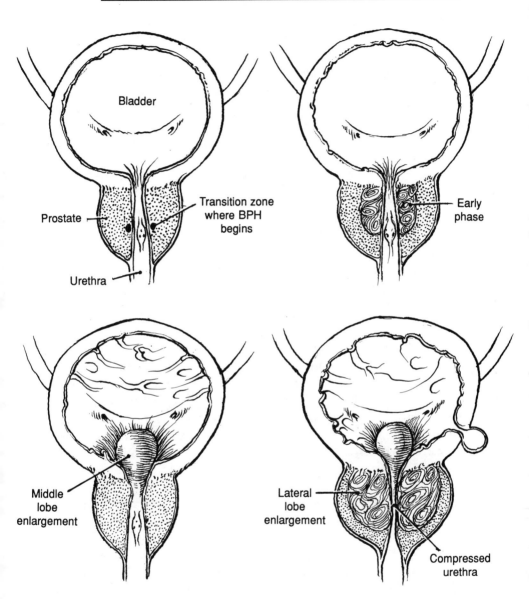

BPH takes place in the tiniest, yet most strategically located, area of the prostate—the transition zone, a ring of tissue around the urethra. As the tissue expands, nodules begin to develop, forming lobes at certain characteristic sites. This illustration shows how the configuration of BPH can affect a man's symptoms. Middle lobe enlargement acts like a cork in a bottle, and this cork tends to plug the bladder neck—which can cause major problems of obstruction. In lateral lobe enlargement, these lobes compress the urethra on two sides—but can swing open and shut like double doors during urination, without producing much obstruction.

In BPH as in real estate, *location* of growth makes all the difference—the *size* of the prostate may have nothing to do with the degree of obstruction. For example, in lateral lobe enlargement, the tissue compresses the urethra from the sides. However, these lateral lobes can become quite large without producing much obstruction—during urination, they just swing open and shut like double doors in a saloon. In middle lobe enlargement, which is sometimes described as a "cork in a bottle," the tissue acts as a moveable plug that can flip to block the bladder neck and cause major symptoms of urinary obstruction—even though the prostate may actually feel small from the outside.

Because these symptoms are the most urgent, men with middle lobe enlargement are much more likely to seek medical relief for BPH than, say, men with simple lateral lobe enlargement. What's more common? Evidence from studies suggests that about 50 percent of men with BPH have middle lobe enlargement, 20 percent have growth in the lateral lobes, and 30 percent have both lateral and middle lobe enlargement.

A Bad Combination:
Different Cell Types, plus Tightening Muscle

BPH involves different kinds of cells, and their growth seems to be stimulated by many factors. (This is frustrating for researchers seeking treatment for BPH, because what works on one group of cells may have little effect on another.)

BPH is not merely a matter of prostate cells on the rampage; the problem involves *two kinds of tissue*. One is glandular tissue, made up of epithelial cells, which secrete fluid that becomes part of the semen. The other is smooth muscle tissue, made up of stromal cells, which contract automatically to launch these secretions out of the prostate and into the urethra. This is the same kind of tissue found in the walls of the intestines and in blood vessels; the actions of this tissue are involuntary responses to signals from the nervous system. Because this dynamic, nerve-rich tissue is easily stimulated, it seems to be set off by the glandular cell build-up in BPH, and it responds with varying degrees of tension. So, together, these prostate cells act as a "double whammy" on the urethra: As the glandular tissue enlarges and begins to clog the urethra, the smooth muscle tissue tightens, and clamps the urethra.

Figure 9.2. *The "double whammy"—growing cells, tightening muscles*

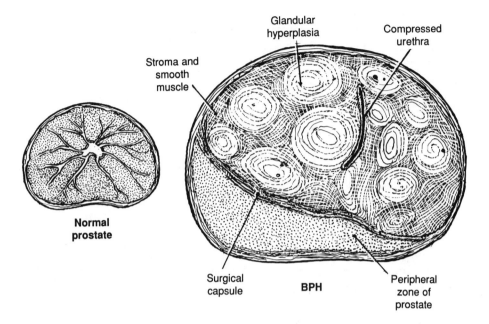

Here are cross-sections of two prostates—one with BPH, one without. What a difference! Look at the lumpy growths of glandular tissue in the prostate with BPH. Several things are happening all at once, and the compressing effect on the poor urethra is easy to see. One kind of tissue involved is glandular—made up of epithelial cells that secrete fluid (which becomes part of semen). In BPH, this tissue starts to form bulbous minilobes. Meanwhile, there's also smooth muscle tissue—made up of stromal cells, which contract automatically to launch these secretions out of the prostate and into the urethra. Smooth muscle tissue seems to be set off by the glandular cell buildup in BPH, and it responds with varying degrees of tension. So, as the glandular tissue enlarges and begins to clog the urethra, the smooth muscle tissue tightens, and clamps it.

What Sets All This in Motion?

There probably isn't one clear-cut explanation for BPH; it involves too many disparate factors. But we do know that the development of BPH has at least two prerequisites—the testes, and aging. And new research suggests that a third condition, family history, may also be important.

The testes, housed in the scrotum, are the main source of the male hormone, or androgen, called testosterone, which is responsible for secondary sex characteristics, like post-puberty body hair and deepening of the voice, and for fertility. Testosterone acts on the prostate, but it's not the only thing that makes the prostate grow. In fact, as it turns out, testosterone is not even the primary troublemaker in BPH; it just initiates the process. The trouble starts when testosterone is *converted* by an enzyme called 5-alpha-reductase to DHT (dihydrotestosterone). DHT is the major androgen, or male hormone, inside the prostate cell. (The thermostat that regulates all this activity is the hypothalamus, located in the brain.)

Where Aging Comes In

As a man grows older, characteristic changes begin to occur in the prostate. There is a cell build-up in its innermost core; the transition zone begins to grow. But the body's hormone levels aren't growing along with the prostate; in fact, there's a *drop* in the amount of testosterone in the blood; DHT levels remain fairly steady, and there's only a slight increase in estrogen. So why is the prostate getting larger? One reason, scientists believe, is that the aging prostate becomes more susceptible to these hormones. In laboratory experiments, scientists have shown that estrogen adds more power to testosterone's punch, making it more effective. At the same time, the aging prostate becomes more sensitive to smaller amounts of testosterone. So some researchers believe that *estrogen plus aging equals a prostate easily influenced by testosterone,* even when there's less of it in the body. In other words, the threshold is lowered.

What's Happening to Urine Flow?

Think of arteries "hardening" as years and years of cholesterol build-up take their toll; eventually, blood has a hard time maintaining its normal pressure and flow as it makes its way through them. BPH doesn't involve a plaque-like accumulation—the build-up here involves an increase in cells, spongy glands and muscles—but what's happening to the flow of urine is roughly the same, and that can be linked to the gland's increased size and weight.

The Estrogen Connection

Another hormone that's being implicated as a factor in BPH is estrogen. Male hormones, such as testosterone, can be converted to estrogen by an enzyme called aromatase. By itself, estrogen doesn't make the prostate grow significantly. Researchers have learned, however, that estrogen stimulates the body's receptors for androgen, or testosterone. Among other things, this enhances the action of DHT in the body; it also stimulates stromal cells, and inhibits cell death. This can lead to BPH.

But another big surprise in recent research is the discovery that growing prostates aren't making scads of new cells. How can this be? If there's not a huge increase in cell *birth,* what's making the prostate grow? Apparently, something's also happening to cell *death;* the cells in question are leading abnormally long lives, and this is resulting in a cellular overcrowding, or population explosion.

Finally, scientists are beginning to investigate the role of substances called growth factors, which serve as switches that activate processes to promote cell division in this balance of cell birth and death. Investigators have found higher levels of some growth factors in tissue with BPH than in normal tissue. Current thinking is that these growth factors have a major impact on the stromal, or smooth muscle, cells. (These growth factors are produced by cells in the prostate and act locally, either on the cell of origin or on adjacent cells. One, such as basic fibroblast growth factor, is known to stimulate glandular cells to grow. Others, such as transforming growth factor–beta, stimulate the stromal and smooth muscle cells.)

Spurred by the growth factors, these cells somehow revert to a more primitive state, which allows proliferation of the lumpy masses of lobes in the prostatic tissue surrounding the urethra. Whatever stimulates the stromal cells also seems to restrain other cells, particularly the epithelial cells, the tiny factories that make the prostate's secretions. This would explain two of BPH's more significant characteristics: The build-up in cells and the drop in prostatic secretions.

IS BPH AN INHERITED DISEASE?

Doctors have just started asking this question, but early evidence from several studies at Johns Hopkins suggests that the answer is yes. Some men get BPH because they've lived long enough for their prostates to enlarge to the point where treatment is needed. But a small number of men—about 7 percent—get it because they have inherited a gene that predisposes them to prostate enlargement. Men who develop BPH at a younger age—in their forties, fifties and early sixties—are more likely to have inherited this gene.

In one Johns Hopkins investigation, scientists studied men aged 64 and younger with notable prostate enlargement. They also studied their relatives and family histories. (The theory behind the age cut-off here is that early age of onset tends to be a marker for hereditary disease.) They found that the male relatives of these men were four times as likely as other men to require a prostatectomy to treat BPH—in other words, they were more likely to develop BPH that was severe enough to need major treatment. And brothers of these men were six times as likely as other men to need surgery to treat BPH.

WHY DOES THE PROSTATE GROW?
THE SHORT ANSWER

Nobody knows what causes BPH; that's why doctors are unable to prevent it, or even to make it go away completely once the disease process has begun. Briefly, here's what we do know: *Hormones play a major role,* but their presence may only be permissive—they may simply provide the necessary soil for the disease to take root and grow. *Aging is crucial* to the development of BPH; as men age, the prostate becomes more sensitive to hormones. *Family history is important,* particularly in families where men develop BPH at a relatively young age. *The balance between epithelial and muscle cells* is also important for the development of the disease, as is the role of growth factors, but in what ways? For doctors to fill in these blanks, much more research is needed. Basically, BPH is a different disease in every man. Its many symptoms—and how a man responds to treatment—depend on an intricate interplay of factors, including the site and configuration of the enlarged lobes, the ratio of smooth muscle and glandular tissue involved, and how all these things affect the bladder.

BPH Causes Urinary Trouble.

Obstructive Symptoms

Weak flow

Hesitancy in starting urination; a need to push or strain to get urine
to flow

Intermittent urine stream (starts and stops several times)

Difficulty in stopping urination

"Dribbling" after urination

A sense of not being able to empty the bladder completely

Not being able to urinate at all

Irritative symptoms

Frequent urination, especially at night

A strong sense of urgency in urination; inability to postpone
urination

Sleep disrupted by the need to urinate

Urgency incontinence

DO I HAVE BPH? TELLTALE SYMPTOMS

BPH affects the urethra first, then the bladder. As BPH begins to impede urine flow, men may experience symptoms that can be broken down into two categories: *Obstructive and irritative.* The first category is just what it sounds like—symptoms resulting from a mechanical obstruction, from the prostate squeezing the urethra. These include the following: A weakened urinary flow or stream; hesitancy in starting urination and difficulty in stopping; intermittency, when the urinary stream starts and stops repeatedly; "dribbling" after urination; a sense of not being able to empty the bladder completely; and occasionally, urinary retention—when the bladder stays completely or partly full.

Early on in BPH, men experience few symptoms because the powerful bladder muscle compensates for the narrowed urethra by making more vigorous contractions and forcing urine through the prostate. But over time, this extra effort takes its toll on the bladder. The mechanical obstruction means the force is diminished for each length of muscle fiber—the bladder becomes less efficient, thus the decreased flow rate and obstructive symptoms.

But as this is happening, the muscle hypertrophies—it gets larger—and there's a marked increase in the smooth muscle tone. Here's where the second category of symptoms comes in. The bladder wall becomes thick and doesn't stretch like it used to; the bladder itself doesn't hold as much, becomes unstable and overly reactive, and causes a need to urinate more often—unfortunately, sometimes spontaneously. These irritative symptoms can include urge incontinence (when a man knows he has to urinate, but can't make it to the bathroom in time); and nocturia, which is frequent urination during the night. The major cause of nocturia from BPH is a thickened bladder that doesn't hold as much as it once did. Another cause is leftover urine from a never-emptied bladder, which greatly reduces the bladder's functional capacity. (Imagine a glass that's capable of holding a pint of fluid, but which is always half-full. This means the glass must be emptied every half-pint—twice as often as before!)

When the prostate's pressure on the urethra gets to be too great for the bladder's compensatory muscle power, a man loses the ability to empty his bladder completely during urination. Sometimes this leads to symptoms that go beyond merely annoying and require treatment—such as repeated urinary tract infections (UTIs) caused by stagnant urine; or damage to the bladder and kidneys from the backup of urine. Sometimes, in acute urinary retention, a man suddenly becomes unable to urinate at all.

Making the Diagnosis

Some men go right to a specialty physician, a urologist, for help with urinary problems, but most men start out with a generalist—their family practitioner or internist. Most likely, all of these doctors will approach your symptoms the same way—there should be a digital rectal examination (discussed below) and a prostate-specific antigen (PSA) blood test. Most family physicians will go ahead and treat a problem such as a urinary tract infection. However, if your family doctor suspects that something else is causing this infection—if it keeps coming back, for example, or if it's accompanied by other symptoms, you may be referred to a urologist for more specific testing. You should also be referred

Differential Diagnosis of Lower Urinary Tract Symptoms:
Besides BPH, What Else Could Be Causing This?

Obstructive Symptoms

Stricture
Cancer
Neurogenic bladder*
Medication

Irritative Symptoms

Infection—bladder or prostate
Bladder tumor
Bladder stone
Neurogenic bladder*

*This is bladder trouble caused by a neurological problem, such as Parkinson's disease.

to a urologist if you are diagnosed as having BPH, prostatitis, or prostate cancer, or if you need urologic surgery or other procedures such as cystoscopy.

First, the Medical History

Because by itself an enlarged prostate causes no problems, all of the symptoms of BPH are secondary, resulting from obstruction of the urethra and bladder and, occasionally, of the ureters and kidneys as well. Most likely, your doctor will begin by taking your medical history, and it's critical that you give an accurate description of your symptoms. *Now is not the time to be embarrassed or reticent about your urinary problems.* Remember, BPH happens to most men; you are not alone.

To help you recognize how often a day you urinate, and the nature of your symptoms, you may want to keep a symptom diary for a few days before your appointment, noting when you urinate, how long it lasts, whether it's characterized by a weak stream, hesitancy, and so on.

There are two important goals for this visit to the doctor: First is to get help for these bothersome symptoms. Second, and equally important, is for your doctor to rule out any other problems—such as a bladder infection, or a blockage (also called a stricture) in the urethra—that may be causing the trouble.

For example: As men grow older, many have trouble making it through the night without one or more trips to the bathroom. But this symptom has many possible causes; so by itself, this might not mean BPH. Among other things, it can be caused by the body's need to eliminate excess urine that accumulates during the day. Many older people—for a variety of reasons—develop swelling in their legs. At night, when the legs are elevated, the fluid that caused the swelling is reabsorbed and excreted by the kidneys. Also, it's recently been recognized that many of the symptoms associated with BPH simply happen because the bladder is aging. (In fact, many symptoms that previously were thought to be suffered only by men, and thus were attributed to BPH, are also present in women as they age.)

Urinary retention—difficulty in emptying the bladder completely, or in urinating at all—also can be triggered by many things, including consuming alcohol; having prostatitis; and taking such medications as antihistamines, antidepressants, tranquilizers, or decongestants. It could even mean prostate cancer, although in most cases, prostate cancer is regrettably "silent," producing no symptoms until it becomes considerably advanced. Two other symptoms, however—trouble starting urination, and a slow or weak stream—almost always signal obstruction.

The lower urinary tract can also be affected by neurological disorders such as diabetes mellitus; multiple sclerosis; Parkinson's disease; and spinal stenosis, pressure on the spinal cord that impairs the brain's ability to communicate with the bladder. These and other diseases can give rise to obstructive and irritative symptoms like those in BPH. (Parkinson's disease makes it particularly tricky to treat the symptoms of BPH. For more on this, see Chapter 10.) The term "neurogenic bladder" refers to a bladder affected by such conditions.

So, because other conditions can mimic the obstruction produced by BPH, a good medical history is vital even if you have what seems like a classic case. An injury to the urethra (from an episode of gonorrhea many years ago, perhaps, or from having a catheter inserted into the bladder during a surgical procedure, such as a coronary artery bypass) can produce a urethral stricture—a scar that narrows the urethra—*that has nothing to do with the prostate,* yet produces urinary problems just as BPH does. Blood in the urine, or pain in the bladder or penis could point to a bladder tumor; it could also indicate that a stone has developed in the bladder, prostate, or kidney. And having a history of other urologic problems—recurrent tract infections or prostatitis, for example—could mean one of these old adversaries has returned, in a different guise.

You will also be asked to score your symptoms on a questionnaire (such as the one in table 9.1). *Be honest;* your answers will help your doctor determine whether your symptoms are mild, moderate or severe, and the impact they're having on your life.

Next, the Physical Exam

Your doctor will probably begin with the outside first, checking your abdomen for swelling (to see whether the bladder is emptying completely), and to make sure the kidneys feel normal—and that they're not palpable. (Normally, kidneys cannot be felt in a physical exam through the abdomen.) Also, your doctor will probably examine your testicles, to make certain that both are present and that they're normal in size.

Because of the prostate's location—below the bladder, and just in front of the rectum—it can't be seen or examined from the outside. So the first step in examining it is usually the *digital rectal examination,* in which a doctor's gloved, lubricated finger is inserted into the rectum to feel for lumps, enlargement, or areas of hardness that might indicate the presence of cancer. Because BPH affects only the innermost core of the prostate, your doctor may find nothing out of the ordinary here. It's important to keep in mind that the *size of the prostate often has nothing to do with the degree of symptoms.* Some men with major prostate enlargement have no urinary tract trouble, while other men with seemingly minor enlargement suffer many symptoms of obstruction. Again, it depends on the site of enlargement in the prostate (see above). Some men, for example, may have middle lobe growth, but hardly any lateral lobe enlargement. Because the middle lobe can't be felt by a doctor's finger, a man may have what feels like a very small prostate, yet have big trouble with urinary retention.

In addition to providing important information about the prostate, the exam also allows your doctor to check the tone of the anal sphincter. This can be abnormal in patients with neurological diseases—such as spinal stenosis, multiple sclerosis, Parkinson's disease, and diabetes mellitus—affecting the lower urinary tract. If your doctor suspects one of these conditions, you may also need to undergo a limited neurological examination, in which your doctor checks your arms and legs for feeling, strength, reflexes, and muscle tone.

Table 9.1 *The American Urological Association Symptom Score*

Circle your score for each question

Question	Not at all	Less than 1 time in 5	Less than half the time	About half the time	More than half the time	Almost always
1. During the last month or so, how often have you had a sensation after you finished urinating of not emptying your bladder completely?	0	1	2	3	4	5
2. During the last month or so, how often have you had to urinate again less than 2 hours after you finished urinating?	0	1	2	3	4	5
3. During the last month or so, how often have you found you stopped and started again several times during urination?	0	1	2	3	4	5
4. During the last month or so, how often have you found it difficult to postpone urination?	0	1	2	3	4	5
5. During the last month or so, how often have you had a weak urinary stream?	0	1	2	3	4	5
6. During the last month or so, how often have you had to push or strain to begin urination?	0	1	2	3	4	5
7. During the last month or so, how many times did you most typically get up to urinate from the time you went to bed at night until the time you got up in the morning?	0 (None)	1 (1 time)	2 (2 times)	3 (3 times)	4 (4 times)	5 (5 times)

Total your score: Total symptom score = sum of questions 1 to 7: _____

In this test, symptoms are classified as mild if the score is 0 to 7, moderate if the score is 8 to 19, or severe if the score is 20 to 35. Your score will help your doctor determine the right treatment for your symptoms.

Diagnosing BPH: What to Expect from the Doctor

A questionnaire, so you can rate your symptoms
A thorough review of your medical history
A physical examination
A digital rectal exam, to evaluate the prostate gland
A urine test, looking for blood or signs of infection
A blood test, to check your kidney function and PSA level

Your doctor may also check for other signs of extreme urinary obstruction, including evidence of weight loss; swelling of the hands and face; pallor or anemia; a buildup of fluid in the lungs; an enlarged heart; and tenderness under the ribs, on either side of the spine (these are quite rare). A *routine urinalysis* (microscopic and chemical examination of the urine) and *urine culture* can test for the presence of blood in the urine and check out the possibility of an infection. A *blood test*—either a serum creatinine or a Blood-Urea-Nitrogen (BUN) test—may be included to check your kidney function. Your doctor may also want to look at your level of PSA. By comparing a baseline PSA level with each subsequent PSA test result, your doctor can monitor your PSA levels over time for any indication of prostate cancer.

The PSA test has generated controversy among doctors, because by itself it's not enough to make a definite diagnosis of prostate cancer, and it's not always accurate. For example, the PSA level can be high in men with BPH who don't have prostate cancer, or normal in men who really do have prostate cancer. (For more on PSA, see Chapter 3.)

A note on these and other tests: They're not painful or time-consuming; they're useful for determining whether or not you have BPH, the degree of your symptoms and any complications. But they're not fortune-tellers. They can't predict the course your condition will take, or which treatment is necessarily best for you.

Other Tests

In addition to the tests mentioned above, your doctor may order other tests, including:

Uroflowmetry. Your doctor may decide to measure the speed of your urinary stream and the amount of urine you pass. This is accomplished as you urinate into an electronic machine (while you're alone in a testing room). To ensure an accurate result, it's important that you urinate at least five or six ounces. This test will identify men whose maximum flow rate is not markedly diminished—*and who may not benefit from treatment.* The normal peak urinary flow rate is fifteen cubic centiliters or more per second.

Residual Urine Measurement. This determines whether you're emptying your bladder completely—and if not, how much urine you're leaving behind. This can be done by an ultrasound examination of the lower abdomen, performed immediately after urination, or by passing a small catheter into the bladder and measuring the amount directly. If it turns out that you do indeed have large amounts of residual urine, watchful waiting (see Chapter 10) may not be a good treatment option for you. These measurements may also be a helpful way to follow the course of your disease and bring to light any change in obstruction.

Urodynamic Studies. Your doctor may want to do these studies if your history or the physical exam suggests that the primary cause of your symptoms—perhaps from a neurologic condition—is bladder dysfunction, not BPH. *Cystometry* is a means of measuring bladder pressure and function. It's performed by threading a small catheter into the penis, through the urethra and into the bladder to monitor pressure changes as the bladder is filled with water. Also helpful are *pressure-flow studies,* in which bladder pressure is monitored as you urinate, again via a small catheter. (Note: Any time a catheter is inserted into the urethra, there's a slight risk of a urinary tract infection developing a few days later. Be sure to tell your doctor about any subsequent fever or discomfort.) Pressures within the bladder are compared to the rate at which the urine flows from the body. Pressure flow studies can be helpful in determining whether men with high peak urinary flow rates are obstructed. Some men with significant obstruction can produce reasonable urinary flow rates because they can generate high bladder pressure; these men will have

Opposite: Here are two kinds of cystoscopes—one rigid (*a*), one flexible (*b*)—which may be used before an invasive procedure such as surgery or balloon dilation. The cystoscope, a tiny, lighted tube, works like a periscope on a submarine. It is inserted in the tip of the anesthetized penis and threaded through the urethra into the bladder; this allows your doctor to check the bladder, prostate, and urethra for abnormalities.

Figure 9.3 (a and b). *Two ways to see inside*

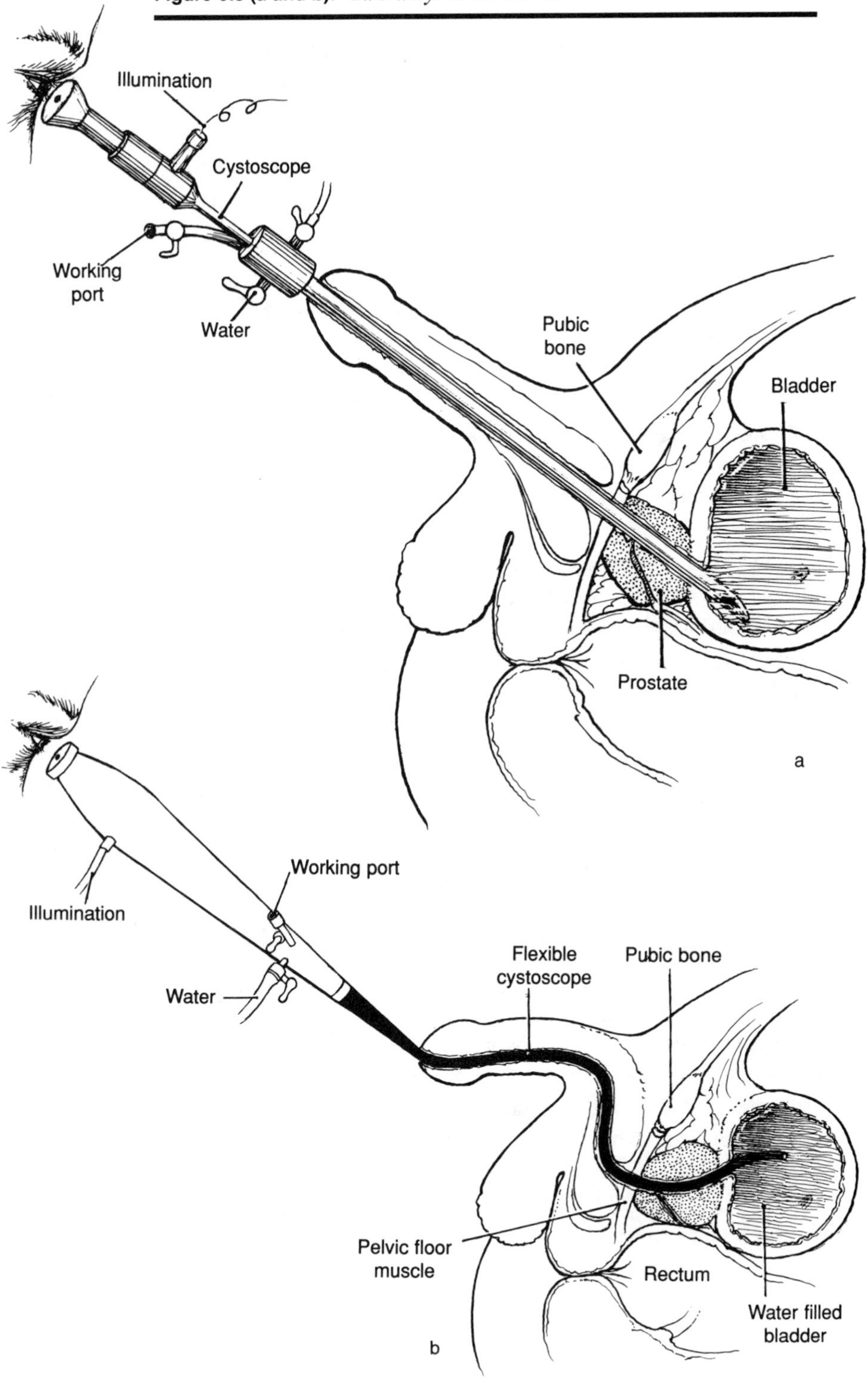

relief of symptoms if their obstruction is treated. But in some men, low urinary flow rates are caused by diseased bladders that do not generate much pressure. These men do not benefit from relief of obstruction.

Ultrasound, a painless method of imaging, creates a picture with high-frequency sound waves—like sonar on a submarine. It may be done either from the outside, through the abdomen, or transrectally, via a wand inserted in the rectum. Though not recommended for most men with BPH, it can be valuable in checking for such problems as obstruction of the kidney, stones, or a hidden tumor in the upper urinary tract, in estimating how well the bladder is emptying, and determining the size of the prostate.

Cystoscopy also may be needed, especially if your symptoms are severe, if you have blood in your urine or a history of repeated infections, or if your doctor suspects that you have a stricture or other out-of-the-ordinary prob-lem. This procedure is uncomfortable but not painful. A cystoscope is a tiny, lighted tube that works like a periscope on a submarine. It is inserted in the tip of the anesthetized penis and threaded through the urethra into the bladder; this allows the doctor to inspect the bladder, prostate and urethra for abnor-malities such as stones, enlargement, or strictures. With cystoscopy, your doc-tor may also be able to see thickened muscle bands in the bladder—these indicate a condition of bladder obstruction that has evolved over months or years—and rule out the presence of such other conditions as a bladder tumor, bladder stone, or urethral stricture. (Note: As with the catheter used in pres-sure flow studies, this test carries a slight risk of a urinary tract infection developing from the urethral irritation caused by the inserted tube. Some men also experience blood in the urine or temporary inability to urinate.) Cysto-scopy is often used to assess the situation before an invasive procedure such as surgery.

Intravenous Pyelogram (IVP), an X-ray view of the urinary tract, can also determine urinary obstruction or the presence of tumors in the kidney. It works like a glow-in-the-dark picture: A special dye is injected, making urine visible and its path from the kidneys and out of the body easily traceable—and any blockage easy to see. Some men have severe allergic reactions to this dye, so this test is not routinely used. (Unfortunately, there is no way to predict who will have such a reaction.) It's usually reserved for evaluating men who have blood in their urine.

THE SHORT STORY

The term *benign prostatic hyperplasia,* or BPH, refers to enlargement of the inner portion of the prostate. Like wrinkles and gray hair, this is something that happens almost inevitably as men get older—it's present in 50 percent of men in their fifties, and in 80 percent of men in their eighties. (However, if BPH is almost a certainty for most men, its annoying symptoms don't have to be. Treatment options are discussed in detail in Chapter 10.)

It's important to note that the key word here is *benign. BPH is not prostate cancer.* If it weren't for the fact that the prostate encircles the urethra (the tube that carries urine from the bladder through the prostate to the penis), BPH might never require treatment. But over time, as BPH progresses, the prostate tissue begins to squeeze the urethra and interfere with urine flow.

This is a complicated process. Part of the problem is that *glandular tissue* in the prostate begins to enlarge, and lumpy nodules in this tissue begin sprouting up like mushrooms. Meanwhile, to make matters worse, *smooth muscle tissue* in the prostate begins to tighten. So together, these kinds of prostate cells act as a "double whammy" on the urethra: As the glandular tissue enlarges and begins to clog the urethra, the smooth muscle tissue contracts, and starts to clamp down on the urethra.

What sets all this in motion? Scientists aren't entirely sure. But it is clear that two important factors are aging—BPH hardly ever occurs in men younger than 40—and the testicles. Studies have shown that BPH never occurs in men who lose their testicles before puberty. It may be that hormones produced by the testicles play a major role, or their presence may only be permissive—they may simply provide the necessary soil for the disease to take root and grow.

There also seems to be a genetic component to the disease. Scientists have recently discovered a new, hereditary form of BPH; a small number of men inherit a gene that predisposes them to prostate enlargement. One day, as scientists learn more about the genetics of BPH, they may at last understand its true causes—and then perhaps this discovery will make it possible to prevent BPH from developing at all.

Do you have BPH? There are some telltale symptoms. These include: A weak urinary stream, hesitancy in starting to urinate, and difficulty maintaining and stopping the stream (this can include a small amount of "dribbling" afterward). Also, many men with BPH have to urinate frequently, especially at night, and often with a strong sense of urgency. If not treated, these symptoms can lead to some serious problems, including urinary retention—when the bladder stays completely or partly full—and even kidney damage.

Men who have any of these symptoms should see a doctor to determine exactly what the problem is. It's important to know if you have BPH. It's equally important to make sure you don't have a more serious condition such as prostate cancer, urinary tract infection, bladder cancer, bladder stones, a neurogenic bladder (a bladder affected by a neurological disease), or a urethral stricture (scar tissue that blocks the urethra); all of these can mimic BPH.

The doctor's evaluation will include a detailed medical history, a physical, including a digital rectal exam; a urinalysis (examination of urine for bleeding and infection); and blood tests to check the level of PSA (an enzyme produced by the prostate) and to evaluate kidney function. Depending on your symptoms, you also may need other tests including a measurement of urinary flow rate (uroflowmetry), a check for residual urine in the bladder, an evaluation of the upper urinary tract with ultrasound or X-rays, cystoscopy (a "periscope" view of the urethra and bladder), and, for some men, bladder pressure tests to rule out neurological conditions.

After the diagnosis of BPH has been confirmed, the next step is to decide, with your doctor, what to do about it. That brings us to the subject of Chapter 10.

10

When BPH Needs to Be Treated

WHEN DO I NEED TREATMENT?

Many men would much rather suffer the inconvenience of BPH than seek medical or surgical help. However, there are times when symptoms can no longer be ignored and treatment is needed. These include:

A "Backed-Up" Bladder, Impaired Kidney Function, or Overflow Incontinence. Sometimes, when the bladder is too full for an extended period and is not emptying completely, the mounting pressure can cause the urine to back up in the kidneys—which can lead to severe damage if left untreated. The first step here is simply to drain the bladder, by means of a catheter threaded into the urethra through the penis. For most men, function of the upper urinary tract (kidneys and ureters) improves right away. Some men may be given oral replacement of fluids and key minerals to flush the body of impurities and prevent dehydration once the pressure is relieved. The fate of the lower urinary tract (recovery of function in the bladder, prostate, and urethra) is less certain, and depends on how much—*and for how long*—strain has been placed on the bladder.

Acute Urinary Retention, the Inability to Urinate. Don't wait on this one; the consequences of not urinating can be grave, and may lead ultimately to kidney failure. Acute urinary retention may be caused by a range of conditions, including acute prostatitis, prostate cancer, an over-distended bladder, and even some medications—most commonly, cold remedies that contract the smooth muscle in the prostate (just as they decongest the nose by constricting the same kind of muscle tissue there). The good news is, this often takes care of itself after a catheter has drained the bladder.

Recurrent Urinary Tract Infections, associated with residual urine. Sometimes, when urine lingers too long in the body—if the bladder is not completely drained for months—it becomes infected. And if the fundamental problem, urinary obstruction, is not solved, it's difficult to get the infection cleared up.

Bladder Stones, also associated with residual urine. These form when crystals of uric acid or calcium precipitate into the urine. It is possible just to treat the stones—uric acid stones can be dissolved medically, by drugs that make the urine more alkaline; and many techniques are available to crush calcium-containing stones. *But these measures do nothing to relieve obstruction.* And the fact that a man has developed a bladder stone in the first place usually means he's got a significant problem with urinary obstruction, which needs to be treated.

An Unstable Bladder, with urge incontinence. From half to as many as 80 percent of men with BPH eventually develop bladder instability, producing the irritative symptoms caused by an embattled, strained bladder. In most cases, these go away with surgical relief of the obstruction—again, the results depend on how much of a burden the bladder has borne, and for how long. These symptoms include increasingly frequent or urgent urination, particularly during the night, and most significantly, urge incontinence—a real warning sign that the bladder is in trouble. If this is not treated (by easing the obstruction), it may reach a point where the damage is irreversible and this incontinence is permanent. Or, if a man delays treatment for too long and then has surgical treatment, this urge incontinence can actually get *worse*—because the obstruction has been relieved, now there's even less tissue to hold back these uninhibited contractions when they occur.

Severe, Recurrent Episodes of Bleeding. This could mean a serious medical condition, such as bladder or prostate cancer. If you're passing blood clots in your urine, you should seek treatment immediately. But blood in the urine may also be related to BPH: In some men, there are big veins that cover the enlarged BPH tissue along the urethra; these veins may break open spontaneously. (Such bleeding tends to occur more frequently in men who regularly take aspirin.) Typically, men with BPH-related bleeding report that they pass a small clot when they begin to urinate, and also note bleeding during urination. This bleeding usually stops after several days but may require cystoscopy, so the bleeding vessels can be cauterized. Repeated episodes are usually a good indication for surgery. (Recently, doctors have reported some success with hormonal therapy as a treatment for bleeding. For more on how hormonal therapy works, see Chapter 7.)

Symptoms that Reach the Point of Diminishing Your Quality of Life, However You Define This.   So think about it: Has BPH changed your life? Are you still able to do everything you want to do? Or are you adjusting your life to accommodate your BPH—giving up seats to a baseball game, for instance, so you won't have to endure the long lines in the men's room?

If you're planning your day around trips to the bathroom, consciously or not, it may be time to seek treatment. Once you've reached this point, here's the next question: Do you want treatment badly enough to run the risk of side effects or complications? If your symptoms are mild or moderate and the answer is no, then watchful waiting (see below) is probably the way to go. But if the answer is yes, educate yourself. Learn as much as you can about these options and the risks involved. Talk to other men with BPH—those who have had treatment, and those who've decided to wait. And most importantly, talk to your doctor. Until fairly recently, the only treatments for BPH were surgical, and many men shied away from them. But now, so many options are available for managing BPH that more men are opting for treatment earlier in the course of the disease than ever before.

WHAT ARE MY OPTIONS?

The first option is called "watchful waiting," and *it doesn't mean "do nothing." It means "wait and see."* The course of BPH is often hard to predict; your symptoms could improve, get worse, or stay the same. Beyond watchful waiting, broadly speaking, there are two paths—surgical and medical. (See table 10.1, page 257.) The choice depends on the severity of your symptoms. If you have one or more of the conditions mentioned above that require treatment, your best option is surgery. But if your symptoms are moderate—that is, not severe enough to require surgery—a trial of medical therapy makes sense.

Watchful Waiting

This is the most conservative approach to BPH, and for most men with mild symptoms, it's the best. *Remember, just having an enlarged prostate does not mean you need treatment.* It's only when the symptoms of enlargement become bothersome, or if your urinary function is seriously affected, that you should consider treatment. So, many doctors begin with what's called a "watch-and-wait" approach to the problem. They keep a close eye on your condition, with checkups once or more a year to make sure you're not developing any complications. Sometimes the symptoms of BPH get better on their own. If they don't, then you and your doctor will move on to the next step—deciding what treatment's best for you.

Risks. Like any other treatment option, watchful waiting is also something of a gamble—low-risk, but a gamble all the same. A few men in programs of watchful waiting develop acute urinary retention, the inability to urinate. A few develop urinary tract infections; some see blood in their urine; some go on to develop kidney or bladder damage *without any noticeable change in their symptoms* (this is called silent prostatism). But such complications from watchful waiting are rare indeed. You can lower the odds even further by limiting your fluid intake before bedtime and by refraining from taking certain over-the-counter medications, such as decongestants, which can make your BPH symptoms worse.

SURGICAL TREATMENTS AND PROCEDURES

Prostatectomy

A century ago, a New York surgeon developed a procedure called "simple," or "open," prostatectomy. He reached the prostate through the bladder and used his fingers to remove the overgrown tissue surrounding the urethra, leaving the rest of the prostate intact. (This is not the same thing as a radical prostatectomy, the removal of the entire prostate, which is often used to treat localized prostate cancer.) A refined version of this procedure, which surgeons call suprapubic prostatectomy, is still used today in a small percentage of men with BPH; so is a variation of it called simple retropubic prostatectomy.

But another form of prostatectomy, developed nearly fifty years ago, has eclipsed both operations and is now the main form of surgical treatment for BPH. In this procedure, called transurethral resection of the prostate (TUR; also called a TURP), surgeons reach the prostate by taking a different route— through the urethra. Unlike other forms of prostatectomy, this does not involve a long hospital stay; there's no incision or scar, and the recovery time is shorter. *One major benefit of the TUR—and all forms of prostatectomy—is the opportunity to check the prostate tissue that was removed for cancer after surgery.*

The TUR is available to men who otherwise might not be eligible for surgery. About 95 percent of the prostatectomies performed in this country are done transurethrally. And despite the development of new techniques to relieve urinary obstruction, the TUR remains the gold standard for BPH treatment.

However, the TUR is not for everybody. For example, men with large prostates (with obstructive tissue that's estimated to weigh more than seventy-five grams, or two and a half ounces) probably should have an open prostatectomy. So should some men with large diverticula of the bladder that need to be treated, or men with large bladder stones. (Diverticula are pockets of the bladder lining that poke out like balloons through the bladder wall.) If diverticula or bladder stones need to be removed, this procedure can be "piggybacked" onto (done at the same time as) an open prostatectomy—as surgical "one-stop shopping."

Nor is the open prostatectomy ideal for every man. The average age of men who have a prostatectomy is 70; by this time in life, many men have other health problems that preclude open surgery—such as a history of heart or lung disease, diabetes, or high blood pressure. For most of these men, and for men with a small prostate, the TUR is the best option. The open prostatectomy is generally reserved for younger men, and those with very large prostates who are otherwise healthy and in good cardiovascular condition.

If your health is considered too precarious even for the TUR, there's still help—a catheter can provide immediate relief of an overfull bladder, for example. Early studies show intraurethral stents to be a good option for long-term relief of symptoms. Also, you may be able to take medication to shrink the prostate. These and other options are discussed in this chapter.

Before Open Prostatectomy or TUR

Are you in shape for surgery? Your doctor will want to check you out thoroughly beforehand. Surgery may be delayed if certain conditions, such as a urinary tract infection, need attention, or if a catheter is needed to empty the bladder. Men with urinary retention and an elevated level of creatinine in the blood (indicating impaired kidney function) must also be treated for these conditions before having a prostatectomy. When you give the doctor your medical history, be sure to say so if you've had any unusual problems with bleeding in the past (from dental work, for example). Also, aspirin can cause excessive bleeding; *if you are taking aspirin regularly, make sure you stop at least ten days before the operation.*

Another important point to discuss with your doctor: About 15 percent of men who undergo open prostatectomy need a blood transfusion during the procedure. The best blood for you to receive is your own; if your hospital allows this, it's a good idea to donate several units of your blood ahead of time.

Shortly before surgery, your doctor may want to get a baseline evaluation of your upper urinary tract to spot anything out of the ordinary. One way of doing this is with ultrasound, which can help detect hydronephrosis (distention of the ureters and renal pelvis, caused by an obstruction downstream) and pick up any unusual masses in the kidneys. This painless, noninvasive technique will also give doctors a pretty good indication of the size of your prostate and the state of your bladder—whether there's any residual urine there. And at the time of surgery, your doctor will probably use a cystoscope—a lighted tube, inserted into the tip of the anesthetized penis—to check for any other surprises in the bladder, such as a stone or tumor that needs to be removed.

What Happens to the Urethra?

In all forms of simple prostatectomy, a chunk of the urethra between the bladder neck and the external sphincter is removed along with the overgrown BPH tissue. So, if the urethra is cut during surgery, how can a man have normal urinary function afterward? The answer is that nature does a pretty good job of helping the body heal itself.

Remember, the whole prostate is not removed—just the innermost part that lines the urethra. The outer shell remains. This shell is lined with small prostatic ducts and, during the first six weeks after surgery, these ducts produce cells that help the normal lining regenerate. (This same regeneration explains why, over time, some men will need more than one operation to keep BPH under control.) The regeneration process is similar to what happens in a split-thickness skin graft, used to treat someone who's been badly burned. In this procedure, part of the healthy skin is removed and transferred to a severely burned area of the body. The part of the skin that stays behind then renews itself from its reservoir of hair follicles and ducts.

Open Prostatectomy: The Suprapubic Approach

Anesthesia

You will be anesthetized; this can happen several ways. Most likely, you'll have either spinal or epidural anesthesia. With both forms, you remain conscious and aware of the procedure, even though you can't feel it. In *spinal anesthesia,* you'll receive a shot of local anesthetic in the small of your back through the dura, the membrane lining the spinal cord, and into your spinal fluid. Within minutes, you'll feel numb, relaxed and heavy from your waist to your toes. After surgery, you'll be asked to lie flat in bed until the numbness goes away and you can move your legs again. *This is important; sitting up too soon can cause a severe headache. Epidural anesthesia* is like having an IV tube hooked up to your back, instead of to a vein in your arm. A local anesthetic enters the body through a tiny plastic tube, inserted between the vertebrae of your spine near the small of your back. The epidural anesthetic (often used to provide pain relief in pregnant women during labor) bathes the area outside the membrane lining the spinal cord, temporarily numbing the nerves in your lower body. Unlike spinal anesthesia, which comes in one dose, epidural anesthesia can be given continuously. The area of numbness can be adjusted; so can the degree of pain relief. After surgery, this tube can also be used to administer pain relief for the first few days.

During Surgery

To reach the prostate (see figure 10.1), a urologist makes an incision in the skin and muscles of the lower abdomen to expose the lower part of the bladder, which is opened next. The surgeon's index finger reaches into this incision in the bladder and through the bladder neck to remove the tissue at the prostate's innermost core, the part compressing the urethra. The surgical description for what happens here is that the tissue "enucleates." For the most part, what this means is that the tissue separates from the surrounding tissue like a walnut from its shell. (At some places, however, a few cuts must be made so some stubborn bits of tissue can be removed along with the rest.)

Because it allows access to the bladder, this procedure is ideal if any problem there, such as a bladder stone or a large bladder diverticulum, needs attention. With the patient's permission (given before surgery), some surgeons perform a vasectomy during this operation to prevent the development of inflammation in the epididymis. (Epididymitis can result from damage to the ejaculatory ducts, which allows infected urine to "back up" into the vas deferens.) A vasectomy involves cutting the vas deferens, so sperm can no longer exit the urethra during ejaculation but are reabsorbed into the body.

The prostate tissue the surgeon has removed is sent to a pathologist, who will examine it for the presence of hidden cancer. The average hospital stay for this surgery is five to seven days.

Afterward

You'll receive fluids intravenously (through your veins) the day of surgery, but you should be able to eat normal meals the next day. You'll probably be given a stool softener or mild laxative to keep you from straining and to make the first bowel movement after surgery easier. A Foley catheter, inserted in the penis (and anchored by a tiny balloon in the bladder) during surgery, will remain in place until the bleeding has stopped. In addition to removing urine from your body, the catheter also keeps the bladder irrigated to help prevent infection or a blood clot from developing. Another catheter is inserted during surgery; this one is called a suprapubic tube because it's placed directly in the bladder and exits through the lower abdomen. It will be taken out between three and five days after surgery. Your incision probably will have staples, not stitches, and these will be removed one week after the operation—probably on your return visit to the doctor's office. When you get home, take it easy but don't just sit around the house—gradually resume your usual exercise and activity. You should feel fully recovered within four to six weeks.

Complications

Like any surgical procedure, open prostatectomy is not without risks, the chief one being blood loss that requires a transfusion. All surgery involving anesthesia carries the risk of death, but this is extremely rare. The serious surgical complications that sometimes befall patients in the over-50 age group, such as a heart attack, pneumonia, or a blood clot in the lung, are also extremely rare. To help prevent such aftereffects, however, *it's crucial to get moving again as soon as possible after surgery*—so be sure to walk, move your legs in bed, and do breathing exercises.

Other complications include epididymitis, if a precautionary vasectomy wasn't performed during surgery; and bladder spasms (painful, uncontrollable contractions of the bladder, forcing urine out in spurts around the catheter)— which may be largely attributable to the presence of a catheter, and which should improve once the catheter is removed.

After the catheter is removed, some men may have trouble with stress incontinence—when urine leaks during certain physical activities, like running or playing golf. This may be temporary, and may resolve itself during the first few months after surgery. In rare cases, however, it is permanent, either as a result of damage to the urinary sphincter during the operation, or as the inevitable consequence of years of bladder damage, persistent bladder instability and urgency incontinence—when urine leaks as a man who urgently has to go to the bathroom is trying to get there.

The most common aftereffect of open prostatectomy is retrograde, or "dry," ejaculation. Impotence (difficulty achieving or maintaining an erection) may affect as many as 15 to 20 percent of men. (This is an unverifiable statistic; it's tough to try to quantify impotence, because so many factors are involved. For more on impotence, see Chapter 8.)

Also seen, but rarely (in 2 percent of men), is a constriction of the bladder neck, called a bladder neck contracture, which is caused by scar tissue from the surgery. This can be reopened in outpatient surgery by a urologist. (Using a cystoscope, the urologist makes a few tiny cuts to relax the tight scar tissue.)

In rare cases, men may also develop a urethral stricture (scar tissue in the urethra). Most urethral strictures respond well to dilation—stretching the urethra, in one or two sessions. Stubborn strictures can also be treated with tiny incisions, like those done to ease bladder neck contractures.

Open Prostatectomy: The Retropubic Approach

Similar to the suprapubic operation in terms of anesthesia and recovery, the retropubic approach is preferred by many surgeons because it allows better access to the prostate and a more accurate approach to the urethra.

Figure 10.1 (a, b, c). *The suprapubic approach*

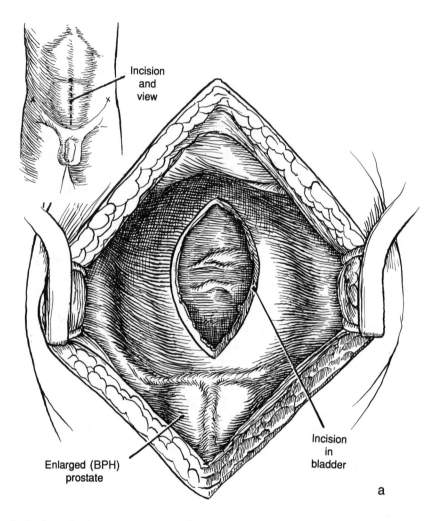

Incision and view

Incision in bladder

Enlarged (BPH) prostate

a

In this form of open prostatectomy (*a*), the surgeon reaches the prostate by making an incision in the skin and muscles of the lower abdomen to expose the lower part of the bladder, which is opened next. The surgeon's index finger reaches into this incision in the bladder (*b*) and through the bladder neck to remove the overgrown tissue at the prostate's innermost core, the part compressing the urethra. After surgery (*c*), the excess tissue is gone, leaving a cavity around the urethra.

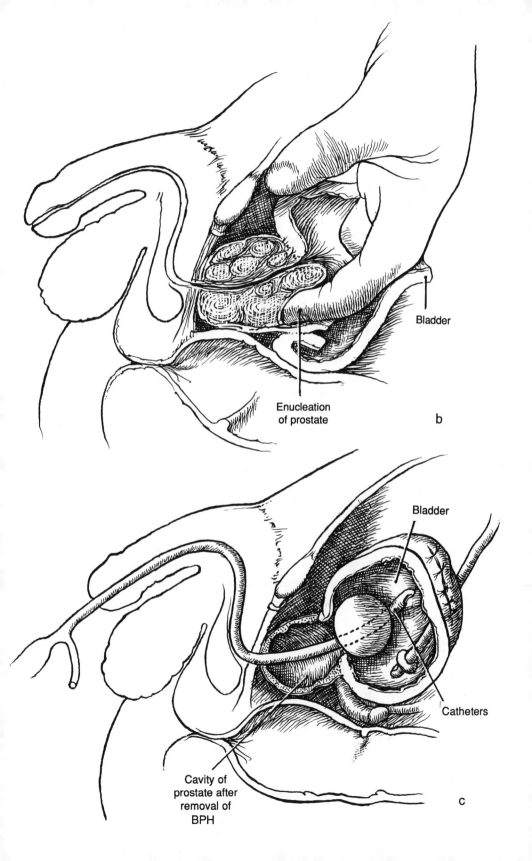

Bladder

Enucleation
of prostate

b

Bladder

Catheters

Cavity of
prostate after
removal of
BPH

c

What Happens

In retropubic prostatectomy, surgeons go directly through the top of the prostate, rather than through the bladder—first making an incision in the lower abdomen, and then separating the abdominal muscles. Instead of opening the bladder, the surgeon moves it aside, and there, beneath the pubic bone, is the prostate.

A small incision is made in the outer capsule of the prostate, and (as in suprapubic prostatectomy) the surgeon's index finger is inserted to remove the overgrowth of prostate tissue compressing the urethra. To avoid the development of epididymitis, many surgeons go ahead and perform a vasectomy during this procedure (see above). The prostate tissue removed during surgery is then sent to a pathologist for examination.

Transurethral Resection of the Prostate (TUR)

What Happens

The prostate's innermost core is removed, usually after spinal anesthesia (see above), without opening up the abdomen. This operation, called a TUR procedure, is a proven, effective way to improve BPH symptoms quickly, and keep them at bay for years. In a TUR procedure, surgeons reach the prostate via the urethra by placing an instrument like a cystoscope through the penis. This instrument, called a resectoscope, shines a powerful light that allows surgeons to view the prostate as they chip away at excess tissue. (This tiny instrument even has its own "windshield wiper," which irrigates the lens and keeps the area clear for surgeons to see.) The prostate's core is removed in fragments, by means of electrosurgical cautery. These tissue chips amass in the bladder, and at the end of the procedure, they're flushed out, collected and sent to a pathologist for examination. Because the resectoscope is threaded through the urethra, no skin incision is needed.

After Surgery

A Foley catheter is inserted into the urethra and the bladder is continuously irrigated with a salt solution for the first twenty-four hours to prevent blood clots from forming. This catheter is usually removed in two to three days. The average hospital stay is one to three days. Most men have little or no pain after a TUR. When pain does occur, it's usually because of bladder spasms, involun-

Figure 10.2. *The TUR procedure*

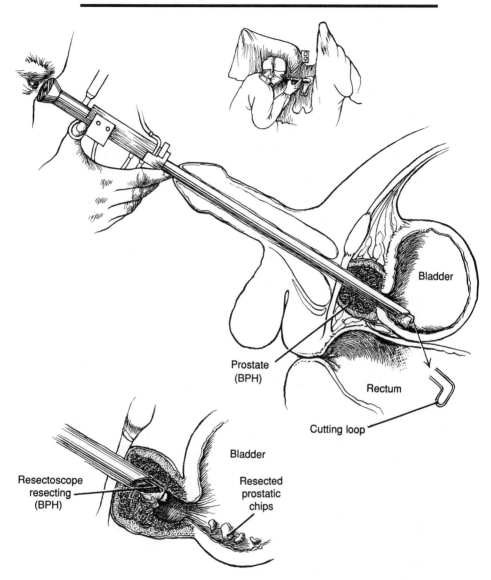

Despite an explosion of new treatments for BPH, this remains the gold standard—the TUR. Here's how it works: Surgeons reach the prostate via the urethra. An instrument called a resectoscope, threaded through the penis, shines a powerful light that allows surgeons to view the prostate as they chip away at excess tissue. (This instrument even has its own "windshield wiper," which irrigates the lens and keeps the area clear for surgeons to see.) The prostate's core is removed in tiny fragments. Tissue chips amass in the bladder; at the end of the procedure they're flushed out, collected and sent to a pathologist for examination.

tary contractions of the thickened bladder around the Foley catheter. These usually go away when the catheter is removed. You should be feeling fully recovered in about three weeks.

Complications

Bleeding.   Bleeding after surgery can be caused by too much activity, including straining to go to the bathroom. Your doctor will probably give you a stool softener or mild laxative to make that crucial first bowel movement after surgery easier. Also, you'll probably be advised to steer clear of aspirin and strenuous activity for the first four weeks after surgery to avoid a delayed episode of bleeding. With the TUR procedures, there's a lower risk than with open prostatectomy of bleeding during and after surgery that requires a transfusion. (In one study, 7 to 14 percent of men who underwent TUR needed transfusions.) Bleeding seems to be associated with the size of the prostate and duration of surgery; a larger prostate generally means more tissue to remove, and thus a longer time spent in the operating room.

The "Rollerball" Variation.   In a brand new approach to TUR, surgeons use an electrocautery "rollerball" instead of the cutting loop. Overgrown tissue is vaporized, not chiseled away, so there are no leftover chips. The technique is highly promising: It appears to have minimal complications, little bleeding, and shorter catheterization and hospital stays. And, while it offers many advantages of laser prostatectomy and other high-tech procedures, it's far less expensive. There are many good reasons to believe the rollerball may soon become the technology of choice.

TUR Syndrome.   This, too, occurs very rarely—in about 2 percent of patients. It's caused when the body absorbs excessive amounts of the irrigating fluid used during the TUR procedure. Its symptoms are nausea, confusion, vomiting, high blood pressure, a falling heart rate, and visual problems. TUR syndrome is temporary and is quickly reversible with diuretics or a saline solution, which help restore the body's normal fluid and mineral balance.

Perforation of the Prostate or Bladder.   Another rare complication, this also occurs in 2 percent of patients. Its symptoms are nausea, restlessness, vomiting, and pain in the lower abdomen or back that can be felt despite the anesthesia. This is generally taken care of by stopping the operation and draining the bladder with a catheter. The injury can be allowed to heal on its own, or in severe cases it can be repaired surgically.

Inability to Urinate. The most common problem right after surgery—experienced by 6.5 percent of men in one study—is the inability to urinate. Sometimes this goes away in a few hours. If it doesn't, your doctor may want to investigate to make sure no excess tissue is remaining in your prostate. You might also need to have cystometry (see Chapter 9) to check bladder function. Sometimes the trauma of surgery causes the bladder to become slack; the temporary placement of a catheter, giving the bladder a few days' respite, seems to help bring the bladder tone—and, with it, the ability to urinate—back to normal.

Urinary Tract Infection. The presence of bacteria in the urine, sometimes associated with fever, may develop in as many as 10 percent of men who have a TUR, and is easily treated with antibiotics. Men over age 80 are more likely to have problems with urinary retention and urinary tract infection than younger men.

Bladder Neck Contracture. Rarely—in fewer than 3 percent of men who have a TUR—scar tissue develops at the neck of the bladder, just above where it empties into the prostatic urethra. This generally happens within the first four to six weeks after surgery. After experiencing a good urinary stream for several weeks, some men notice a sharp change—the stream is poor again, like it was before surgery. What's happened is that scar tissue is blocking the urethra, just as the tissue in BPH did, except the dam in the river has moved upstream. This can be diagnosed with a cystoscope in an outpatient procedure. By making a few tiny incisions, your urologist can open the scarred tissue and restore urine flow.

Urethral Stricture. Another rare complication, occurring in fewer than 3 percent of men after a TUR, this is caused by trauma to the urethra—sometimes from a catheter, and sometimes from the resectoscope.

Incontinence affects from 2 percent to 4 percent of men who have a TUR. It can have several causes: One is damage during surgery to the external sphincter—the valve that opens and shuts at the junction between the prostate and urethra (see figure 5.1). Another is a bladder that's been damaged and rendered hypersensitive by months or years of urinary obstruction from BPH; it might be that surgery has come too late to undo the years of damage. A third possibility is that there's some residual prostatic tissue blocking the urethra, which either is holding the external sphincter open or is obstructing the urethra, producing overflow incontinence.

Most men experience temporary urgency and stress incontinence after the catheter is removed; it takes the urethra hours to days to recover from being stretched or irritated by having the catheter inside. Persistent stress incontinence (leaking urine when you stand up or exercise) is rare, and total incontinence is almost unheard of. There's also something you can do to help control stress incontinence—Kegel exercises, which strengthen the external sphincter. The best way to do them is when standing to urinate: Try to start and stop your urinary stream by contracting the muscles in your buttocks. There are other methods of performing Kegel exercises, but by doing them this way you can be sure you're exercising the right muscles.

If incontinence doesn't get better over time, your doctor may do cystometry to determine the state of the bladder, or check with a cystoscope to make sure there's no residual prostatic tissue blocking the urethra. Some drugs may also help: If you have urgency incontinence, for example, anticholinergic drugs can help stop involuntary bladder contractions. For stress incontinence, drugs that cause smooth muscle tissue to contract—such as nasal decongestants, or even an antidepressant that often makes it more difficult to urinate (a drug called imiprimine)—can help. If incontinence persists for more than a year, or is severe, your doctor may suggest further treatment—possibly placement of an artificial sphincter. In this procedure, a rubbery cuff is positioned around the urethra and connected by tubing to a reservoir for fluid that's installed in the abdomen, and to a small pump, placed in the scrotum. The pump transfers fluid from the reservoir to inflate the cuff (and block the urethra), and a valve next to the pump can be released to deflate the cuff and allow urine to pass through the urethra. The artificial sphincter is an elaborate device; but there are several simpler solutions that involve injecting material (collagen) into the tissue around the urethra or bladder neck. It's possible that with further refinements, these techniques will be sufficient for managing incontinence in almost all men who develop it.

Impotence has been reported in as many as 10 percent of men after a TUR, but this is the most difficult to document of all the postsurgical complications. *In some older men, impotence just develops spontaneously, whether or not they've had surgery.* And there are so many variables to consider—self-consciousness; the presence or absence of a sexual partner; even a man's perception of his sexual ability before and after surgery. For example, when some men who reported trouble with erections after surgery were studied, doctors found they could still have erections during their sleep—which suggests at least part of the problem could be psychological. It's safe to say that if a man was having trouble achieving or maintaining an erection before the TUR, surgery probably hasn't helped the situation. And that a man who was sexually active before surgery probably will continue to be. (For a discussion of impotence after prostate surgery, see Chapter 8.)

"Dry" Ejaculation may happen in as many as 75 percent of men after TUR. It has nothing to do with sexual performance, and does not change the pleasant sensation of orgasm.

Results

It's important to understand that *no form of prostatectomy stops BPH; these procedures only treat the disease that's present.* It's a bit like mowing the lawn, in that, depending on how fast the prostate grows back, the procedure may have to be performed again.

In a recent study of more than 400 men who had the TUR procedure, *symptoms improved markedly in 93 percent of those with severe manifestations of BPH, and in 79 percent of those with moderate problems.* None of the men died as a result of the procedure, none had a heart attack, and only 5 percent reported impotence. In other research on men who've undergone the TUR, the improvement in urinary flow has been shown to last longer than seven years after surgery in most men.

Despite generally excellent results, TUR has come under fire recently. Some research has suggested that it's less effective, in the long run, in fighting urinary obstruction than open prostatectomy. One such study examined the long-term progress of men in Denmark, England, and Canada, who underwent either open prostatectomy or TUR: 13 percent of those who had TUR needed a second procedure, as opposed to 3.5 percent of men who'd had open prostatectomy. (The proportion of men having had a TUR who need a repeat TUR amounts to about 1 percent to 2 percent a year.) However, from this and other studies, it's clear that, given the choice, many men would *rather* have two TURs over ten years than one open prostatectomy.

In the same controversial study, investigators raised another issue: The statistics suggested that, four or five years after surgery, TUR might be associated with a higher likelihood of death from heart attacks than open prostatectomy. (The likelihood of a man dying from a TUR itself is almost nonexistent—less than 0.5 percent.) Further research, however, brought an explanation—that *men undergoing open prostatectomy were healthier to start with*. Men with heart disease and a large prostate were excluded from undergoing open prostatectomies; the more complicated nature of this procedure demanded healthier patients. With the simpler TUR procedure, however, *nearly all men*—including those with heart disease—were still considered eligible for surgery. Thus, the increased number of deaths from heart disease four or five years after surgery can be fully explained by the fact that *more men with heart disease underwent a TUR than underwent open prostatectomy*.

TUR Versus Watchful Waiting. In a recent Department of Veterans Affairs study involving 556 men at several medical centers, researchers systematically compared men who underwent TUR to men with moderate to severe BPH symptoms who opted for watchful waiting. The average age of patients was 66; the study lasted three years.

In this study, the TUR patients were the clear winners in terms of symptom improvement and quality of life. They had "significantly fewer treatment failures, fewer crossovers to alternative treatment, and less bother from urinary symptoms," the researchers noted. (Some men in the watchful waiting group eventually decided to have a TUR to relieve symptoms.) Men in the TUR group also had a greater improvement in their symptom scores, urinary flow, and quality of life. (Interestingly, spouses or "significant others" were also asked to evaluate their mates' quality of life, and their reports confirmed the patients' own assessments.)

The researchers concluded that TUR was safe, that it did not cause incontinence and impotence, and that it was associated with very few short- or long-term complications in men who didn't have any serious health problems; reoperation rates were also low. Based on these findings, they determined that TUR was superior to watchful waiting in reducing symptoms and improving quality of life in men with moderate to severe BPH. However, they also noted that watchful waiting didn't cause significant harm to anyone—and therefore, that for men with tolerable symptoms a conservative approach is certainly reasonable.

Transurethral Incision of the Prostate (TUIP)

What Happens

In terms of anesthesia, recovery, and mode of access to the prostate, this procedure is similar to the TUR: An instrument called a resectoscope lights the way for surgeons to see the prostate; the resectoscope is threaded through the urethra, so no skin incision is needed. The difference is that, *instead of removing the excess prostate tissue, surgeons just make two tiny longitudinal cuts in it.* (See figure 10.1.) These incisions extend from the bladder neck down into the prostate, and they break the ring of tissue's stranglehold on the urethra—giving it "breathing room." Like the TUR, this procedure is preferable for men whose prostates are not grossly enlarged, and is the procedure of choice for men in whom the prostate is smaller than thirty grams, or one ounce.

It is also better suited to younger men, mainly because of one key advantage: The TUIP is more likely to preserve normal ejaculation than TUR. (This has nothing to do with sexual function or performance; it means simply that these men are more likely able to father a child. Otherwise, there's no noticeable difference in orgasm between the two procedures.) Men who undergo TUR report a slightly better urinary flow rate than men getting the TUIP procedure. And it's not certain whether the effects of TUIP last as long as those of TUR. The re-operation rate is about the same for both procedures, about 1 to 2 percent a year.

One concern with TUIP is that it produces no resected tissue chips—and thus, no way of checking for prostate cancer; some doctors recommend going ahead and performing a biopsy of the prostate during this procedure, as long as they're "in the neighborhood." The average hospital stay for TUIP is one to three days.

LESS INVASIVE PROCEDURES

Balloon Dilation

For more than a century, doctors have tried to find mechanical means—using catheters, for example—of opening up the urethra constricted by BPH. In this technique, originally designed for expanding clogged arteries, a balloon is passed into the narrowest part of the urethra and then inflated to stretch the

Sexual Problems after Prostatectomy and Other Procedures

The good news is that, *for most men, surgery for BPH has no effect on sexual function or performance.* One aftereffect of prostatectomy that may take some getting used to is a phenomenon called "dry," or retrograde, ejaculation. It's pretty much what it sounds like— semen is not expelled out the urethra when a man reaches sexual climax. Instead, it goes the other way—back into the bladder. This happens because part of the bladder neck is usually resected along with the prostate tissue, so the bladder neck does not contract at the time of ejaculation—and there's nothing to prevent semen from heading in that direction. For most men, this does not alter the pleasant sensation of orgasm. Also, having semen in the bladder does no harm; it is eliminated from the body the next time a man urinates.

This "dry" ejaculation is the most common sexual side effect, and it has *nothing to do with* a man's ability to have an erection or to reach a sexual climax. If you are not planning to father children, this is nothing to worry about.

Some 10 to 15 percent of men who have BPH surgery report problems with impotence, or difficulty with erections. Even this does not have to be a permanent problem. There are many options to help men with impotence (see Chapter 8), now more than ever before.

opening, and thus improve urine flow. (See figure 10.4.) This procedure has a lot of advantages: It's safe and simple, can be done on an outpatient basis using a local anesthetic, and so far has shown no signs of causing impotence or retrograde ejaculation. Even the most high-risk patients, those in precarious health, are eligible and can get immediate relief of symptoms.

But does it work, and for how long? The answer is, symptoms may improve at first, but the results don't last. One study found a 50 percent improvement in urinary flow at one month; however, this improvement disappeared after one

Figure 10.3. *The TUIP procedure*

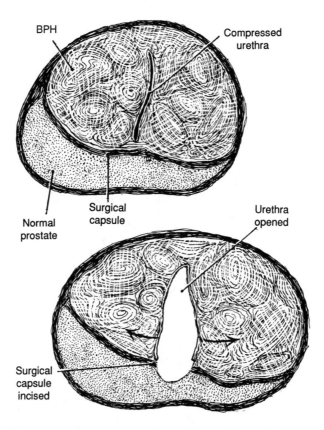

BPH

Compressed
urethra

Surgical
capsule

Normal
prostate

Urethra
opened

Surgical
capsule
incised

In BPH, lobes of prostate tissue become a binding ring around the urethra. In the TUIP procedure, this ring is cut, so the lobes spring apart—instantly creating more space around the urethra.

year. Current studies suggest that balloon dilation is not a long-term cure, that
the urethra does not stay open for years, as it does with prostatectomy. (As one
urology textbook puts it, "It would appear that the objective, long-term results
will be measured in months, rather than years.") Much more research is
needed. Also, not everyone is a good candidate for this procedure; for example,
it's not recommended in men with a decompensated bladder, middle lobe
enlargement, or an active urinary tract infection. Finally, the procedure does

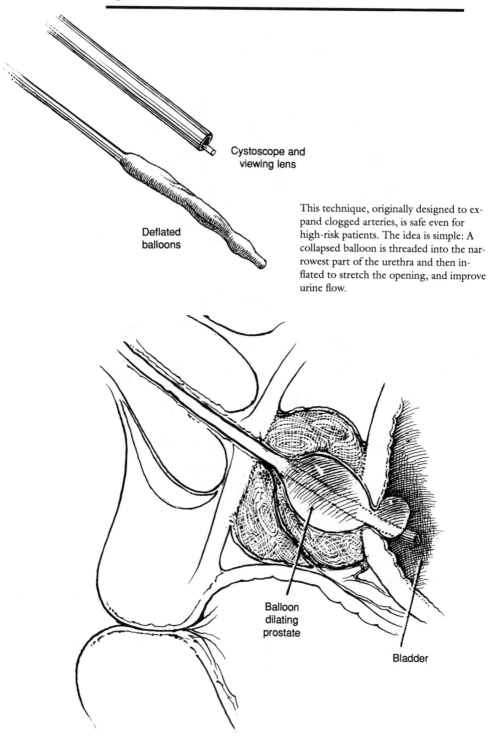

Figure 10.4. *Balloon dilation*

Cystoscope and viewing lens

Deflated balloons

This technique, originally designed to expand clogged arteries, is safe even for high-risk patients. The idea is simple: A collapsed balloon is threaded into the narrowest part of the urethra and then inflated to stretch the opening, and improve urine flow.

Balloon dilating prostate

Bladder

not yield any tissue samples for a pathologist to inspect for prostate cancer, so a digital rectal examination and PSA blood test are as important now as ever.

NEW TREATMENTS, AND HOW TO EVALUATE THEM

The last several years have seen an explosion of new information and strategies for managing BPH; many more advances lie on the horizon. It's tough for anyone—including doctors—to assimilate the sometimes confusing, often conflicting reports of the latest innovations in treating BPH.

So what are you supposed to do? When you read about a breakthrough in the newspaper or hear about it from a friend, how should you evaluate it?

Here are some basic principles:

Beware of the Placebo Effect.   This is the first "grain of salt" to take into consideration in any study. Researchers are always wary of the placebo effect, an inexplicable improvement in the so-called "control" group who are taking "sugar pills," which they believe to be real medication. In almost every study of a drug or treatment for any disease, there is some improvement in the control group. This phenomenon is almost always attributable to a boost in mental health that comes from taking part in a study, or from the belief that some new medication is making a real difference in symptoms. (However, it also reminds us never to underestimate the powerful effect of a positive attitude on physical symptoms!)

With BPH, there is a tremendous placebo effect to any form of treatment. In one series of studies that included a placebo group, 30 percent to 75 percent of placebo-treated men reported subjective improvement in their urinary symptoms—this means that they believed their symptoms were better—and as many as 15 percent to 20 percent reported significant improvement in urinary flow rates.

Look at the Study.   If you can, ask your doctor for a copy of the study, or at least get the reference to the medical journal in which it was published. Before you accept any results, make sure the new drug or technique has been evaluated in a *randomized, controlled study* that lasted at least one year. If it's a medical (as opposed to surgical) or minimally invasive form of treatment, the trial should include a placebo-treated group of patients for comparison. If it's a more invasive form of treatment, the results should always be compared to the accepted gold standard—in this case, the TUR. Is there a noticeable improvement in benefits?

Next, make sure that both *subjective and objective* results were measured. (Remember, encouraged by being involved in a study, a man might feel that his flow rate has improved more than it actually has.) All participants in the study should at least have completed symptom scores and had uroflow measurements taken. Ideally, the study should be stratified according to age, risk factors and severity of obstruction. Endoscopic treatment techniques preferably should be compared only to TUR and, if feasible, these studies too should include a placebo-procedure group.

Ask about the Complication Rate, and the Need for Retreatment.
Consider the cost. How long will the treatment be effective? Although a technique appears to be safe and can easily be done as an outpatient procedure, if it has to be repeated at frequent intervals (as in balloon dilation), it's not going to be very valuable to most people. The study should include a clear analysis of side effects and costs, and these should be compared with established surgical therapies and with watchful waiting. *A final word,* and in the excitement over new breakthroughs this can be easy to forget: *BPH doesn't kill people.* Fortunately, many effective and safe treatments are already available. BPH isn't an incurable, devastating disease. And because of this—because we're not desperately racing the clock for a cure—we can be careful not to rush into new technologies until we're sure they are safe and effective.

NEW TREATMENTS: WAVES OF THE FUTURE?

The treatments in this section all have something in common: Waves. They all channel a form of energy—heat, radio frequency, ultrasound, microwaves, and light—to kill cells. Energy waves are generated, focused, aimed, and fired at the overgrowth of BPH tissue surrounding the urethra. Some waves work like a shotgun, blasting holes in the prostate. Others are as sensitive as a scalpel, delicately nibbling away at BPH tissue until the urethra is free.

As yet, none of these treatments can be classified as standard therapy. *They're still too new; long-term results are not yet available.* It's not certain how long their effect on BPH will last, and whether men will need to have repeat procedures.

But some of these alternative treatments are highly promising. They include:

Thermal (Heat) Therapy

This group of procedures can be divided into three categories based on temperature. The normal body temperature, 98.6 degrees Fahrenheit, is 37 degrees centigrade. *All of the temperatures discussed below are in centigrade.*

Hyperthermia, the mildest approach, uses temperatures that are *less than 45 degrees*—which probably isn't hot enough to accomplish major relief of obstruction. In *thermotherapy,* tissue is heated to temperatures *greater than 45 degrees*—at which point some cellular protective mechanisms are overwhelmed, and normal cells are destroyed. To make sure *only* the BPH tissue is destroyed, temperatures in the region are monitored closely during this treatment. *Thermal ablation* techniques can produce the hottest temperatures of all—*above 60 degrees*—and are usually performed using high-intensity focused ultrasound, transurethral microwave therapy, interstitial radio frequency waves, and lasers.

An important fact about thermal therapy is that—except for contact laser prostatectomy—the BPH tissue in the targeted area is killed *but not removed.* One problem with this is that many men experience acute swelling immediately after these procedures and may need a catheter until the dead tissue is re-absorbed by the body, or is sloughed into the urethra and washed away in urine. (Another problem is the lack of tissue samples for pathologists to examine.) This marks a big difference from surgical procedures such as TUR, where the obstructive tissue is extracted, and the patient generally can urinate well immediately afterward.

As noted, temperatures in hyperthermia range from 41 degrees to 45 degrees. *As heat treatment goes, these temperatures are rather lukewarm.* Hyperthermia is not painful, and it can be performed as an outpatient procedure; it usually involves multiple treatments. It can be done in two ways—transrectally, by a probe inserted into the rectum, and transurethrally, by an instrument inserted through the penis into the urethra.

The technique has only recently undergone randomized, placebo-controlled studies, in which patients were treated without knowing whether the heat generator was activated. The largest recent study has demonstrated *no significant objective improvement in urinary flow rates.*

Why is this? For more than a century, doctors have known that heat can kill cancer cells. Hyperthermia as a treatment for BPH grew out of techniques used to treat malignancies, including prostate cancer. It can be given to cancer patients along with radiation because rapidly multiplying cancer cells in certain phases of division are particularly susceptible to heat.

The basic problem here is that *normal cells respond differently than cancer cells;* and just because a technique works on cancer cells, it doesn't necessarily follow that it will work in normal tissue. BPH tissue—though growing—is benign, not cancerous, and it just isn't that sensitive to these temperatures. Scientists who have looked under the microscope at BPH cells heated to 45 degrees have trouble telling them apart from BPH cells that have not been treated. Hyperthermia isn't hot enough to kill BPH tissue. The tissue reacts, certainly, but the results are not permanent, and the injured tissue eventually recovers. *So at this point, using temperatures less than 45 degrees should be considered an ineffective solution to a long-term BPH problem.*

Transurethral Microwave Thermal (TUMT) Therapy

This form of treatment uses microwaves to produce temperatures hotter than 50 degrees and "zap" the tissue in the prostate's innermost core, thereby creating space around the urethra. These temperatures are hot enough to do some good; they are able to destroy the smooth muscle and glandular cells in BPH tissue. What grows back over the next few months is a different mixture of cells that include collagen.

TUMT works by miniature remote control: A tiny antenna that targets BPH tissue surrounds a catheter that goes through the penis and into the urethra. The microwave generator is situated nearby, in the rectum. (The device is called the Prostatron.) The degree of power is controlled by different software programs that can produce a range of temperatures.

At Temperatures below 60 Degrees C. The technique produces significant improvements in urinary symptom scores and in urinary flow rates, but little change in pressure-flow urodynamic studies—which suggests that the ultimate improvement in obstruction may not be great. The procedure can be performed under local anesthesia.

Figure 10.5. *Using microwaves to "zap" the prostate*

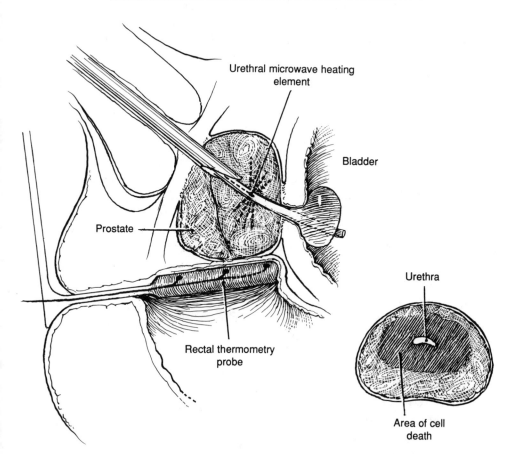

The TUMT approach uses microwaves to generate heat and destroy tissue around the urethra, giving it some breathing room. It works by miniature remote control: A tiny antenna that targets BPH tissue surrounds a catheter that goes through the penis and into the urethra. The microwave generator is situated nearby, in the rectum.

At Really Hot Temperatures—from 60 to 75 Degrees (this may be needed in cases of severe obstruction)—the treatment can create gaping cavities where tissue used to be. This can cause irritative symptoms that last until the tissue in the prostatic urethra dies and then is sloughed and reabsorbed by the body, or washed away by urine. (When all the dead tissue is gone, the prostatic urethra should be much less constricted.) The treatment causes inflammation and may require stronger pain-killing medication. Swelling and urinary retention (usually temporary) are also common after the procedure and can be eased with a catheter. Preliminary results are encouraging. However, how long these results will last—and whether or when a repeat procedure will be necessary—is not yet known.

Laser Prostatectomy

Have you ever focused the sun's rays through a magnifying glass? The glass harnesses just a fraction of the sun's colossal energy, but the focused light beam is powerful enough to burn a hole through a leaf or to start a small fire.

A laser is focused light, and it's an awesome source of energy that cuts a path wherever it's aimed. Two distinctive methods—called "non-contact" and "contact"—are available for laser prostatectomy. Although both spring from the same energy source—light—they involve different techniques.

Non-Contact Laser Techniques

Non-contact techniques include the TULIP (Transurethral Ultrasound-Guided Laser-Induced Prostatectomy) device and the side-firing Urolase Fiber. Both produce temperatures from 60 to 100 degrees. (The energy varies with the strength of the beam. Picture a flashlight shining in a dark room. As the beam spreads and diffuses, so does its energy; at its outermost edges, it is least powerful.) The TULIP device features an ultrasound scanner, which gives surgeons a picture of the areas the laser will target and allows for greater accuracy. The side-firing technique is performed through a cystoscope, whose tiny camera allows surgeons to view the procedure on a television monitor. This also is called the VLAP (Visual Laser-Assisted Prostatectomy) procedure. These non-contact techniques use a transurethral probe, inserted through the tip of the penis, that beams the laser at a 90-degree angle directly into the prostate.

Like thermotherapy, non-contact laser prostatectomy does not remove BPH tissue. Instead, space is created around the urethra when the "zapped" tissue dies, sloughs away, and is absorbed back into the body. Because of this, both non-contact techniques cause swelling in the prostate (just as tissue swells around a burn), resulting in obstruction and the need for a catheter for several days in some men. Really hot temperatures (which may be needed for severe

Figure 10.6. *One laser technique*

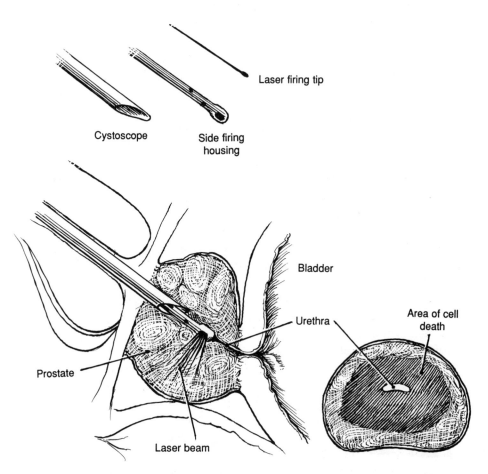

Laser firing tip

Cystoscope

Side firing housing

Bladder

Urethra

Area of cell death

Prostate

Laser beam

This illustration shows a side-firing laser, used through a cystoscope. The laser blasts BPH tissue, which soon dies, sloughs away and is absorbed back into the body—thereby creating extra space for the urethra.

obstruction) can blast holes in the prostate; these can cause irritative symptoms until the tissue has dissolved into tiny particles that are flushed out over time during urination, which will result in the gradual widening of the prostatic urethra.

The Contact Laser Techniques

In a contact laser prostatectomy, the laser probe actually touches—and immediately vaporizes—the BPH tissue, producing temperatures between 500 and 700 degrees. So—poof! The obstructing tissue is gone immediately. Tissue touched by the laser probe instantly turns to steam. Energy from a kind of laser known as Neodynium (Nd):YAG, which penetrates deeply into tissue, is conducted through a flexible fiber (a fiberoptic pipe that conducts the light energy) and is used through a standard cystoscope. This energy can produce temperatures well over 60 degrees, which can either "cook" (and thus kill) tissue or vaporize it altogether. Yet, as powerful and as hot as the contact laser is, it barely penetrates tissue even one millimeter beyond the point of vaporization. There is no delayed sloughing; only the tissue touched with the probe is affected. Essentially, "What you see is what you get." In other words, only the tissue removed the day of surgery is going to be gone from the prostate—no other tissue will die and be sloughed off days or weeks later. This is a key difference between the contact and non-contact laser techniques.

The contact method is more time-consuming than the non-contact technique; in this it is much more like a standard TUR than other laser prostatectomies. The potential advantages over TUR include less bleeding (and therefore a lower risk of a transfusion), no risk of TUR syndrome, less risk of incontinence and urethral stricture, and the possibility of shorter hospitalization and catheterization (a catheter is required for about three days after surgery). Also, symptoms appear to improve earlier than after non-contact laser surgery. One point to consider is the size of a man's prostate: The probes currently being used are small and work best on smaller prostates (with a volume of less than 50 grams or slightly under two ounces). Because there is less bleeding, this form of treatment is ideal for men who are taking anticoagulants.

Laser Prostatectomy: Pros and Cons. One advantage of laser prostatectomy is that surgeons can use smaller instruments, which should produce fewer strictures, scars resulting from injury to the bladder neck or urethra. And, if the bladder neck is not treated, there should be no retrograde ejaculation and no sexual dysfunction. These techniques cause less bleeding, and unlike the TUR they can be performed on an outpatient basis under local anesthesia. Also, there's no fluid absorption (so no risk of TUR syndrome).

To date, the biggest problems with these still relatively new techniques have been prolonged urinary obstruction after the operation in some patients, and the need for a catheter (either in the urethra or a suprapubic tube, attached directly to the bladder) for several days after surgery. Also, it takes longer for laser prostatectomy to improve urinary flow than for TUR. So, laser surgery may not be best for an impatient patient. *The ideal candidate for laser prostatectomy should have a prostate that weighs less than sixty grams or two ounces; should not have urinary retention; and should have mainly obstructive, not irritative, symptoms.*

Another problem is that no tissue samples are available for pathologic study. And if the energy beam creates holes in the prostate, there can be distressing irritative symptoms that persist until the tissue has dissolved and been flushed from the body.

Moreover, lasers may not be as widely available as other forms of treatment because of their cost: Laser fibers are very expensive, and most of them can't be reused. For each laser procedure, the laser fiber alone costs about $800. (The laser machines themselves cost hospitals about $100,000, but they can be used for other procedures.)

Results: Early randomized trials comparing laser prostatectomy to TUR demonstrate that urinary flow rates and symptom improvement are better in patients who have TUR. In these early laser studies, about 10 percent of men needed to be retreated in the first year. Laser treatment of BPH is too new for anyone to make predictions about its long-term effectiveness.

So, the jury's still out; the final verdict on laser prostatectomy won't be given until we know what the true retreatment rates will be. Currently, the results for laser prostatectomy aren't as immediate or as long-lasting—and improvement is not as dramatic—as in TUR. However, unlike TUR, laser prostatectomy doesn't involve hospitalization, and it can be done under local anesthesia. Currently, many men would rather have two TURs in ten years than one open prostatectomy. It may be that, in the future, men will prefer to have two or three treatments with a laser than one TUR. Another point to keep in mind, as a Stanford urologist noted in a recent journal article, is that "all laser devices available today represent first-generation products . . . All will most likely become obsolete in the foreseeable future," as the design of these devices, and the knowledge it takes to use them, continues to improve.

High-Intensity Focused Ultrasound (HIFU)

Ultrasound energy can be focused with exquisite precision to produce temperatures hotter than 65 degrees within a few seconds. The focus is so sharp that

Figure 10.7. *Focused ultrasound at work*

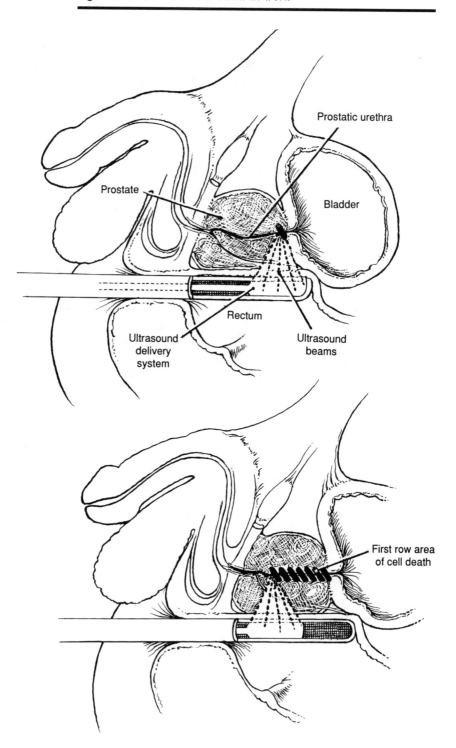

areas outside it—even those a fraction of an inch away—are not heated or damaged. The ultrasound works like a scalpel (and in this precision, HIFU has a key advantage over microwave therapy). The HIFU selectively blasts BPH tissue; like the hottest TUMT therapy, it can form cavities in the prostate. Over time, this tissue liquifies and is reabsorbed by the body or flushed out during urination. With such high temperatures, some form of anesthesia (spinal or local) is needed during the procedure.

There have been very few side effects to this procedure, the main one being temporary urinary retention in most men. Early studies of HIFU in animals and men have been promising. One highly sophisticated HIFU unit currently being tested (called Sonablate) comes equipped with a rectal probe that uses ultrasound to map out the prostatic urethra.

Transurethral Ultrasonic Aspiration of the Prostate (TUAP)

The technique here is often used in operations on other tissue—in eye surgery, for example—and now doctors have begun applying it to BPH. It uses a special ultrasound probe that works through an endoscope, a lighted "periscope" used in exploration and treatment of many diseases. The ultrasound targets tissues high in water content, like BPH tissue, while leaving surrounding tissue in the bladder neck, urethral sphincter, and elsewhere in the prostate un-scathed (this surrounding tissue has a different makeup—more collagen, less water). The probe simultaneously breaks up the BPH tissue and flushes it out of the body; an aspirator device in the instrument vacuums up the tissue fragments.

In one study of fifty-nine men who were followed a year after the procedure, there was no incontinence, and no men reported urinary problems; two men had bladder neck contractures, and one man developed a stricture in the urethra at the tip of the penis. About 85 percent of men reported retrograde ejaculation. Men who may not benefit from this procedure are patients with middle lobe enlargement, because the ultrasound does not work as well in tissue near the bladder neck.

Opposite: Ultrasound energy can be focused on BPH tissue with exquisite precision to produce searing, cell-killing temperatures within seconds. Over time, the dead tissue is reabsorbed or flushed out of the body.

Transurethral Needle Ablation (TUNA)

Radio frequency energy can also be conducted through tiny needles, which are inserted directly into prostate tissue via a special catheter. The needles can riddle the BPH tissue with holes of various sizes to weaken the tissue's grip on the urethra. Experiments using TUNA in animals have been promising, and clinical trials of this technique are under way. The TUNA device is battery-operated, and may be among the least expensive of these techniques.

Pyrotherapy

This is the least invasive of these thermal therapies; in fact, there's not even a probe to enter the body. Here's how it works: Multiple ultrasound waves are focused at a single point some distance away from the power source. Only the concentration point, the target where all these beams intersect, is damaged. The cumulative energy of these waves, entering the body through a broad area, is great enough to cause thermal injury to BPH tissue and to create cavities in the prostate around the urethra. A prototype system (called Pyrotech) has been tested, and clinical trials are under way. However, it is not yet certain whether pyrotherapy will be able to pinpoint the prostate tissue surrounding the urethra as precisely as it needs to—entering the body either through the abdomen or perineum—because the bony pelvis gets in the way; this may turn out to be an insurmountable obstacle.

Cryotherapy

In this treatment, instead of heat, the opposite—extremely cold liquid nitrogen—is used to freeze and kill cells in BPH tissue. Guided by transrectal ultrasound, doctors circulate the freezing liquid nitrogen through three to five metallic probes, which are placed in the prostate gland through the perineum. A special catheter works like a hot water bottle to keep the urethra from freezing. There are no long-term studies to determine the effectiveness of this procedure. (For more on cryotherapy, see Chapter 6.)

Intraurethral Stents

Stents are tubes, implanted and left in place to hold open a space that otherwise would collapse or be compressed—in this case, in the urethra where it's

Figure 10.8. *Holding the pathway open*

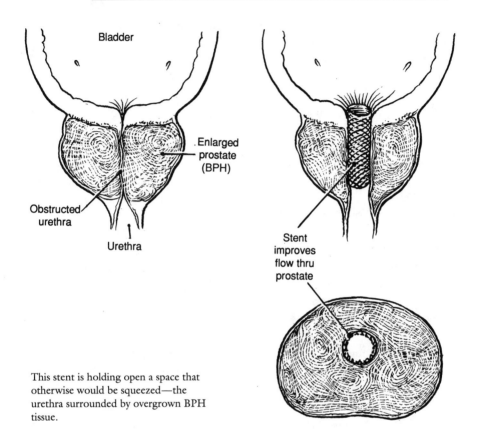

Bladder

Enlarged
prostate
(BPH)

Obstructed
urethra

Urethra

Stent
improves
flow thru
prostate

This stent is holding open a space that
otherwise would be squeezed—the
urethra surrounded by overgrown BPH
tissue.

choked by the prostate. The tubes are not visible and can be implanted quickly,
in outpatient surgery that lasts about fifteen minutes. They are a good option
for older men who are too ill to be eligible for other procedures. They're also a
major addition to the meager range of alternatives formerly available to these
men. Until recently, this consisted mainly of bladder catheters, left in place
indefinitely, whose presence in the body over time leads to urinary tract infection, sepsis, bladder stones, and even kidney damage.

With the stents, there's no need for a urinary catheter, and the procedure
can be performed under local anesthesia. There's hardly any bleeding during

or after the operation, minimal recovery time, and sexual function is not impaired.

The stents come in several models. The newest ones are made of nickel-titanium alloys, which are flexible and have an intrinsic memory—they expand when heated, and become flaccid and increasingly malleable when cooled. They're easy to install and, when positioned correctly, will expand when irrigated with warm water. If it becomes necessary to remove them, these stents can be irrigated with cold water, which cause them to contract and become malleable again. They're designed to be incorporated into the body, to meld with the epithelial tissue lining the urethra—a feat that takes the body about three to six months to accomplish, as the tissue knits a thin blanket of cells to cover the tube. Why is this coverage necessary? It's like greasing a pan before cooking so nothing will stick to it—except the "grease" here is the body's own cells. (During this time, bicycle riding and other activities that put pressure on the perineum should be avoided.)

One drawback of the stents is that no prostate tissue is removed and sent to a pathologist for examination. Also, the possibility exists that, over time, the epithelial tissue lining the urethra could do such a good job of covering the tube that it might overgrow the stent, and surgery to correct this may be needed. Stents aren't a good option for men with BPH in the middle lobe; the site of enlargement interferes with the coverage of epithelial cells.

Results.   Long-term results with permanent stents are not available. Temporary stents made of nickel alloy appear to be well tolerated, with few problems of becoming encrusted with stones. The permanent stents made of nickel-titanium alloy have been used for both the treatment of BPH and of urethral strictures. These also appear to be associated with fewer problems such as encrustation and urinary tract infection.

Complications with the stents are few and, in most cases, seem to resolve themselves over time. Most men experience irritative symptoms—some incontinence, a sense of urgency to urinate, and a need to urinate frequently—and some discomfort in the perineum for days to weeks after the operation. Anticholinergic drugs may be prescribed to help slow a too-frequent need to urinate. A few men in one study reported painful ejaculation the first time they had sex after the operation, but this went away with later sexual activity.

Sometimes the stents don't work out—if the irritative symptoms persist, or if the epithelial cells fail to cover the tubes adequately, causing them to become

Table 10.1 *How to Select the Appropriate BPH Treatment Option*

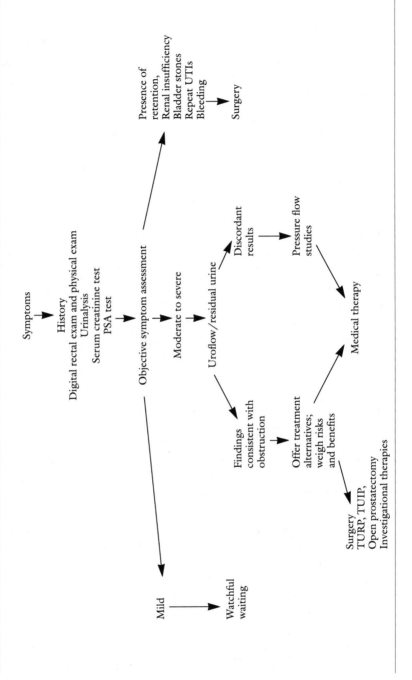

clogged. In these and other studies, when this happened the stents were re-moved intact, without harming the urethra or the bladder's external urinary sphincter. Stents can also be repositioned, and sometimes just a slight adjust-ment in their placement can resolve such symptoms as incontinence and uri-nary retention.

MEDICATIONS FOR BPH

From a medical standpoint, most of the drugs used to treat BPH are still very new. There have been no long-term studies of how well they work, and how they compare to surgical treatments for BPH. When a patient with BPH really needs treatment, surgery is still the option most urologists prefer, for several reasons. One is that pills must be taken daily; their effect ends soon after you stop taking them, and a prescription might well mean taking these pills for life. Also, it may take weeks on medication before any improvement is noticeable. The TUR procedure, particularly, has faster and more effective results than any medications for BPH currently available. Nonetheless, because surgery is not an option for all men—and because many men have symptoms that are annoy-ing but not severe enough to warrant surgery—the availability of drugs means more treatment alternatives than ever before. And perhaps just knowing there's something out there besides surgery will encourage some men who until now have been reluctant to seek help for their symptoms.

Drugs currently being developed and used to treat BPH attack the problem in two ways: One strategy is targeted at shrinking the prostate by interfering with the hormones that cause certain prostate cells to enlarge and accumulate (see "What Makes the Prostate Grow?" in Chapter 9). The other is aimed at keeping the prostate muscle tissue from tightening around the urethra.

DRUGS THAT MAKE THE PROSTATE SHRINK: 5-ALPHA REDUCTASE INHIBITORS AND LHRH AGONISTS

5-alpha Reductase Inhibitors (Finasteride, Proscar)

A drug called finasteride acts by shrinking the prostate and decreasing the obstructive symptoms of BPH. But it may do more than simply ease the symptoms of BPH—*it may halt its progression.*

Table 10.2 *Major Endocrine Factors That Stimulate the Prostate*

Gland	Location	Hormone	Action	Inhibitor
Hypothalamus	Brain	LHRH	Releases LH and FSH from the pituitary	Estrogen
Pituitary	Brain	LH	Acts on testicles to cause testosterone secretion	LHRH agonists (Lupron, Zoladex)
Testicle	Scrotum	Testosterone	Prostate growth	Inhibitors of androgen synthesis
Prostate	Pelvis	DHT	Prostate growth	5-alpha reductase inhibitors, such as finasteride

Finasteride works by thwarting a hormonal process without affecting levels of testosterone, the hormone responsible for a man's libido and sexual function. Scientists have learned that the trouble in BPH starts *after* testosterone is converted by an enzyme called 5-alpha-reductase into a substance called *DHT,* which is the active form of male hormone within the prostate. Finasteride stops testosterone from changing to DHT by blocking this enzyme. So the amount of DHT in the bloodstream and prostate tissue drops; but because testosterone levels in the blood remain unchanged, impotence is not a problem for most men who take finasteride. The drug causes a significant reduction in the tissue surrounding the urethra, which is responsible for obstruction.

In one study of 1,600 men with BPH, finasteride shrank prostate size over a two-year period by an average of 25 percent, improved urinary flow significantly in 31 percent of the patients, and brought some relief of symptoms in 71 percent of these men. Finasteride achieved this benefit with very few side effects—the main one being the development of impotence, which occurred in only 3.4 percent of men and was reversible when the men stopped taking the drug.

Results from this and other studies show that while this drug is helpful, it's not for everybody. The gains in urine flow, for example, are much higher in men who undergo the TUR procedure, and for men with minimal symptoms, these gains would hardly be noticeable. However, the drug might prove helpful in men with moderate to severe symptoms of BPH—for example, those with a weak urinary stream, hesitancy in starting urination, or who are making so many nighttime trips to the bathroom that they're losing sleep.

The bottom line: Currently, a man taking finasteride has about a 30 percent chance of seeing a significant improvement in his symptoms—and this will come *only* after six months to a year of taking the drug. Finasteride is not a fast-acting treatment for BPH. Its major advantage is that it causes the prostate to shrink—and in control studies, it appears that once the prostate does shrink, it tends to stay shrunk. Perhaps most exciting is that it may prevent the disease of BPH from progressing.

However, there's another point worth noting: About 10 percent of men who undergo prostatectomy for the treatment of BPH are found to have some cancer in the bits of prostate tissue that are removed. This is one of the advantages of having surgery for BPH; you can rule out the presence of prostate cancer. But in men taking medicine to treat BPH, the presence or absence of prostate cancer is less easily determined.

One concern with finasteride is that it lowers concentrations of prostate-specific antigen (PSA) in the blood by 50 percent. Why is this a problem? In recent years, the PSA blood test has become an important means of checking for prostate cancer, and finasteride could obscure the results of this test in the men who are taking the drug. Therefore, before embarking on a long-term course of finasteride, it's vital to have a digital rectal exam and PSA blood test and, if your PSA is high (see discussion of PSA in Chapter 3), a prostate biopsy to rule out the presence of cancer.

Once a man is on finasteride, his PSA levels should drop about 50 percent during the first year and then remain constant. If his PSA levels fall to less than 50 percent, or if they start to rise while he's on the drug, something's not right, and there are two possibilities. One is that he's not taking the drug regularly or properly. The other is far more serious—he could have prostate cancer. In any event, a change in PSA levels definitely needs to be investigated.

LHRH Agonists (Lupron, Zoladex)

Testosterone is made in the testes, but it's the pituitary gland that really calls the shots: The pituitary gland transmits a chemical signal, called luteinizing hormone (LH), which motivates the testes to make testosterone. But LH can be blocked by a synthetic analog (a chemical look-alike that acts differently) of another of the body's chemical messengers. This messenger is called LHRH (for luteinizing hormone-releasing hormone; it's also called GnRH, for gonadotropin-releasing hormone).

Here's how it works: LHRH, made in the brain by the hypothalamus, is

Finasteride and Prostate Cancer

Can finasteride help prevent malignant growth in the prostate? In other words, can it stop prostate cancer from forming? The National Cancer Institute has launched a multimillion-dollar study to find this out. For seven years, this massive project will follow 18,000 men, aged 55 and older, who are otherwise healthy (men with any prostate ailment, benign or otherwise, are not eligible). All of the men will take daily pills; half of them will get finasteride, the rest will get a placebo. All of the men will have regular physical exams, including a digital rectal exam and PSA test, during the study period. And, at the end of the study, all of the men will have a prostate biopsy. The study is double-blind—neither the men participating in the study nor the physicians treating them will know who's getting the finasteride until it's over.

Why do scientists think a BPH drug can have an effect on prostate cancer? One reason is that finasteride lowers a man's levels of PSA, an enzyme made by the prostate used as an indicator for prostate cancer (see Chapter 3). Another assumption is tied to the fact that finasteride works by interrupting a hormonal process (it blocks an enzyme called 5-alpha-reductase, which changes the male hormone testosterone into a substance called DHT—the active form of male hormone within the prostate). Prostate cancer is intrinsically linked to hormonal activity. So maybe, some scientists speculate, by thwarting the prostate's normal hormonal pattern, prostate cancer can be stopped before it ever has a chance to begin.

However, other scientists doubt that finasteride will have any effect in preventing prostate cancer. First, there's no evidence that DHT is the hormone responsible for the growth of prostate cancer. In fact, the levels of 5-alpha reductase activity are actually *lower* in prostate cancer than in normal tissue. Also, there's no supporting evidence from laboratory experiments to suggest that finasteride will work; in one animal tumor model, in fact, finasteride has no effect at all. And finally, finasteride's effect in men who already have prostate cancer is marginal at best—which makes it unlikely that it will have any effect in preventing the disease.

dispatched in signal pulses—like Morse code or flashes of light—to the nearby pituitary gland. These pulses tell the pituitary to make LH. The powerful synthetic analogs called LHRH agonists work by providing *prolonged* stimulation—by turning on the light and *keeping* it on, for example, instead of just flashing the light. So these drugs trick the pituitary: Because the pituitary receives no flashes, or pulses, it thinks no signal is being sent. And it doesn't make LH. It's like a chess game, and LHRH agonists effectively put LH—and therefore, testosterone—in checkmate.

Why is it so important to stop production of testosterone? Testosterone, not in itself the prime culprit of BPH, represents just one step in a chain of chemical interactions involved in BPH—but it's a big one. One of the most convincing demonstrations is the study in which scientists achieved a "chemical castration," by suppressing testosterone in patients with BPH. They found that prostate size decreased by an average of 25 percent, reaching a plateau after about four months. When they reversed the chemical castration—by allowing testosterone production to resume—prostates returned to their former size.

That's how LHRH agonists work, by shutting down testosterone. They do help BPH symptoms—in the above study, for example, one-third of the men had improved rates of urinary flow—and they may be an option for men who are not candidates for surgery. But as with any medication that must be taken regularly (as shots once a month), beginning this kind of therapy means assuming the cost of medication for years. Also, improvement is not immediate; it takes weeks or months before the prostate begins to shrink.

LHRH agonists are not standard therapy for BPH, mainly because in cutting the body's levels of testosterone they cause impotence, hot flashes and weight gain. For BPH, such results are considered extreme and cause most men (except for those who are already impotent) and their doctors to wonder which is worse—the disease or the treatment. However, for an elderly man who has urinary retention and is not a candidate for other forms of treatment, an LHRH agonist may be successful and may act quicker than finasteride.

Of course, in prostate cancer—for which these drugs are mainly used—it's a different story. Potency assumes a lower rung on the ladder of priorities in the face of a life-threatening disease.

DRUGS THAT RELAX THE PROSTATE

Alpha Blockers

Remember the two kinds of tissue involved in BPH? One is glandular and is made up of epithelial cells, which secrete fluid that becomes part of the semen. The other is smooth muscle tissue—the stromal cells, whose automatic contractions squeeze this fluid out of the prostate and into the urethra. In BPH, these kinds of tissue act together as a one-two punch: As the glandular tissue enlarges and begins to clog the urethra, the smooth muscle tissue tightens like a fist, and clamps it. But something else is happening with these two kinds of tissue: The balance between them is shifting. *In the normal prostate, there are two stromal cells for every epithelial cell; in BPH, it's five to one.* Researchers have described BPH, on a cellular level, as a "stromal process." In other words, it's a smooth-muscle problem. And one way to make the passage of urine easier is by taking a drug that relaxes this muscle tissue.

This concept is still relatively new in terms of mainstream drug treatment for BPH (although scientists have been studying alpha blockers and their effect on BPH symptoms for more than fifteen years). But medical researchers have studied smooth muscle tissue, in blood vessels and intestinal walls, for decades. They know, for example, that its actions are involuntary responses to signals from the nervous system. That certain neurotransmitters—chemical messengers which target receptors on the wall of the prostate's smooth muscle cells—are responsible for making this tissue contract. That other chemical messengers, designed to *block* these transmitted signals, can make this clenched tissue relax. And that the distribution of these alpha-1 adrenoceptors—they seem to be particularly abundant in the bladder base and prostate—makes alpha-blocking drugs ideally suited for relieving the obstructive symptoms of BPH. The drugs can selectively target and relax muscle cells in the prostate and bladder neck, while ignoring the cells involved in voluntary control of urination.

This promising class of drugs got its start as a treatment for some forms of hypertension, which can involve the same kind of smooth muscle contractions (in blood vessels, not the prostate) as those in BPH. In 1981, the Food and Drug Administration approved an alpha blocker called prazosin (Minipress), for treatment of high blood pressure. Prazosin has a relatively short half-life in the body, and must be taken more than once a day. In 1986, terazosin (Hytrin), an alpha blocker with a longer half-life, was approved by the FDA for treatment of hypertension. Recently, an FDA panel recommended that terazosin be approved for treatment of BPH. Other alpha blockers such as doxazosin (Cardura) are available, and still others are being investigated for use as potential BPH drugs.

In a recent multi-center study, terazosin was given in various doses, ranging from two to ten milligrams daily, to more than 200 men. (Men who had "absolute indications" for prostatectomy—the conditions mentioned above—were not included in the study, and should not be considered eligible for this treatment.) Only the men receiving 10 milligrams, the largest dose, had a significant improvement in urinary flow rate and obstructive and irritative symptoms, and the study suggested that larger doses could be given to bring about even greater results. The study proved the drug to be safe and effective in most men. It also found that some of the side effects, such as dizziness, were less of a problem if the drug was taken at night—which might be best anyway, as bedtime is often when BPH is at its most annoying. In another study, symptoms improved in 72 percent of men with BPH for at least two years of treatment with terazosin.

The change in symptoms and improvement in urinary flow with alpha blockers isn't as dramatic as it is after prostatectomy, and alpha blockers aren't recommended for men with severe symptoms. On the other hand, alpha blockers create fewer side effects than prostatectomy—and they're all reversible when men stop taking the drug. One advantage of alpha blockers is that they work almost immediately, unlike finasteride, which must be taken for months before any change is noticeable. A drawback is that alpha blockers don't change the course of BPH—they work like cold pills, just treating the symptoms, not the underlying cause of the illness. If your doctor prescribes an alpha blocker, you'll probably be checked regularly over the first few weeks to fine-tune the dosage of the drug. Then you should be seen every few months to have your prescription refilled and your symptoms checked.

Side Effects. Alpha blockers improve urine flow by relaxing clenched smooth muscle tissue. Because their effect is not limited simply to the prostate, they may not be best for men with a history of significant heart disease or blood pressure problems. But they don't seem to have any adverse effects on blood pressure or heart rate in men who are otherwise healthy. They are vasodilators —they open up blood vessels, making a wider channel for blood to go through, which means they reduce blood pressure. Their side effects can include dizziness, heart palpitations, lightheadedness or even fainting, nasal congestion, and fatigue, especially during the first few doses. These symptoms tend to improve over time as the body adjusts to the drug. They also seem to be diminished in men who take the drug at night.

ON THE HORIZON: DRUGS OF THE FUTURE?

Currently, major medical therapy for BPH falls into two main categories—one class of drugs to shrink the prostate, and another to relax the smooth muscle. Which is better? It probably depends on each man's particular makeup of prostate cells. It's assumed that men with more epithelial cells will respond better to finasteride, and that men with an overgrowth of smooth-muscle cells may respond better to alpha blockers.

These two types of drugs are currently being tested against each other in a large randomized study being carried out by the Veterans Administration.

They're also being tested—and this may revolutionize drug treatment—*in combination.* Using finasteride and alpha blockers together makes a lot of sense. Indeed, it's possible that the second generation of medical therapy for BPH will involve medication that combines a drug like finasteride with an alpha blocker.

Another exciting possibility is a group of drugs that are called "subtype-selective." Scientists recently have learned that the 5-alpha reductase enzyme, which converts testosterone to DHT, has two subtypes: Type I, which is predominant in the liver and hair follicles, and Type II, which is present in the prostate, and which is blocked by finasteride. However, finasteride only lowers levels of DHT in the blood by about 80 percent. Scientists now are working to develop a new inhibitor that will block both types of the enzyme. It's possible that this will produce better results. Also, there appear to be subtypes of the alpha-1 adrenoceptors and inhibitors that specifically inhibit one type or the other. It may be that a particular subtype is present in the prostate, but not on other types of smooth muscle. If this is true, it might be possible to develop a highly selective inhibitor, one that will block a specific subtype without causing side effects elsewhere in the body.

OVER-THE-COUNTER MEDICATIONS

Permixon

Permixon is a drug made up of fatty acids, extracted from the fruits of palm trees. According to its manufacturers, it has been found to have an anti-androgenic effect—that is, to block the effects of male hormones like testosterone—in rats and mice. These results, however, have not been confirmed by others. Comparisons of this drug to placebos and finasteride have not found it to be of substantial help for men with BPH. In one British study, seventy men with BPH were given either Permixon or a placebo. In *both* groups, 60 percent of men had a progressive, nearly identical improvement in urinary flow rates. *That was the problem—the results were the same in men taking Permixon and men taking nothing but sugar pills.*

"The most remarkable feature of the results," the British researchers wrote, ". . . is a demonstration that dramatic improvements, even in such quantifiable variables as urinary flow rate, can result from placebo treatment." However, they concluded, "it is clear that the results obtained offer no support to the suggestion that Permixon is of benefit in prostatic hypertrophy."

In another study (done by scientists at Merck, which makes finasteride) finasteride was compared to a host of over-the-counter plant extracts that included Permixon, Bazoton, Talso, Strogen Forte, Prostagutt, Tadenan, Remigeron, and Harzol. None of the over-the-counter drugs was found to have any significant inhibition of the 5-alpha-reductase enzyme or anti-androgen effect that could cause the prostate to shrink.

Prostex

Prostex, another over-the-counter medication, is made up of three pure amino acids (glycine, alanine and glutamic acid), according to its manufacturers, who claim the drug works by relieving swelling caused by edema (fluid retention) in the prostate and pelvic tissues. The problem here is that, because this swelling is not a cause of BPH, there is no evidence to suggest that treating edema will improve BPH symptoms.

To the best of our knowledge, there currently is no over-the-counter medication that's effective in treating BPH. However, it is humbling to realize that one of the most effective medications for the heart, digitalis, is derived from a plant leaf, and one of the newest and most promising anti-cancer drugs, taxol, comes from the bark of the Western yew tree. So, because we don't know the cause of

BPH, we can't dismiss these medications out of hand. The makers of these over-the-counter medications have been strongly encouraged to carry out adequately controlled, randomized trials, so their value can be truly assessed.

WHY ISN'T MEDICAL THERAPY BETTER?

For years, doctors considered BPH to be a simple disease. The prostate was enlarged, it obstructed the bladder. The obstructing tissue was removed, and the patient got better. This simplistic approach to the disease was possible in an era when there was only one form of treatment for BPH—surgery.

However, as medical therapy has become a reality, it's now clear that BPH is a complicated disease, involving hormones and other factors, appearing in various kinds of cells, taking many shapes, and affecting every man differently. In some men, BPH manifests itself mainly in glandular epithelial cells; under the microscope, their prostate tissue looks like a sponge. In other men, BPH tissue consists mainly of smooth-muscle and stromal cells, with very few glands. In some men, prostate enlargement presents itself in big lateral lobes; other men produce a middle lobe that can seal off the bladder neck like a cork in a bottle. Finally, in addition to all these considerations, the response of the bladder is crucial: If the bladder's in fairly good shape and is able to respond to the obstruction, a man is likely to respond well to any kind of drug treatment. But if the bladder muscle is stretched out and is no longer able to contract forcefully, it might be that no drug can improve urinary flow—no matter how well it relieves the obstruction.

In the not-too-distant past, when the only option was surgery, treatment was simple. By producing a "surgical strike," and eliminating the critical tissue that was causing the obstruction, results were good—despite the causative factors, the makeup of tissue, type and degree of obstruction, configuration of the prostate, or even the bladder's response. By removing the obstructing tissue, the bladder outlet was opened so wide that often even the weakest bladder was able to empty.

Contrast that with the current approaches to medical management of BPH: Treating patients with hormonal therapy to shrink the prostate can only be expected to work in cases when a hormonal factor plays a big role in the disease, and when the glandular tissue is primarily responsible for the obstruction.

Conversely, using smooth-muscle relaxants can only be expected to work well in men with mostly smooth-muscle tissue in their prostate, and a predominantly dynamic form of obstruction. Also, because drugs provide only modest relief of obstruction, neither approach can be expected to be very effective in men with a weak bladder muscle.

Why Diuretics Don't Help

Diuretics work by altering the way the body metabolizes sodium; the kidneys absorb less water, so more of it leaves the body in the form of urine. For most people, diuretics mean more frequent urination and a more forceful stream. But they can be disastrous for a man with BPH. Imagine a clogged pipe. Turning on the faucet full-blast isn't going to make the obstruction go away. Instead, the water's just going to back up, or overflow (and, in the case of BPH, distend the bladder). The only way to get rid of the clog is to dissolve it with chemicals, or to extract it from the pipe.

A   W O R D   O N   P A R K I N S O N ' S   D I S E A S E   A N D   U R I N A R Y   T R O U B L E

Together, BPH and Parkinson's disease can add up to a diagnostic nightmare for a physician, because Parkinson's disease can mimic the symptoms of BPH in three ways: One, it can produce a poorly sustained bladder contraction that leads to a drop in urinary flow rate and symptoms of urinary hesitancy. It also heightens the tone of the external urethral sphincter, which can lead to residual urine and obstructive symptoms. And, Parkinson's disease can make the bladder muscle spastic or hyper-reflexive, which can cause irritative symptoms.

When BPH is suspected in a man with Parkinson's disease, a doctor needs to be extremely conservative in treating the symptoms. The consequences of treating BPH symptoms in men with Parkinson's disease are serious; in fact, one urologist believes, *even persistent residual urine and recurrent urinary tract infections should not warrant a TUR in this group of men.* Still another complicating factor is that men with Parkinson's disease are often taking several medications that can have significant side effects on the lower urinary tract.

So what to do? Probably the safest course of action is to start with an alpha-blocking drug, which works in two ways (a more thorough description appears earlier in this chapter): First, alpha blockers reduce resistance in the bladder outlet. They also decrease residual urine, and therefore the threshold for bladder instability and irritative symptoms. In Parkinson's disease, the same factors that cause rigidity can affect the bladder's ability to contract and the pelvic floor's ability to relax when a man tries to urinate. One possibility, if this is happening to you, is to work with a physical therapist to learn techniques for relaxing your pelvic floor muscles, which might make urination easier.

WEIGHING THE ODDS: A LOOK AT FOUR TREATMENTS

Which BPH treatment is right for you? With all of them—even watchful waiting—there's a risk of complications. *Be your own advocate; learn as much as you can.* Before committing to one of these treatments, you owe it to yourself to find answers to some basic questions, including:

*What are the odds that my symptoms will improve?

*How long will the effects of the treatment last—will I need to do this again?

*What are the risks of complications, and *which complications* are likely to result?

To help you decide which treatment's right for you, table 10.3 breaks down the risks and benefits of the most important BPH treatments.

Symptom Improvement. The top row of table 10.3 shows your best odds for symptom improvement lie in the TUR procedure. But even the TUR is not an ironclad guarantee; the ranges for all of these are pretty wide. One surgical rule of thumb: Generally, the worse your symptoms before treatment, the more dramatic the improvement—if the treatment works.

Immediate Complications. The highly conservative numbers in the second row of table 10.3, derived from treatment studies of men with BPH, encompass *every* health problem the men reported—including problems that were not actually due to the BPH treatments. So, with that in mind, look at the figures: *In most cases, complications do not occur.* And even when they do, most complications are not serious. Some of them are—particularly bleeding that requires transfusion, a risk of surgery. Among the most common complications is retrograde ejaculation. This may occur in as many as 70 percent of men after

Table 10.3 *Comparison of BPH Treatments*

	Watchful Waiting	Alpha Blockers	Finasteride	TUR
Chances of symptom improvement for at least one year	31–55%	59–86%	54–78%	75–96%
Risk of immediate complications	None	3–43%	14–19%	5–31%
Immediate risk of incontinence	None	None	None	0.7–1.4%
Risk of impotence	Probably no additional risk; however, without any treatment, one out of fifty men age 67 and older, per year, loses ability to get an erection.		Can cause impotence in about 5% of men; this is reversible and should disappear when the drug is stopped.	3–35%; however, doctors think the risk for most patients is 5–10% and actually may be no higher than with watchful waiting.
Need for future treatment	15–65% over 3 to 5 years	6–54%	Unknown	9–11% 5 to 8 years after treatment
Loss of work and activity time during first year of treatment	1 day	3.5 days	2 days	7–21 days

Source: The U.S. Department of Health and Human Services, Public Health Service, Agency for Health Care Policy and Research.

TUR, and in a few—about 7 out of 100—men on alpha blocker drugs. Some men taking alpha blockers report dizziness, tiredness and headaches. About 5 percent of men taking finasteride report some kind of sexual problem, such as a diminished sexual drive, a decrease in the amount of semen they make, or trouble achieving or maintaining an erection. Note: Although watchful waiting doesn't carry any *immediate* complications, over time, symptoms may get worse or new symptoms may develop as the disease progresses and the urethral obstruction becomes more severe. Only TUR clearly reduces the risk of future problems with obstruction.

Incontinence. As the third row of table 10.3 indicates, over the short run, the risk of uncontrollable urine leakage is extremely rare, even with surgery.

However, over time, BPH *itself* can cause incontinence; that's one long-term risk of watchful waiting. And men taking alpha blockers or finasteride may run some risk of incontinence over the long run.

Impotence.   Discussed in the table.

Need for Future Treatment.   The ranges indicated in the fifth row of table 10.3 are so wide because doctors really don't know the long-term success of some treatments. Some men who opt for nonsurgical treatment wind up getting surgery later to relieve bothersome symptoms. And some men who do get surgery may need it again after several years if the prostate grows back.

Loss of Work and Activity Time.   The sixth row of the table includes time spent at the doctor's office and in the hospital.

WHICH TREATMENT FOR BPH? ONE MAN'S STORY

When he was 66 years old, Bill realized he had a problem that wasn't going away—urinary trouble. For more than a year, he'd noticed a big change in the way he was urinating; his stream was weak, no matter how hard he tried to force the urine out. He couldn't cut off his stream, he couldn't keep it going—it started and stopped—and there was a problem with dribbling. "I was never totally blocked," he says, "but it was bothering me." Particularly annoying were the frequent nighttime trips to the bathroom. "I realized something had to be done."

So he went to a urologist. "Bill had significant outlet obstructive symptoms," his urologist recalls. "His prostate weighed forty-one grams (more than an ounce); he had a urinary flow rate of five milliliters per second, and his symptom score was 14." (His BPH symptoms were scored from a minimum of 1 to a maximum of 4 for four symptoms: Hesitancy, decreased stream, dribbling, and intermittency. On this test, the best possible score is 4; the worst is 16.)

Not anxious to rush into surgery, Bill agreed to take part in a short-term study of an LHRH agonist to see if the drug could make a difference in his symptoms. After six months, his prostate had shrunk to thirty grams, or one ounce; his urinary flow rate had increased to fifteen milliliters per second, and his symptom score had dropped to 9.

Although his symptoms were better, the LHRH agonist "was a pain in the neck," Bill says. "It was not a very pleasant experience. I'm one of the few men who had hot flashes, like a woman has during menopause—now when women say they have hot flashes, I know what they mean!" The hot flashes diminished after a few weeks, but the drug also produced other undesirable hormonal effects; one was some mild swelling of the breasts. The other was worse: "My potency was pretty much knocked out."

Bill stopped taking the drug after six months when the study was over, and a year later he was back in the doctor's office. His prostate had grown again and now was at forty-three grams; his urinary flow rate had dropped back down to five milliliters per second. His symptom score, however, was only 10, so he decided to wait a while before taking the next step—his doctor recommended a TUR. It took just over a year for Bill's symptoms to worsen until he was ready for surgery.

During the TUR, his urologist removed eleven grams of tissue—the same amount by which Bill's prostate had been reduced on the drug therapy. "The important thing is that this was a strategic strike," his doctor notes; "the tissue was removed just in the area that was obstructing the urethra." A year later, Bill's urinary flow rate was 17.5 milliliters per second and his symptom score was 5.

"If I had the whole thing to do again, I wouldn't take the LHRH agonist," Bill says. "I'd have the TUR again in a minute. I feel fine. My urination is okay. It's not as strong a stream—not like it was when I was 20—but it's a heck of a lot better than it was; I may have to get up once during the night, but only occasionally."

Bill's recovery from surgery was uneventful, with only mild discomfort for a couple of days after the operation, and he's had no problems with potency or incontinence. He does have dry ejaculation, but he says, "It's not a problem—not when you're my age and you've had six kids!"

THE SHORT STORY

You suspected it for a long time, and now you know for sure: You've got BPH. What should you do? Do you need to be treated, and if so, how? With surgery, medication, or another form of treatment? Or, should you just wait a while, and see whether your symptoms get worse?

If your symptoms are mild and you can live with them, you should consider watchful waiting. This doesn't mean "do nothing." It means "wait and see."

However, if you have any of the following problems, you need surgery now: Kidney damage, recurrent or persistent episodes of urinary retention (not being able to empty the bladder completely, or worse, not being able to urinate at all), recurrent urinary tract infections, bladder stones, repeated episodes of bleeding when you urinate, or severe urgency that leads to incontinence—when urine leaks because you can't make it to the bathroom in time.

A lot of men with BPH, consciously or not, plan their day around trips to the bathroom. What about you? Has BPH started to intrude on your life? Can you still do everything you want to do? If not, do you want treatment badly enough to run the risk of side effects or complications? If you're somewhere in between these two extremes of BPH mentioned above, there are many options for you to consider. Read about them in this chapter, weigh the risks and benefits of each, and discuss them with your doctor.

Surgery is the "gold standard" treatment for BPH symptoms. In 95 percent of men, it can be accomplished in a minimally invasive way—without an incision—in a procedure called transurethral resection of the prostate (TUR). The TUR is safe, effective, and has few side effects. If your prostate is very large, however, you may need to have the kind of surgery that requires an incision. And if your prostate is very small, you may be eligible for a simpler form of the TUR, called a transurethral incision of the prostate (TUIP).

In addition to these tried-and-true forms of treatment are many new techniques for treating BPH. One of these is balloon dilation, although its popularity seems to be waning—mainly because its effects don't appear to be long-lasting. Other new treatments channel energy—heat, radio frequency, ultrasound, microwaves, and light—to kill the overgrowth of prostate cells surrounding the urethra. Some of these energy waves work like a shotgun, blasting holes in the prostate. Others are as sensitive as a scalpel, delicately nibbling away at BPH tissue until the urethra is free. Among these new techniques are transurethral microwave thermal therapy (TUMT), lasers, high-intensity focused ultrasound (HIFU), transurethral needle ablation (TUNA), and pyrotherapy. The goal of these techniques is to achieve the same result as with a TUR but with less anesthesia, less bleeding, and a shorter hospital stay.

Preliminary evaluation of these techniques suggests the relief of obstruction they bring may not be as pronounced as that achieved with TUR, and it's not clear whether this relief will be as long-lasting. However, as these new techniques evolve, it's likely that their results will improve.

An attractive option for older patients, or men in poor health who aren't candidates for more aggressive therapy, is mechanical—special tubes called stents that hold the prostate open to relieve the squashed urethra.

There's also medical therapy—new drugs designed to attack the problems of BPH in a couple of ways. One strategy is targeted at shrinking the enlarged prostate; the other is aimed at keeping smooth muscle tissue in the prostate from tightening around the urethra.

A drug called finasteride shrinks the prostate by blocking the formation of a powerful hormone called DHT. Because finasteride doesn't affect the body's production of the male hormone testosterone, impotence is a rare complication. About one-third of men taking finasteride have a significant improvement in symptoms, but this doesn't happen right away; it generally takes six months to a year for the drug to reach its maximal effect.

Drugs called alpha blockers relax the smooth muscle tissue within the prostate. For many men, they can provide immediate relief. Because these drugs can also lower blood pressure, the dose needs to be increased gradually, and these medications are best taken at night.

The degree of improvement in symptoms is similar to the results achieved with finasteride.

Which BPH treatment is right for you? Be your own advocate; learn as much as you can about the disease itself, and about the pros and cons of each treatment. Before committing to any treatment, you owe it to yourself to find answers to some basic questions, including: What are the odds that my symptoms will improve? How long will the effects of the treatment last? And, what are the risks of complications? All of these specifics are discussed in this chapter.

11

Prostatitis

Inflammation of the Prostate

What is prostatitis? The answer is easy: It's inflammation of the prostate. But that's the only simple thing about this annoying and sometimes debilitating condition. One urologist calls prostatitis the most imprecise diagnosis in all of medicine. Another ranks it among the most frustrating: "As a doctor, you never want to tell somebody you can't *cure* him, particularly when we live in an age when medical technology is supposed to be so great. And prostatitis *sounds* so simple. It is not a complicated disease."

Sadly, many clinicians tend to give up if their patients don't respond quickly to prostatitis treatment. They may send these men to other doctors, or simply tell them, "Learn to live with it." At the same time, most men with chronic prostatitis don't really understand what's happening to them and are not satisfied with their treatment.

Much has been learned about prostatitis in recent years. Doctors now know, for example, that the disease comes in several distinct varieties, each with its own causes and features. And getting the diagnosis right is critical in determining the best form of treatment.

True, no doctor can promise to make prostatitis go away for good. It is not always curable. *But prostatitis is treatable. Most men can get medical relief from their symptoms.* It is not contagious; men can continue a normal sex life without worrying about giving the disease to someone else. And, having prostatitis does not mean you're at a greater risk of getting BPH or prostate cancer. (On the other hand, it doesn't mean you're *not;* a man over 40 still needs to have his prostate checked at least once a year.)

WHAT IS IT?

Prostatitis is a broad name for a disease that can be either acute (intense, but for a finite interval), or chronic (of indefinite duration). It is either bacterial (caused by bacteria) or not bacterial. (Some doctors refer to bacterial prostatitis as "infectious." This simply refers to an infection caused by bacteria; it does not mean you can "catch" it or give it to someone else.)

The disease is common in men but extremely rare among boys before puberty. How common is it? Statistics are hard to come by, but a National Health Center for Health Statistics study between 1977 and 1978 found 76 annual doctor's office visits per 1,000 men for genitourinary tract problems. Of these visits, about 19 were for prostatitis.

Prostatitis is an umbrella diagnosis that spreads to encompass three conditions—acute and chronic bacterial, and nonbacterial, prostatitis—although a fourth ailment, called prostatodynia, is often lumped into this category.

Both *acute and chronic bacterial prostatitis* are associated with urinary tract infections (UTIs), positive cultures that pinpoint the bacteria's location to the prostate, and an abundance of inflammatory cells in prostatic secretions. Acute bacterial prostatitis comes on suddenly, accompanied by fever and symptoms that demand prompt treatment (see below). Chronic bacterial prostatitis typically manifests itself by repeated urinary tract infections; these keep returning when the culprit—a persistent form of bacteria—defies the antibacterial drugs intended to kill it. The bacteria usually go away for a while after antibiotics, but then they come back. The hallmark of chronic bacterial prostatitis is that, when the infection returns, it's caused by the same type of bacteria that caused the previous infection. One reason bacterial prostatitis is so closely linked to urinary tract infections is that they often are caused by the same nasty bacteria—most commonly, by varieties of *E. coli*. (These bacteria also cause urinary tract infections in women.) Also, the bacteria generally are enteric—the kind commonly found in the intestines. In most cases, just one variety of bacteria is involved, but some infections involve two or more types.

In *nonbacterial prostatitis,* there is a similar excess of inflammatory cells in the prostatic secretions, but no history of urinary tract infections, and negative cultures. Still another ailment, *prostatodynia* (which means "painful prostate") is a good mimic, often manifesting itself by the same symptoms, but patients have no history of urinary tract infections, and they have negative cultures and normal prostatic secretions.

WHICH KIND DO I HAVE?

This is a key question: Medical treatment varies for each type of prostatitis. Nonbacterial prostatitis, for example, can't be helped by antimicrobial (bacteria-killing) drugs such as antibiotics. But bacterial prostatitis can't be treated *without* them. Therefore, making the right diagnosis is crucial.

Acute Bacterial Prostatitis hits suddenly, with the impact of a freight train, and it's impossible to ignore. *Its symptoms include:* Chills and fever; blood in the urine; pain in the lower back and perineum (area between the scrotum and rectum); extreme pain, burning, urgency or difficulty urinating, which can lead to urinary retention; and usually an accompanying urinary tract infection. Symptoms of such intensity are frightening, and often they mandate an urgent visit to the doctor's office or emergency room. Sometimes men need to be hospitalized for a few days. (It's important to note here that *this is no time for stoicism;* men who have these symptoms need to seek medical help immediately.) The good news is that this condition is the easiest to treat; often it responds dramatically to antimicrobial drugs, and often it never returns.

If the condition does not begin to respond to treatment within a few days, something else might be involved—namely, a prostatic abscess. This is a localized accumulation of pus—like a pimple—under pressure in the prostate. If this is suspected, your doctor should order further tests, such as a prostate ultrasound or MRI (described in Chapter 3), to find out for sure. And if an abscess *is* present, it can be drained, via a needle passed into the prostate from the rectum or perineum, or it can be removed by a procedure commonly used to treat BPH, called transurethral resection of the prostate (known as TUR; for more on this, see Chapter 10).

Chronic Bacterial Prostatitis is also caused by bacteria, and is treated by antimicrobial drugs. It can be a recurring illness, coming back periodically for years after an initial episode of acute bacterial prostatitis. *Its symptoms include:* Difficult, frequent, urgent, burning or painful urination; and pain in one or more of these sites—the lower back, perineum (the area between the rectum and scrotum), penis, scrotum, and pubic region. A doctor might suspect that a patient has chronic bacterial prostatitis when a urine test shows bacteria in the absence of any other symptoms (although other problems, such as infected kidney stones, also might show up in this way). The symptoms of chronic bacterial prostatitis usually don't manifest themselves until sufficient amounts of bacteria have built up.

Chronic bacterial prostatitis is one of the most common causes of a repeated urinary tract infection in men, as the same bacteria tend to be involved in both problems. The disease is linked so intrinsically with urinary tract infections that many doctors believe that if you don't have a urinary tract infection, and if you've never had one, you probably don't have chronic bacterial prostatitis. One reason the situation remains chronic is that, even though the urine becomes free of bacteria and the symptoms of a urinary tract infection go away after treatment, the bacteria persist in the prostate because many antibiotics are not as effective there; these drugs do not diffuse well in the prostatic tissue.

Another explanation for lingering bacterial prostatitis may be the presence of infection in tiny stones, called calculi, in the prostate. Prostatic calculi (the prostate's version of gallstones or kidney stones) are quite common—about 75 percent of middle-aged men and 100 percent of elderly men have them. They can be detected with an imaging process called transrectal ultrasound (for how this works, see Chapter 3). They're usually small, found in grapelike clusters, and, most important, *harmless*. But when they get infected—as they often do in men with chronic bacterial prostatitis—prostatic calculi can cause an infection to persist, and symptoms of urinary tract infections and prostatitis to return again and again. (What causes calculi? Molecular analysis has shown that these stones contain ingredients generally found in urine but not prostatic secretions—which suggests they form when urine somehow "backs up," or refluxes, into the prostate.)

When a man has both prostatic stones and a history of chronic bacterial prostatitis, it's pretty safe to assume that the stones are infected. The significance of this is that *infected calculi have never been cured by medication alone,* although antibiotics can certainly treat the symptoms. The only way to cure infected prostatic stones permanently is to remove them surgically, by a procedure known as transurethral resection of the prostate (TUR—see Chapter 10).

Nonbacterial Prostatitis, as far as we know, does not involve bacteria. It is the most common form of prostatitis, and it's a diagnostic puzzler: Nobody knows what causes it, and antibiotics don't make it go away. Its symptoms are often indistinguishable from those of chronic bacterial prostatitis: Difficult, frequent, urgent, burning or painful urination; and acute or vague pain in areas including the lower back, perineum (the area between the rectum and scrotum), penis, scrotum, and pubic region. Most men who get nonbacterial prostatitis never have had a urinary tract infection. White blood cells appear in the prostatic fluid, but the urine shows no evidence of infection.

Prostatodynia produces symptoms that are basically identical to those of nonbacterial prostatitis; the difference is made in diagnosis (see below). Prostatodynia can be caused by many things, particularly muscle spasms in the bladder neck, prostatic urethra, perineum, or pelvic floor.

DIAGNOSIS

Doctors generally base any diagnosis at least in part on the patient's medical history and physical examination. But these aren't always helpful in diagnosing prostatitis. Many men with the chronic and nonbacterial forms of this disease often have a history of problems centered around the prostate—numerous occasions of pain or spasms in the region, for example, Also, because the urethra, bladder, and prostate are so closely associated, it can be difficult to pinpoint the source of a problem in that region; the symptoms often overlap.

Clearly, the easiest form of prostatitis to diagnose is the acute bacterial form (the fever and chills are a big tip-off). But for the other kinds, and for prostatodynia, other tests are needed. Because of the prostate's location—below the bladder, and just in front of the rectum—it can't been seen or examined from the outside. So the first step in examining it is usually the *digital rectal examination,* in which a doctor's gloved, lubricated finger is inserted into the rectum to feel for lumps or enlargement, or anything else unusual. This examination may be uncomfortable, but it doesn't hurt and it's generally brief, lasting less than a minute. (For more on this, see Chapter 9.)

One important test for prostatitis is *prostate massage.* This is also done during a digital rectal exam, as a doctor vigorously massages or presses on the prostate to express, or force, fluid out of the prostate and into the urethra. This fluid then is collected on a glass slide and examined under a microscope in the doctor's office. The purpose of the test is to look for such signs of infection or inflammation as abnormally high levels of white blood cells. This can be done while you wait and, like the digital rectal examination, it's usually more uncomfortable than painful. (One exception: In acute bacterial prostatitis, the rectal examination will have found a remarkably tender prostate that is also swollen, warm and firm. In this case, a doctor should not continue with prostatic massage; it would be too painful, and could lead to the release of bacteria into the bloodstream, causing sepsis. Because a urinary tract infection often accompanies acute bacterial prostatitis, the harmful bacteria can be targeted by a simple urine test.)

The key step in diagnosing prostatitis is a urine test, which is done in three parts (and which sounds much more complicated than it is; actually, it doesn't take long—less than five minutes). In what's called a *three-glass urine collection* method, you will be asked to collect your first ounce of urine in one container, then to take a midstream sample in another. (The first urine to come out contains fluid from the urethra; urine collected in midstream comes from the bladder.) Next, continue urinating in the toilet until your bladder is *almost* empty. Now is the time for the prostate massage, and your doctor will collect on a glass slide any prostatic fluid that's expressed. Finally, in the third container, you will collect the remaining urine, which contains fluid from the prostate.

An examination of expressed prostate fluid by itself is not enough to make a good diagnosis. Comparing the urine samples with the prostatic fluid enables the doctor to determine the *site* of infection (the urethra, bladder, or prostate), if there indeed *is* an infection. And cultures of this urine will show the type of bacteria that's causing it. Then, having pinpointed the bacteria, the doctor can identify the drug that best targets that particular kind of infection.

In chronic bacterial prostatitis, the digital rectal examination may be normal, but white blood cells and bacteria will be spotted in the urine or prostatic fluid. In nonbacterial prostatitis, the expressed prostate fluid contains high levels of white blood cells, and shows other signs of inflammation, but the cultures are negative. *In prostatodynia, however, this fluid is normal* on microscope examination and culture. Signs of inflammation then, are the litmus test for ruling out prostatitis.

What Else Could It Be?

Say you have some of these symptoms and they go away. Everything's fine, right? Maybe. But you should still have your prostate checked out. Other causes for these symptoms could be serious, and include:

A urinary tract infection that does not involve the prostate;

Benign prostatic hyperplasia (BPH), or enlargement of the prostate;

Urethritis, or inflammation of the urethra, often caused by an infection. Not seeking treatment for this condition could result in a urethral stricture or a nasty infection that progresses back into the vas deferens and involves the epididymis (for a look at the anatomy involved, see Chapter 1).

In rare instances, urinary problems such as those manifested in prostatitis could indicate something even more serious, such as bladder cancer; they also could mean a stricture or blockage in the urethra, an infected kidney stone or early signs of diabetes.

There are causes of prostatitis other than the ones we've covered here; these are not only extremely rare, but they're secondary to another disease, such as gonorrhea or tuberculosis. In some parts of the world (but hardly ever in the United States), prostatitis can be caused by parasites or fungal infection.

TREATMENT

For acute bacterial prostatitis, doctors approach first things first—they get the fever down and stabilize the patient; some men may need to be hospitalized for a few days. Other treatment may include bed rest; drinking plenty of fluids (to keep the body well hydrated—this helps the body's defense mechanisms); analgesic drugs such as aspirin to relieve pain; temporarily abstaining from sex; stool softeners (because the prostate is directly in front of the rectum, straining to have a bowel movement could make the already tender prostate hurt even worse); and, in some cases, the temporary insertion of a catheter (a flexible, lubricated tube inserted in the urethra via the tip of the penis) to drain the bladder, if a man is unable to urinate, or if he's retaining urine.

The good news: The intense inflammation of the tissue gives many drugs ready access to the normally not-so-accessible prostatic fluid. That's why this condition responds so dramatically to antibiotics. The bad news: Many men are undermedicated; they are not prescribed an adequate dose of antibiotics.

Many doctors prescribe antibiotics such as ciprofloxacin (one of a new class of antibiotics called fluoroquinalones) for a week to ten days. *This is not long enough.* Ten days of treatment may ease all signs of infection, and a man may feel "back to normal" within that time. But infections in the prostate are insidious. This is due in part to something called the blood-prostate barrier; it serves the same function as a bouncer at a bar—it's designed to protect the prostate from harmful substances. Yet despite its good intentions, it often keeps out the very drugs needed to stop infections in the prostate. This barrier breaks down during bacterial prostatitis—acute as well as chronic. And while these defenses are weakened, says a University of Maryland urologist who is an expert in prostatitis: "This is the time to hit hard, to knock it out the first time."

A man with acute bacterial prostatitis should stay on antibiotics for six weeks, even if his symptoms get better right away. Bacterial prostatitis could be compared to another stealthy infection too easily harbored by the body—tuberculosis—in that if it's not obliterated right away, it becomes much more difficult to cure. Somehow, over time, the bacteria become tougher to eliminate. Eradicating acute bacterial prostatitis the first time around, by relentless treatment with antibiotics, is the best way to avoid developing chronic bacterial prostatitis.

The same holds true for patients with chronic bacterial prostatitis. Again, says the University of Maryland urologist, "Any treatment with antibiotics will help somebody initially; a week to ten days' worth will get you through the first episode. Then a few months later, the infection might come back." In many cases, the infection goes away *every time* with treatment; if, a few months later, it returns, it will vanish again after another round of antibiotics.

For men with nonbacterial prostatitis, the anti-UTI antibiotics are useless: If there's no infection, and thus no bacteria, why take bacteria-killing drugs? No reason. (However, some doctors try fourteen days' worth of drugs, such as erythromycin and tetracycline, commonly used to treat *other* kinds of pathogens, as a first step. There is no real information on whether this is effective.) For the most part, all doctors can do currently for this kind of prostatitis is try to give relief from the symptoms.

The University of Maryland urologist tells his patients that having non-bacterial prostatitis is like having arthritis or bursitis: "It's a chronic condition; we can treat the symptoms, even if we can't figure out what causes it." Muscle relaxants, such drugs as alpha blockers (originally marketed as anti-hypertensive drugs, also used to treat BPH—see Chapter 10), have been helpful in alleviating the muscle tension in the prostate, and making urination easier. Some doctors recommend anti-inflammatory drugs and the use of hot sitz baths, where the patient sits in (or sometimes over a fine spray of) soothing, warm water. Also, many men have found that diet has an effect on nonbacterial prostatitis, and that some foods—particularly, spicy dishes, red wine and caffeine—seem to aggravate their symptoms.

HOW DID THIS HAPPEN?

Sometimes there's a clear cause-and-effect relationship at work in prostatitis—the insertion of a urinary catheter, for example, during a medical procedure. This causes more trauma in the urinary tract for some men than for others.

Other risk factors include a recent bladder or kidney infection; an enlarged prostate (BPH, in which the prostate grows to constrict the urethra and can have a harmful effect on the urinary tract); and rectal intercourse, also associated with trauma to the urinary tract.

In bacterial prostatitis, the question is, how did the bacteria get into the urinary tract? In the instances mentioned above, bacteria may be able to invade the prostate from the urethra when infected urine "backs up" into the prostate ducts. (During unprotected rectal intercourse, too, rectal bacteria can be picked up by the penis and drawn into the urethra, and then can make their way into the urinary tract.)

But for nonbacterial prostatitis, and prostatodynia, the basic answer is that nobody knows. There have been severe cases in which men have had their prostates removed—*and yet the symptoms failed to go away.* Which leads to the question of whether nonbacterial prostatitis and prostatodynia are really happening in the prostate at all? "Prostatitis is a catch-all term," says the University of Maryland urologist. "Too often, any time a patient comes in with pelvic pain, rectal pain, lower back pain—the doctor says, 'You've probably got a touch of prostatitis.' But a lot of men are told they have prostatitis when they've really got something else."

And, because the disease—in all its forms, particularly the nonbacterial kind—is poorly understood, "a lot of patients get shrugged off by their doctors," the urologist continues.

There are as many different reactions to prostatitis as there are cases of it; how men cope depends, in large part, on their response to illness and discomfort in general. "Some men can't seem to stand it," the urologist says. "But other men, as long as they know it isn't cancer, can live with it."

WHEN PROSTATITIS DOESN'T GO AWAY: ONE MAN'S STORY

For many men, the symptoms of prostatitis appear suddenly and then go away with treatment. For these men, prostatitis is an awful episode to endure and then put behind them; it does not require a lifetime adjustment. But for Alan, a 52-year-old Baltimore attorney with perhaps a "worst-case" scenario of nonbacterial prostatitis, the situation is distinctly different.

His trouble began three years ago. He'd had some minor prostate "episodes" before that, he says, but nothing like this. Then, after seeking treatment for a headache, he was prescribed a migraine medication, in a class of drugs called tricyclic antidepressants. "What it [the drug] did, was slow down my urine flow terrifically." Within a couple of days, Alan began noticing some new symptoms: "I found I was spending a lot of time going to the bathroom, and I developed some stinging, and a lot of nonspecific symptoms like headaches— just not feeling well. The first time I had sex after that [developing these symptoms], it was painful, and I was sore for a day or two afterward," with pain in the lower abdomen, scrotum and perineum.

Eventually, Alan was diagnosed as having nonbacterial prostatitis. "The symptoms ebb and flow, but they haven't disappeared," he says. These include reduced urine stream; occasional difficulty starting and stopping urination; generalized pain in the perineal region, usually beginning about twelve to fifteen hours after sexual intercourse and lasting two to three days; and "just feeling lousy." He's also been awakened by muscle spasms in his perineal region, but he can't pinpoint an exact location. He tried abstaining from sexual intercourse, but that didn't help.

At first, Alan had what he describes as "menopausal-type" feelings, accompanied by a lot of anxiety: "When this first came on, because of that fear of losing something very special to me, I think there was a heightened sense of sexual drive or desire, which was of course immediately frustrated by the inability to do anything about the symptoms." And he thought, "Is this going to be a permanent impairment, will this limit sexual activity and the free expression of physical love in my marriage? Is this going to be the end of a chapter in my life?"

Alan's suggestions for men with his condition: "First, just try to have a positive outlook on being able to live with this situation. With time, there comes a better ability to adjust and accept what is really a very annoying and irritating condition."

He was treated early on by an internist, who described Alan's problem as "prostatosis," a vague, unhelpful term that means simply "a condition of the prostate." Another word of advice: "Don't let anybody tell you it's all in your head." Alan even consulted a psychiatrist, who confirmed that prostatitis is "a real, live condition that could not be explained solely by psychological causes."

"Sometimes the symptoms are worse than others," Alan says; "I can't deter-

Table 11.1 *Is It Prostatitis?*

Type	Definition/Cause	Symptoms
Acute bacterial	Caused by bacteria; is intense but finite	Chills and fever; blood in the urine; pain in the lower back and perineum; extreme pain or difficulty urinating, usually accompanied by a UTI
Chronic bacterial	Caused by bacteria; of indefinite duration; may go away and return	Associated with repeated UTIs. Difficult, frequent, urgent, burning or painful urination, and pain in one or more of these sites—the lower back, perineum, penis, scrotum, and pubic region
Nonbacterial	Not caused by bacteria; not associated with UTIs; cause unknown	Difficult, frequent, urgent, burning or painful urination; and acute or vague pain in areas including the lower back, perineum, penis, scrotum, and pubic region
Prostatodynia	Painful prostate; may be caused by muscle spasms in the bladder neck, prostatic urethra, perineum or pelvic floor; not associated with UTIs; cause unknown	Difficult, frequent, urgent, burning or painful urination; and acute or vague pain in areas including the lower back, perineum, penis, scrotum, and pubic region

Table 11.2 *What Kind of Prostatitis Do I Have?*

Type	History of UTIs	High WBCs in Prostate Fluids	Positive Cultures	Responds to Antibiotics
ABP	Yes	Yes	Yes	Yes
CBP	Yes	Yes	Yes	Yes
NP	No	Yes	No	Rarely
P	No	No	No	No

Note: The choices are acute bacterial prostatitis (ABP), chronic bacterial prostatitis (CBP), nonbacterial prostatitis (NP) or a related condition, and prostatodynia. Some factors your doctor will consider in making a diagnosis include: A history of urinary tract infections (UTIs), a high white blood cell (WBC) count, and positive urine cultures. This will determine your treatment— as the last column indicates, it's pointless to treat prostatodynia with antibiotic drugs; they're rarely helpful in nonbacterial prostatitis. They do work in both forms of bacterial prostatitis, however, and you should stay on the drugs for six weeks.

mine what makes them different. There just isn't any clear-cut pattern. I guess part of this experience has been simply accepting the condition."

THE SHORT STORY

Prostatitis is a term that refers to inflammation of the prostate. It's an annoying and sometimes debilitating condition. It's also, too often, an imprecise diagnosis. There are actually four conditions lumped under the umbrella name of *prostatitis*. Each one has distinct characteristics and responds differently to treatment; that's why getting the right diagnosis is so important.

Two common forms of prostatitis are caused by infections produced by bacteria: *Acute bacterial prostatitis* hits suddenly, with the impact of a freight train, and it's impossible to ignore. Its symptoms include chills and fever, blood in the urine, pain in the lower back and perineum, extreme pain, burning, urgency, or difficulty urinating. If ignored and left untreated, it can lead to more serious problems such as urinary retention—the inability to urinate—and formation of an abscess within the prostate. The good news is that treatment with antibiotics is usually successful, and relief is as dramatic as the symptoms were. Important: Antibiotics must be taken for six weeks, even after the symptoms have disappeared. The reason is that, if it's not obliterated right away, acute bacterial prostatitis becomes much more difficult to cure. Eradicating acute bacterial prostatitis the first time around, by relentless treatment with antibiotics, is the best way to avoid developing chronic bacterial prostatitis.

Chronic bacterial prostatitis is also caused by bacteria, and also treated by antibiotics. It can be a recurring illness, coming back periodically for years after an initial episode of acute bacterial prostatitis. Its symptoms are usually milder versions of those in the acute form. Here, too, treatment with antibiotics should continue for six weeks.

Nonbacterial prostatitis is the most common form of prostatitis, and it's a mystery. Nobody knows what causes it, and antibiotics don't make it go away. Men with this form of prostatitis may have many of the same symptoms as in chronic bacterial prostatitis, and white blood cells may be present in fluid made by the prostate—but as far as we know, it doesn't involve bacteria.

Prostatodynia has basically the same symptoms as nonbacterial prostatitis; the difference is made in diagnosis. Prostatodynia can be caused by many things, particularly muscle spasms in the bladder neck, urethra, perineum, or pelvis.

Treatment for nonbacterial prostatitis and prostatodynia is largely symptomatic. Muscle relaxants and other drugs have been helpful in easing the muscle tension in the prostate and making urination easier. Some doctors recommend anti-inflammatory drugs and sitz baths, and many men have found that diet has an effect on nonbacterial prostatitis, and that some foods—particularly, spicy dishes, red wine and caffeine—seem to aggravate their symptoms.

Even if prostatitis is not always curable, it is treatable. Most men can get medical relief from their symptoms. It is not contagious; men can continue a normal sex life without worrying about giving the disease to someone else. And, having prostatitis does not mean you're at a greater risk of getting BPH or prostate cancer.

Where to Get Help

The first thing you need to know is that you're not alone. Whether it's BPH, prostate cancer or prostatitis, there are sources of good information available to help you. Here are a few of them:

American Cancer Society
1599 Clifton Rd., Atlanta, GA 30026
1-800-ACS-2345

Cancer Care, Inc.
1180 Avenue of the Americas, New York, NY 10036
(212) 221-3300 or (212) 302-2400 (social services)

National Cancer Institute Cancer Information Services
Public Inquiries, Office of Cancer Communication
National Cancer Institute
9000 Rockville Pike, Bethesda, MD 20892
1-800-4-CANCER

National Hospice Organization
1910 North Fort Myer Dr., Suite 307, Arlington, VA 22209
1-800-658-8898

National Kidney and Urologic Diseases Information Clearinghouse
(For information about BPH and prostatitis—but *not* prostate cancer)
Box NKUDIC, Bethesda, MD 20892
(301) 654-4415

Prostate Cancer Support Network (PCSN)
(Provides services for several support groups, self-help organizations, and their members, including "USToo")
300 W. Pratt St., Suite 401, Baltimore, MD 21201
1-800-828-7866

Prostate Health Council
American Foundation for Urologic Disease
300 W. Pratt St., Suite 401, Baltimore, MD 21201
1-800-242-2383

Sexual Function Health Council
American Foundation for Urologic Disease
300 W. Pratt St., Suite 401, Baltimore, MD 21201
1-800-242-2383

Glossary

A guide to medical language of the prostate, from A to Z. Most of the words here are nouns; where we thought it necessary, we indicated a term's part of speech.

Ablation—"getting rid of." *Cryoablation*, for example, means "using freezing temperatures to get rid of prostate cancer." *Hormonal ablation* means "getting rid of the hormones that nourish a prostate tumor."

Acid phosphatase—an enzyme that, like PSA, is secreted by the prostate. Elevated acid phosphatase levels can signal that something is wrong with the prostate.

Acute bacterial prostatitis—a form of prostatitis associated with urinary tract infections, positive cultures that identify bacteria in the prostate, and an abundance of white blood cells in prostatic secretions. Acute bacterial prostatitis comes on suddenly, accompanied by fever and symptoms that demand prompt treatment.

Adrenal androgens—weak male hormones made by the adrenal glands. These include androstenedione, dehydroepiandrosterone (DHEA), and dehydroepiandrosterone sulfate (DHEAS), plus small amounts of testosterone. They are minor players, believed to make up only 5 percent or less of the total androgen stimulation to the prostate. Their total effect on the prostate is a controversial issue.

Age-specific PSA levels—a new way to evaluate PSA tests, using a man's age to determine the significance of his PSA reading.

Figure G.1.

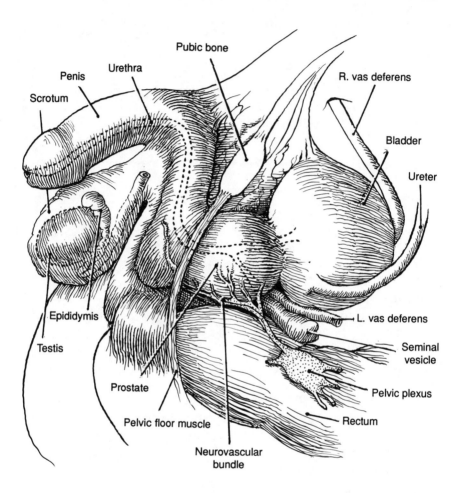

Pubic bone

Urethra

Penis

Scrotum

R. vas deferens

Bladder

Ureter

Epididymis

Testis

Prostate

Pelvic floor muscle

Neurovascular bundle

L. vas deferens

Seminal vesicle

Pelvic plexus

Rectum

Alpha blockers—drugs, originally designed to treat hypertension, that act on the prostate by relaxing smooth muscle tissue.

Analgesics—painkillers.

Analog—a synthetic look-alike of a drug or body chemical.

Anal stricture—tight scar tissue that can interfere with a bowel movement.

Anastomosis—the site where two structures are surgically reconnected after an organ has been removed. After radical prostatectomy, this refers to the connection between the reconstructed bladder neck and urethra.

Androgen-dependent, or -sensitive cells—cells in prostate cancer that are nourished by hormones, which can diminish dramatically when the hormones that nourish the prostate are shut off.

Androgen-independent, or -insensitive cells—cells in prostate cancer that are *not* nourished by hormones, and therefore don't respond to hormone therapy.

Androgens—male hormones such as testosterone.

Antiandrogens—drugs such as flutamide, used in hormone therapy to treat prostate cancer. These drugs block the effects of testosterone and DHT on the prostate cell by neutralizing their effect (they prevent testosterone and DHT from binding to the androgen receptor).

Antibiotics—drugs that kill bacteria.

Anticholinergic drugs—a group of drugs whose side effects include hindering urination. These may help some men with incontinence.

Anticoagulants—medications that hinder the blood from clotting.

Antimicrobial drugs—bacteria-killing drugs, such as antibiotics.

Arterial (adj.)—relating to the arteries.

Artificial sphincter—an implanted device used to treat incontinence that has persisted for a year or longer and shows no signs of improving on its own.

Asymptomatic (adj.)—experiencing no symptoms. A man with asymptomatic prostate cancer doesn't notice anything out of the ordinary, he feels fine.

Balloon dilation—a safe, although not very long-lasting, technique to treat BPH. The idea is simple: A collapsed balloon is threaded into the narrowest part of the urethra and then inflated to stretch the opening, and thus improve urine flow.

Benign—harmless; not cancerous, not fatal.

Benign prostatic hyperplasia—see *BPH*.

Biopsy of the prostate—a means of sampling prostate tissue so it can be checked for the presence of cancer. This is often done using a spring-loaded biopsy gun, a tiny device that's attached to a urologist's finger, and with the help of transrectal ultrasound.

Bladder—a hollow, muscle-bound reservoir that functions as a holding tank for urine.

Bladder neck contracture—constriction of the bladder neck, caused by scar tissue. This can impede urine flow.

Bladder spasms—painful, uncontrollable contractions of the bladder.

Bladder stones—tiny formations, made when crystals of uric acid or calcium precipitate into the urine.

Bloodless field—a surgical term that means controlling bleeding within a patient, to give surgeons a better field of vision as they perform an operation.

Blood-prostate barrier—a membrane that prevents many substances—including antibiotics—from entering the prostate. This barrier breaks down during bacterial prostatitis, permitting most antibiotics to enter.

Bone scan—also called radionuclide scintigraphy. In a bone scan, doctors inject into the bloodstream a radioactive tracer, a chemical that's attracted, like a magnet, specifically to bone. The bone scan is an excellent means of finding out whether prostate cancer has spread to bone.

BPH—benign prostatic hyperplasia, or enlargement of the prostate. A benign condition that results in most older men when prostate tissue begins to grow around the urethra, gradually compressing it and hindering urine flow.

BUN test—the blood-urea-nitrogen test, a blood test to check kidney function.

Calculi—See *prostatic calculi.*

Capsule of the prostate—the outer wall of the prostate gland.

Castrate range—the level to which testosterone drops after orchiectomy. This is an important point of comparison in monitoring hormone therapy, as certain drugs are judged by their ability to reduce testosterone to this range.

Castration—See *orchiectomy.*

Catheter—a tube used for drainage or irrigation, most commonly to drain urine out of the bladder.

Cell division—how the body's cells multiply. A single cell divides in two. Then those two cells divide in two, and so on.

Chemical castrators—drugs that accomplish the same effect as orchiectomy, that is, lowering testosterone to the critical "castrate range."

Chemotherapeutic drugs—a host of cell-killing drugs used to treat many forms of cancer.

Chronic bacterial prostatitis—a form of prostatitis associated with urinary tract infections, positive cultures that identify bacteria in the prostate, and an abundance of white blood cells in prostatic secretions. This can be a recurring illness, coming back periodically for years after an initial episode of acute bacterial prostatitis.

Clinical stage of prostate cancer—an estimate, the stage a doctor believes a man's cancer to be, based on factors such as the digital rectal exam, the PSA test, transrectal ultrasound and needle biopsy. Pathologic stage is much more certain, but this can only be determined when a pathologist examines actual prostate tissue after surgery.

Clonal selection—the process whereby the most poorly differentiated, rapidly growing, aggressive cells overtake the slower well-differentiated cells as a tumor progresses.

Contact laser prostatectomy—a form of treatment for BPH in which the laser probe actually touches—and immediately vaporizes—the BPH tissue.

Corpora cavernosa and corpus spongiosum—spongy chambers in the penis that become engorged with blood during an erection.

Creatinine test—a blood test that checks for impairment of kidney function.

Cryoablation, cryotherapy—using extremely cold liquid nitrogen to freeze the entire prostate, causing cancer cells within the gland to rupture as they begin to thaw.

CT (computed tomography) scan—a circular series of X-ray pictures taken by a machine that goes around the body. A computer puts the pictures together, generating images that, as in MRI, are like slices of anatomy.

Cystometry—a test to measure bladder pressure and function, done by passing a small catheter through the urethra into the bladder. Changes in pressure are monitored as the bladder fills with water.

Cystoscope—a tiny, lighted tube that works like a periscope on a submarine. In cystoscopy, it is inserted in the tip of the anesthetized penis and threaded through the urethra into the bladder; this allows the doctor to inspect the bladder, prostate and urethra for abnormalities.

Deep venous thrombosis—blood clots that form in the legs' deep veins, a potential complication of major surgery such as radical prostatectomy. At best, these clots can be painful. At worst they can be fatal, if a chunk of a blood clot in the leg breaks free and shoots up to the lungs. These should be treated immediately.

DES—See *estrogens.*

DHT (dihydrotestosterone)—the active form of male hormone in the prostate. It is made when testosterone is transformed by an enzyme called 5-alpha reductase.

DIC—disseminated intravascular coagulation, a blood-clotting disorder that develops in some men with advanced prostate cancer.

Differentiation of prostate cancer cells—how cancer cells look under the microscope. Well-differentiated cells have distinct, clearly defined borders and clear centers, and their growth is relatively slow and orderly. Everything about poorly differentiated cells is murkier, not so well-defined. As cancer progresses, these poorly differentiated cells seem to melt together and form solid, nasty blobs of malignancy. These are the most aggressive cells in a tumor, and they are given a high grade (8, 9, 10) in the Gleason scoring system. Well-differentiated cells are called low-grade (2, 3, 4). Moderately well-differentiated cells fall right in between (5, 6, 7), and it's hard to predict what these cells will do.

Digital rectal exam (DRE)—a very important part of the physical examination, in which a doctor's gloved, lubricated finger is inserted into the rectum to feel for lumps, enlargement, or areas of hardness that might indicate the presence of cancer. It is uncomfortable but not painful, and it's generally brief, lasting less than a minute.

Diuretics—drugs that work by altering the way the body metabolizes sodium; this causes the kidneys to absorb less water, so more of it leaves the body in the form of urine. For most people, diuretics mean more frequent urination and a more forceful stream. They can be disastrous for a man with BPH.

Diverticula—pockets of the bladder lining that poke out like balloons through the bladder wall. (A single one of these is called a diverticulum.)

DNA—the "genetic blueprint," vital information contained in the nucleus of every cell.

Dorsiflexion exercises—pumping the feet up and down to exercise the calf muscles, a good exercise immediately after surgery.

Double-blind study—a study in which neither the doctor nor the patient knows who's receiving placebo, the standard medication, or the new medication being tested.

"Dry" ejaculation—also known as retrograde ejaculation. This is a complication of some prostate procedures including TUR. For most men, this has no effect on the pleasant sensation of orgasm. Dry ejaculation is pretty much what it sounds like—semen is not expelled out the urethra when a man reaches sexual climax. Instead, it goes the other way—back into the bladder. This happens because part of the bladder neck—a muscular valve, whose job is to slam shut at the time of ejaculation, forcing semen out the urethra—often is resected along with the prostate tissue. When this area is damaged or missing, there's nothing to prevent semen from heading the wrong way.

Edema—swelling caused by fluid retention.

Ejaculate (noun)—This is semen, the fluid that exits the body during ejaculation, or sexual climax. *Ejaculate* can also be a verb.

Ejaculation—emission of semen at the climax of sexual intercourse.

Enucleate (verb)—to remove. In an open prostatectomy, the surgeon's fingers enucleate, or dig out, prostate tissue around the urethra. For the most part, the tissue separates from the surrounding tissue like a walnut from its shell.

Epididymis—the "greenhouse" where sperm mature and are stored until orgasm.

Epididymitis—an infection of the epididymis. This may occur after a surgical procedure that damages the ejaculatory ducts, allowing infected urine to "back up" into the vas deferens.

Epidural anesthesia—a local anesthetic administered through a tiny plastic tube, inserted between the vertebrae of the spine, near the small of the back. The epidural anesthetic bathes the area outside the membrane lining the spinal cord, temporarily numbing the nerves in the lower body. Unlike spinal anesthesia, which comes in one dose, epidural anesthesia can be given continuously. The area of numbness can be adjusted; so can the degree of pain relief.

Epithelial cells—cells in the glandular tissue of the prostate, which secrete fluid that becomes part of semen.

Erectile dysfunction—the inability to have an erection sufficient for sexual intercourse.

Estrogens—female hormones. Estrogens block a signal transmitted by the pituitary gland called luteinizing hormone (LH), which stimulates testosterone. Oral estrogens, taken as hormone therapy by men with prostate cancer, reduce testosterone to the crucial castrate range. The main oral estrogen is DES (diethylstilbestrol).

Excise (verb)—to cut out, to remove surgically.

External-beam radiation therapy—a curative treatment for prostate cancer. It involves beaming X-ray energy into a prostate tumor from the outside, a few minutes at a time, over the course of several weeks.

Fascia—a thin blanket of connective tissue.

5-alpha reductase—enzymes in the prostate that convert testosterone to DHT.

5-alpha reductase inhibitors—drugs that block the formation of DHT. This causes the prostate to shrink and improves the obstructive symptoms of BPH. These drugs do not affect levels of testosterone, the hormone responsible for a man's libido and sexual function.

Fluoroscopy—an X-ray image that appears live on a TV screen instead of as a still photograph.

Foley catheter—a catheter inserted in the penis and threaded through the urethra to the bladder, where it's anchored in place with a tiny, inflated balloon. It removes urine from the body; it can also be used for irrigation, to prevent blood clots.

"Following expectantly"—See *watchful waiting.*

Frozen sections—In a staging pelvic lymphadenectomy, lymph nodes are removed, then rushed to a pathologist for frozen-section analysis to check for cancer. This is pretty much what it sounds like—the tissue is frozen, then sliced into very thin sections to be examined under the microscope.

FSH—follicle-stimulating hormone, made along with LH by the pituitary gland. FSH has its major effect on sperm production.

Genetic drift—As a cancer progresses, as its cells double over and over again, the DNA becomes less stable. The cancer develops new mutations; it becomes more aggressive. As the tumor progresses, well-differentiated cells deteriorate into poorly differentiated cells. This downside is called genetic drift.

Gleason score—a way to classify the grade of cancer, based on how it looks under the microscope. Cells that are well-differentiated are given a low grade (2, 3, 4); poorly differentiated cells are given a high grade (8, 9, 10). Moderately well-differentiated cells fall right in the middle. See also "differentiation of prostate cancer cells."

Grade of prostate cancer—See *Gleason score.*

Growth factors—substances that activate processes that promote cell division.

Gynecomastia—tenderness, pain, or swelling of the breasts in men. This is a common, easily treatable side effect of some forms of hormone therapy for prostate cancer.

Hemi-body irradiation—a once-common form of radiation treatment to ease pain in prostate cancer patients with metastases to bone in several places. It involves irradiating large expanses of the body, and comparatively high doses of radiation.

Hereditary prostate cancer (HPC)—HPC is present in families if there are three first-degree relatives (a father or brothers) who develop prostate cancer—or two first-degree relatives, if both developed it before age 55—or if prostate cancer has occurred in three generations in the family (grand-father, father, son). HPC can be inherited from either side of the family.

Heterogeneity—diverse, varied. Not uniform. In prostate cancer and BPH, *heterogeneity* refers to a "melting pot" of cells, all jockeying for position in one area.

HIFU—high-intensity focused ultrasound, a technique used to treat BPH. Ultrasound energy is focused with exquisite precision to produce temperatures hotter than 65 degrees centigrade within a few seconds. The focus is so sharp that areas outside it—even those a fraction of an inch away—are not heated or damaged. The ultrasound works like a scalpel.

Hormone-dependent, -sensitive—See *androgen-dependent, -sensitive.*

Hormone-independent, -insensitive—See *androgen-independent, -insensitive.*

Hormone therapy—the use of hormones to treat advanced prostate cancer. Hormone therapy is aimed at shutting down the hormones that nourish the prostate. Some cells in a prostate tumor are responsive to this, and some aren't. Doctors also say *hormonal therapy, hormone deprivation therapy,* or *anti-androgen therapy,* and may use these terms interchangeably.

Hot flash—a sudden rush of warmth in the face, neck, upper chest and back, lasting from a few seconds to an hour; a side effect of some hormonal treatments for prostate cancer. Although hot flashes aren't harmful to a man's health, they can be bothersome.

Hydronephrosis—distention of the ureters and renal pelvis, caused by an obstruction.

Hyperplasia—an increase in the number of cells in an organ or tissue with the result that the organ or tissue becomes enlarged. In BPH, this enlargement is benign; in other words, it is *not* cancer.

Hyper-reflexive—overly reactive; spastic.

Hyperthermia—the mildest form of thermal therapy for BPH, involving temperatures that are less than 45 degrees centigrade—which probably isn't hot enough to accomplish major relief of obstruction.

Imaging (verb)—seeing and taking pictures inside the body, using various forms of energy including ultrasound, magnetic resonance (MRI) and X-rays.

Impotence—the inability to have an erection.

Incidental prostate cancer—small clusters of cancer cells, an apparently dormant form of cancer that resides in millions of men. In some men, this cancer never poses a danger. In others, however, it eventually does.

Incontinence—unintentional leakage of urine; this is also called urinary incontinence. (Another kind of incontinence, fecal incontinence, means having an unintentional bowel movement.)

"Infectious" prostatitis—a term some doctors use in describing bacterial prostatitis. Bacterial prostatitis is not infectious; men can continue a normal sex life without worrying about giving the disease to someone else.

Interstitial brachytherapy—implanting radioactive "seeds," or minute radioactive chunks of material, in the prostate to kill cancer.

Intrabdominal (adj.)—in the abdomen.

Intraurethral (adj.)—in the urethra.

Invasive (adj.)—Invasive surgery means an incision is involved; the body is physically entered. In minimally invasive surgery, this incision may be a hole as small as a dime, or there may be no incision at all if the body's own passageways—such as the urethra in the TUR procedure—are used. A noninvasive procedure does not invade the body at all; many forms of imaging are noninvasive.

Irritative symptoms in BPH—These include frequent urination, especially at night, a strong sense of urgency in urination, inability to postpone urination, and sleep disrupted by the need to urinate.

IV—an abbreviation for *intravenous,* which means literally, "through the veins." Medication, fluids or nutrition supplements can be administered this way.

IVP (Intravenous pyelogram)—an X-ray view of the urinary tract, which works like a glow-in-the-dark picture: A special dye is injected, making urine visible, and its path from the kidneys and out of the body easily traceable—and any blockage easy to see. Some men have severe allergic reactions to this dye.

Kegel exercises—exercises to strengthen urinary control, done as a man stands to urinate. They involve trying to shut off the urinary stream by tightly contracting muscles in the buttocks.

Kidneys—the body's main filters. They cleanse the body of impurities and, at the same time, salvage and recycle useful materials.

Laparoscopic pelvic lymphadenectomy—dissection of the lymph nodes as a means of staging prostate cancer. Laparoscopic surgery is minimally invasive; there's a tiny incision, and much of the surgery is conducted through "telescopes."

Laser prostatectomy—using the powerful energy from focused light to remove prostate tissue in BPH. There are two distinctive methods, called non-contact and contact laser prostatectomy.

Latent (adj.)—dormant; passive.

Lateral lobe enlargement—a form of BPH that results when prostate tissue compresses the urethra from the sides.

LH—luteinizing hormone, a chemical signal transmitted by the pituitary. LH motivates the testes to make testosterone.

LHRH—luteinizing hormone-releasing hormone (also called GnRH, for gonadotropin-releasing hormone), a chemical signal made in the brain by the hypothalamus. LHRH tells the pituitary gland to make LH and FSH.

LHRH agonists—synthetic look-alikes of the body's chemical, LHRH. These drugs shut down the pituitary's production of the hormone called LH.

Libido—sex drive.

Localized prostate cancer—cancer that is confined within the prostate, and therefore is considered curable.

Local recurrence of cancer—when cancer returns to the prostate or nearby tissue after treatment.

Metastasis, metastases, metastatic—A metastasis is a chunk of cancer that has broken off from the main tumor and established itself elsewhere. A distant metastasis means this new site of cancer is far from its point of origin. *Metastases* is plural, and *metastatic* is an adjective that refers to a *metastasis.*

Middle lobe enlargement—a type of BPH in which a lobe of prostate tissue grows up inside the bladder. When it reaches a critical size, it can block the opening of the bladder neck like a cork in a bottle. This explains how some men with a "small prostate on rectal exam" can develop major symptoms of urinary obstruction.

"Minilap"—mini-laparotomy staging pelvic lymphadenectomy. The Minilap begins with an incision slightly larger than in the laparoscopic pelvic lymphadenectomy. If there's cancer in the lymph nodes, the incision is closed. But if the lymph nodes are cancer-free, this incision is lengthened and the radical retropubic prostatectomy is performed under the same anesthetic.

MRI (magnetic resonance imaging)—a means of imaging that's painless, noninvasive and does not use X-rays. It is time-consuming, however, often lasting about 45 minutes. MRI gives a three-dimensional scan of the body, producing images that are like slices of anatomy.

Neodynium (Nd):YAG laser—a kind of contact laser whose energy penetrates superficially into tissue.

"Nerve-sparing" radical prostatectomy—what some doctors call the anatomical approach to radical retropubic prostatectomy; they're referring to important modifications that reduce blood loss and allow men to remain potent and continent after radical prostatectomy.

Neurogenic bladder—trouble in the bladder caused by a neurological problem such as Parkinson's disease.

Neurotransmitters—chemical messengers, signals sent from a transmitter in one nerve cell to a receptor in another.

Neurovascular bundles—cordlike structures that run down the side of the prostate near the rectum. The bundles contain microscopic nerves that are essential for erection; they also contain arteries and veins that help surgeons identify the location of these nerves. In the past, these nerves were almost always injured during surgery, but were rarely removed completely because doctors didn't even know of—and therefore couldn't appreciate—their existence.

Nitric oxide—a substance released by the nerve endings during penile erection. This causes smooth muscle tissue in the penis to relax.

Nocturia—frequent urination during the night. A man has nocturia if he has to get up several times a night to go to the bathroom; this is often a symptom of BPH.

Nocturnal penile tumescence test—an evaluation to determine whether a man has erections at night while he sleeps.

Nonbacterial prostatitis—a form of prostatitis associated with an excess of white blood cells in prostatic secretions, but no history of urinary tract infections, and no bacteria that can be detected in the prostate. Its cause is a mystery.

Non-contact laser prostatectomy—a procedure to treat BPH that does not remove BPH tissue, but instead creates space around the urethra when the "zapped" tissue dies, sloughs away, and is absorbed back into the body.

Noninvasive (adj.)—not invasive; in other words, there's no incision.

Obstructive symptoms in BPH—These include weak urine flow, hesitancy in starting urination, a need to push or strain to get urine to flow, intermittent urine stream (starts and stops several times), difficulty in stopping urination, "dribbling" after urination, a sense of not being able to empty the bladder completely, and not being able to urinate at all.

Open prostatectomy—a surgical procedure to treat BPH, requiring an incision, to remove the part of the prostate surrounding the urethra. There are three ways to do this—the suprapubic, retropubic, and perineal approaches.

Orchiectomy—surgical castration. A form of hormone therapy, involving removal of all or part of the testicles. This causes testosterone to fall to the "castrate range."

Orgasm—the climax of sexual intercourse.

Overflow incontinence—when urine leaks out because the bladder is too full to hold any more.

Palliate—to ease or relieve. Palliative treatment makes symptoms, and therefore quality of life, better—even though it may do nothing to cure the underlying cause of these symptoms.

Palpable (adj.)—tangible. Palpable cancer in the prostate means there's a lump, lesion or nodule that a doctor's gloved finger can feel during a digital rectal exam.

Pathologic fracture—When cancer invades bones, they become brittle. Brittle bones break. Therefore, men with metastatic prostate cancer are prone to broken bones, called pathologic fractures. Most susceptible are the bones that bear much of the body's weight, in the hip and thigh.

Pathologic stage of cancer—the definitive extent of a man's prostate cancer. (The possibilities include organ-confined cancer, capsular penetration, positive surgical margins, invasion of the seminal vesicles, and/or involvement of the pelvic lymph nodes.) This is determined after prostate surgery when a pathologist examines the actual prostate specimen and dissected tissue from the nearby lymph nodes—instead of merely making guesses about how far the cancer has spread based on test results and a few cells from biopsies.

Pathologist—a doctor who studies cells, tissue and organs, and makes determinations about them—answering such questions as "Is there cancer here?" and "Was all the cancer removed?"

Penile (adj.)—relating to the penis.

Penile implants—bendable, inflatable, or mechanical prostheses that enable an impotent man to have erections and a normal sex life.

Perforation—puncture.

Perineum—the area between the scrotum and rectum.

Peripheral zone—the largest part of the prostate and the area where most prostate cancer occurs.

Periprostatic tissue—tissue just outside the prostate.

Placebo—a sugar pill, often taken by participants in a medical study. Patients taking a placebo are compared to patients taking actual medications.

"Placebo effect"—a phenomenon that happens often in medical studies, in which patients taking a placebo have an inexplicable improvement in symptoms.

Pressure-flow studies—tests to monitor bladder pressure changes as a man urinates.

Proliferation—spread, or growth, as in "proliferation of cancer."

Prostate—A muscular, walnut-shaped gland about an inch and a half long that sits directly under the bladder. Its main function is to make part of the fluid for semen. (Note: "Prostate" is often confused with the adjective *prostrate*, which means "lying face-down, or being exhausted.")

Prostatectomy—an operation to remove all or part of the prostate.

Prostate massage—an important test for prostatitis, done during a digital rectal exam. A doctor vigorously massages or presses on the prostate to express, or force, fluid out of the prostate and into the urethra. It then is collected on a glass slide and examined under a microscope.

Prostate-specific antigen—See *PSA*.

Prostatic (adj.)—relating to the prostate.

Prostatic abscess—localized accumulation of pus, like a pimple, under pressure in the prostate.

Prostatic calculi—the prostate's version of gallstones or kidney stones. They're usually tiny and harmless. But when they get infected, as they often do in men with chronic bacterial prostatitis, they can cause an infection to persist, and symptoms of urinary tract infections and prostatitis to return again and again.

Prostatic urethra—the part of the urethra that runs through the prostate.

Prostatism—a group of symptoms often associated with BPH, including a weak urinary stream, hesitancy in starting to urinate, and difficulty maintaining and stopping the stream, frequently with a small amount of "dribbling" afterward.

Prostatitis—inflammation of the prostate. Four conditions fall into this category: Acute bacterial prostatitis, chronic bacterial prostatitis, nonbacterial prostatitis, and prostatodynia.

Prostatodynia—This means "painful prostate." Patients have no history of urinary tract infections, and no trace of bacteria found in the prostate and normal prostatic secretions. The symptoms of prostatodynia are basically identical to those of nonbacterial prostatitis; the difference is made in diagnosis. Prostatodynia can be caused by many things, particularly muscle spasms in the bladder neck, prostatic urethra, perineum, or pelvic floor.

Prostatosis—a vague, unhelpful term that means simply "a condition of the prostate."

Prosthesis—an artificial replacement for part of the body that is either missing or not functioning properly.

PSA—prostate-specific antigen, an enzyme made by the prostate. Levels of PSA can be checked in a simple blood test; elevated amounts of PSA in the blood can signal prostate cancer.

PSA density—the blood PSA score divided by the volume of the prostate, as determined by transrectal ultrasound.

PSA velocity—PSA's rate of change from year to year.

Psychogenic erectile dysfunction—erection problems that are psychological, not physiological in nature. Doctors make this ruling if a man can't produce an erection during sexual activity, but has several a night while he sleeps.

Pulmonary embolus—a blood clot in the lungs, a potential complication of radical prostatectomy. This is extremely serious, and can be fatal.

Pulsed Doppler evaluation—a test that uses high-resolution ultrasound to evaluate the arteries' blood supply to the penis.

Pyrotherapy—a noninvasive form of thermal therapy used to treat BPH. Multiple ultrasound waves are focused at a single point some distance away from the power source. Only the concentration point, the target where all these beams intersect—the prostate tissue in BPH—is damaged.

Quality of life—Basically, this means how good you think your life is. When "quality of life" is excellent, this means a patient is relatively untroubled by symptoms or pain. When it is poor, this means that pain or symptoms have interfered with a man's ability to function, to pursue his daily activities and enjoy his life.

Radiation "seeds"—See *interstitial brachytherapy.*

Radiation therapy—See *external-beam radiation therapy, interstitial brachytherapy,* and *three-dimensional conformal therapy.*

Radical prostatectomy—the operation to remove the prostate, and the "gold standard" for curing localized prostate cancer. There are two approaches: The radical retropubic prostatectomy, which involves an abdominal incision, and the radical perineal prostatectomy, which reaches the prostate through the perineum.

Radioactive strontium 89—a highly effective radioactive substance, injected into the body, that is specially tailored to ease bone pain in cancer patients.

Radionuclide scintigraphy—see *bone scan.*

Randomize—Doctors use this verb when discussing medical studies in which some men are assigned one treatment or another at random.

Receptors—highly specific "locks" in cells that are opened, or activated, only by certain hormones or chemical signals, which act as "keys."

Regeneration—regrowth.

Resect (verb)—to cut out, to remove surgically.

Resectoscope—an instrument used in the TUR procedure. Threaded through the penis, it shines a light that allows surgeons to view the prostate as they chip away at excess tissue.

Retreatment, reoperation—having to undergo a repeat procedure to treat the same initial problem.

Retrograde ejaculation—see *"dry" ejaculation.*

Retropubic (adj.)—a surgical approach. In retropubic prostatectomy, the surgeon makes an incision in the lower abdomen, separates the abdominal muscles and moves the bladder aside, unopened, to reach the prostate directly (as opposed to the suprapubic approach, in which the prostate is reached by cutting through the bladder).

"Salvage" therapy—This is a medical term for "Plan B." It means a patient is undergoing another form of treatment because "Plan A," the first form of treatment the patient underwent, was not successful in curing the problem. Salvage therapy doesn't always work, and it's often associated with a higher rate of complications.

"Sandwich approach"—a technique to make radiation treatment easier to tolerate, and thus minimize side effects. In a "sandwich approach," the radiation dose is split in two, with a break in between. This gives the bowel and part of the bladder a "breather," a window of opportunity to recover from the shock of the treatment.

Semen—the fluid that transports sperm.

Seminal vesicles—glands that, like the prostate, are "sex accessory glands." Fluid secreted by these glands is critical in ensuring the consistency of semen.

"Sex accessory" tissues—glands such as the prostate, seminal vesicles and Cowper's gland, which produce secretions that become part of the fluid in semen.

Sextant biopsy—an attempt to get a comprehensive picture of the prostate, by taking six tiny samples of cells from throughout the gland—one from the top, middle, and bottom of the gland on the right and left sides.

Silent prostatism—when kidney or bladder damage develops without any noticeable symptoms. This can be a result of BPH left untreated.

Sinusoids—spongy chambers within the penis that become engorged with blood during an erection.

Small-cell carcinoma—a variety of prostate cancer. Cells in these tumors have a make-up similar to other small-cell cancers (of the lung, for example), and they respond to the same kinds of chemotherapy drugs used to treat these tumors.

Spinal anesthesia—a shot of local anesthetic in the small of the back through the dura, the membrane lining the spinal cord, and into the spinal fluid. Within minutes, the patient feels numb, relaxed, and heavy from the waist down.

Spinal cord compression—a very serious problem in men with metastatic prostate cancer. This happens when cancer attacks the spine, causing part of the spinal column to collapse, trapping and sometimes crushing nearby nerves.

"Spot" radiation—This is localized external-beam radiation treatment, targeted at one or several painful bone metastases. It won't prevent new metastases from cropping up in bone, but it can ease pain dramatically in the sites it does treat.

Stage of prostate cancer—Determining the stage means finding out the extent of the disease—how big it is, and how far it has spread. The stage of prostate cancer has a major role in determining what treatment a man should receive. There are two main systems for staging prostate cancer— the Whitmore-Jewett, and the TNM system. See also, *clinical stage* and *pathologic stage*.

Staging pelvic lymphadenectomy—dissection of the pelvic lymph nodes to see whether they contain prostate cancer. This procedure is generally performed just before a radical prostatectomy.

Stents—tubes, implanted and left in place to hold open a space that otherwise would collapse or be compressed. In the case of BPH, they're placed in the urethra to stave off the choking overgrowth of prostate tissue, and to ease obstructed urinary flow.

Stress incontinence—when urine leaks during certain activities, such as running or playing golf.

Stricture—a blockage caused by scar tissue.

Stromal cells—cells found in the prostate's smooth muscle tissue, which contract automatically to launch secretions into the urethra.

Subcapsular orchiectomy—a cosmetic approach to orchiectomy. In this operation, a surgeon opens the lining to the testicles and empties the contents of each testicle. The lining is closed again, and this empty shell is placed back inside the scrotum—so nothing looks different; in other words, no one can tell from outward appearance that there's nothing inside the scrotum.

Suprapubic (adj.)—an approach to the prostate. In a suprapubic open prostatectomy, the surgeon reaches the prostate by making an incision in the skin and muscles of the lower abdomen, then goes through the bladder to reach the prostate.

Surgical margins—This is established when pathologists look at the edges of tissue that has been cut out during surgery. If no cancer appears on these edges and the margin is "clear," or "negative," then it's a pretty good bet that all the cancerous tissue was removed. If the margin is "positive," this means that the surgeon's ability to cut out all the cancer is uncertain.

Sutures—surgical stitches used to close an incision.

Template—a highly sophisticated kind of paint-by-numbers map of the prostate that helps doctors know exactly where to insert radioactive seeds.

Testes, or testicles—Housed in the scrotum, these are a man's reproductive organs and the main source of the male hormone, testosterone, and of sperm.

Testosterone—the male hormone, or androgen, which is important to the prostate and is essential for sex drive and fertility. It also is responsible for such "manly" characteristics as post-puberty body hair and deepening of the voice. Lowering testosterone is a major goal of hormone therapy to treat prostate cancer.

Thermal ablation—the form of thermal therapy that produces the hottest temperatures of all, above 60 degrees centigrade.

Thermal therapy—using heat to destroy tissue.

Thermotherapy—a form of thermal therapy, in which tissue is heated to temperatures greater than 45 degrees centigrade.

Three-dimensional conformal therapy—a technique to increase external-beam therapy's potential, by maximizing the dose of radiation to the prostate tumor while keeping the risk of damaging nearby tissue to a minimum.

Three-glass urine collection—an important test for prostatitis. When a man urinates, the first urine to come out contains fluid from the urethra; urine collected in midstream comes from the bladder. The last collection of urine is taken after a brief prostate massage, and this contains fluid from the prostate.

Total androgen blockade, or ablation—a form of hormone therapy to treat prostate cancer. The theory here is that even low levels of testosterone and DHT—engendered by the adrenal androgens—can stimulate cancer in the prostate, and they must be stopped. This can be accomplished by combining whatever achieves a castrate level of testosterone—surgical castration, estrogen or an LHRH agonist—with an antiandrogen such as flutamide.

Transabdominal (adj.)—through the abdomen.

Transition zone—the innermost ring of the prostate, tissue that surrounds the urethra. This is the site of BPH.

Transperineal (adj.)—through the perineum.

Transrectal (adj.)—through the rectum.

Treatment-planning CT scan—CT images to show the physical terrain of the targeted area, the prostate and surrounding organs, before radiation treatment.

Trilobar enlargement—a type of BPH involving three (two lateral and one middle) lobes, in which obstruction can occur in the bladder neck as well as the urethra.

TUAP—transurethral ultrasonic aspiration of the prostate, a technique used to treat BPH, involving a special ultrasound probe. The ultrasound targets tissues high in water content, like BPH tissue, while leaving surrounding tissue in the bladder neck, urethral sphincter and elsewhere in the prostate unscathed.

TUIP—transurethral incision of the prostate. A surgical procedure used to treat BPH, in which a surgeon makes a few tiny cuts in the binding ring of prostate tissue that's choking the urethra. When this ring is cut, the lobes spring apart—instantly creating more space around the urethra.

TULIP—transurethral ultrasound-guided laser-induced prostatectomy, a treatment for BPH using a noncontact laser. The TULIP laser device features an ultrasound scanner, which gives surgeons a picture of the areas the laser will target and allows for greater accuracy.

TUMT—transurethral microwave thermal therapy. A treatment for BPH that uses microwaves to generate heat and destroy tissue around the urethra, giving it some breathing room. It works by miniature remote control: A tiny antenna that targets BPH tissue surrounds a catheter that goes through the penis and into the urethra. The microwave generator is situated nearby, in the rectum.

TUNA—transurethral needle ablation, a procedure used to treat BPH. Radio-frequency energy is conducted through tiny needles, inserted directly into prostate tissue via a special catheter. The needles riddle the BPH tissue with holes of various sizes to weaken its grip on the urethra.

TUR—transurethral resection of the prostate (also called a "TURP" procedure), the "gold standard" operation to treat symptoms of BPH. It does not require an incision; instead, prostate tissue is reached, chipped away and removed in tiny fragments through the urethra.

TUR syndrome—a rare complication of TUR, caused when the body absorbs excessive amounts of the irrigating fluid used during the procedure. Its symptoms are nausea, confusion, vomiting, high blood pressure, a falling heart rate, and visual problems. TUR syndrome is temporary and is quickly reversible with diuretics or a saline solution, which help restore the body's normal fluid and mineral balance.

Ultrasound—a painless, noninvasive way of imaging that creates a picture with high-frequency sound waves, like sonar on a submarine. It may be done either from outside, through the abdomen, or transrectally, via a wand inserted in the rectum. Transrectal ultrasound can detect differences between cancerous and normal tissue in the prostate.

Ureters—muscular, one-way channels that work like toothpaste tubes, squeezing urine out from the kidneys and onward to the bladder.

Urethra—a tube that, like the prostate, is involved in both the urinary and reproductive systems. It serves as a conduit not only for urine but also for secretions from the ejaculatory ducts and the prostate.

Urethral sphincter—the muscle responsible for urinary control.

Urethral stricture—scar tissue that blocks the urethra.

Urethritis—inflammation of the urethra, often caused by an infection. If left untreated, this can result in a urethral stricture or a nasty infection that progresses back into the vas deferens and involves the epididymis.

Urge, or urgency, incontinence—when a man knows he has to urinate but some urine leaks before he reaches a bathroom.

Urinalysis—microscopic and chemical examination of urine.

Urinary retention—when the bladder stays completely or partly full. Acute urinary retention means someone can no longer urinate. This is a very serious condition, and it requires immediate treatment.

Urodynamic studies—tests that measure urinary flow, pressures and volumes to find out whether urinary trouble is caused by BPH or from a problem with the bladder.

Uroflowmetry—a test to measure the amount of urine a man passes, and the speed of his urinary stream.

Urologist—a physician who specializes in the diagnosis and in the medical and surgical treatment of problems in the urinary and male reproductive systems.

UTI—urinary tract infection. The presence of bacteria in the urine, sometimes associated with fever.

Vacuum erection device—an apparatus that creates suction using an airtight tube, which is placed temporarily around the penis. An attached pump withdraws air, creating a reduced atmospheric pressure—a vacuum—around the penis, causing it to become engorged with blood. The penis becomes erect. Then a constricting ring, like a rubber band around the neck of a balloon, keeps the blood trapped in the penis, so the erection can be sustained.

Vascular (adj.)—involving blood vessels.

Vas deferens—There are actually two of these hard, muscular cords, but doctors often speak of the vas deferens as a single unit. The vas deferens winds its way from the epididymis to the base of the prostate, where it meets with the duct of the seminal vesicle to form the ejaculatory duct.

Vasectomy—a surgical procedure that is a form of male contraception. When the vas deferens is cut, sperm cannot exit the penis through ejaculation but are instead reabsorbed into the body.

Vasodilators—drugs that open up blood vessels, making a wider channel for blood to go through. In the penis, they also cause the smooth muscle tissue to relax and the veins to close; some vasodilators, injected in tiny amounts of the penis, are used to produce erections.

Venous (adj.)—relating to the veins.

Venous leak—a common cause of erection problems. Even though the arteries fill the penis with blood, producing a partial erection, the veins don't clamp down to keep this blood trapped inside the penis, so a full erection can't be achieved.

VLAP—visual laser-assisted prostatectomy, a "non-contact" laser procedure. It uses a transurethral probe, inserted through the tip of the penis, that beams the laser at a 90-degree angle directly into the prostate.

Watchful waiting—the most conservative treatment there is. It means following someone's symptoms closely, but delaying treatment until these symptoms become severe enough to warrant it. Some doctors also call this "following expectantly."

"Wide excision"—During a radical prostatectomy, this means that a surgeon cuts out as much tissue as possible surrounding the prostate in an aggressive attempt to get every last bit of cancer.

Window of curability—a limited period of time in which prostate cancer can be cured, while it's still confined to the prostate. Once cancer spreads beyond the prostate, cure is no longer possible.

X-ray therapy—See *external-beam radiation therapy.*

YAG laser—see *Neodynium (Nd):YAG laser.*

Zones of the prostate—there are five distinct regions of the prostate. The two most commonly referred to are the transition zone and the peripheral zone.

Index